AN OUTLINE OF HUMAN EMBRYOLOGY

AN OUTLINE OF
HUMAN EMBRYOLOGY

HARRY WANG, Ph.D.

Professor of Anatomy, Loyola University
Stritch School of Medicine, Hines, Illinois

WILLIAM HEINEMANN MEDICAL BOOKS LTD

LONDON

First published 1968

SBN 433 34850 X

Printed in Great Britain by Robert MacLehose & Co. Ltd,
The University Press, Glasgow

To my wife
LILY
in appreciation of her sustaining support
during the writing of this book

PREFACE

The place of Embryology in a medical curriculum has been the subject of controversy for years. As one who has been teaching this subject for more than a decade I have not the slightest doubt that it will always play a significant role in the medical curriculum. This view is shared by many who, like myself, have had a direct contact with embryology one way or another, by a majority of the medical students themselves, and by many practising doctors who would not hesitate admitting their inadequate exposure to embryology, and have since regretted that inadequacy. These consentient opinions have instilled in me a strong conviction, which has served as the main driving force behind the writing of this book. Of course, what really stands behind this conviction is the fact that the information concerning the origin of the individual and the orderly development of its organ systems cannot but constitute an overall prerequisite to the study of the human body, structure or function.

I believe there is need for a short treatise on human embryology that will serve either as a textbook or as a reference book. The present volume is written with this purpose in mind. It tells the story of human developmental anatomy simply, directly, and to the point with as few details and as many illustrations as possible so that anyone who has had a course in Introduction to Biology would be able to follow. So, regardless of the format of instruction, whether the subject be taught traditionally, modified or radically curtailed, this book ought to serve the student equally well.

Second, I believe that a foundation of embryological knowledge is to be laid by the student through an understanding of the normal processes of development. Accordingly, the latter have received prime consideration throughout the book. Anomalies and malformations are given adequate attention at the proper places so as to make discussions on their possible causative mechanisms and aetiology as intelligible as possible.

Third, although this book deals primarily with human materials, other forms are occasionally included either for the purpose of pertinent comparisons (e.g., on cleavage patterns, foetal membranes, etc.) or for appreciating significance of evolution as evidenced by the phylogeny of many organ systems. An example of the latter is the unique considerations given to the endocrine tissues and organs. They are brought under one chapter and described from the standpoint of progressive developmental complexities and functions.

Fourth, I have made good use of tables for summarizing and/or itemizing information wherever and whenever possible. This is a further step in an attempt to facilitate the insemination of facts for the time-pressed present day medical student. Also frequent cross references are provided for his convenience,

I hope that this book may be useful also to students of dentistry, clinicians in all branches of the medical science as well as for those preparing for professional examinations. Certain sections of the book contain information that may be of value to the obstetricians. Finally, students of embryology in general may find this book helpful.

A list of books is given below, which I highly recommend to the students for collateral readings.

HINES   HARRY WANG
ILLINOIS

ACKNOWLEDGEMENTS

In the preparation of this book a number of textbooks have been freely consulted. They have proved of immense value and help especially in the matter of illustrations. Besides carrying the traditional acknowledgment with each illustration so utilized, my publisher, William Heinemann Medical Books Limited and I wish to thank the following publishers and authors for their permission to base some of my illustrations on their material:

W. B. Saunders Co.: *Developmental Anatomy* by L. B. Arey; *Introduction to Embryology* by B. I. Balinsky; *Fundamentals of Neurology* by E. Gardner; *The Anatomy of the Nervous System* by S. W. Ranson; *A Textbook of Histology* (7th ed.) by A. A. Maximow and W. Bloom. McGraw-Hill Book Co., Inc.: *Human Embryology* and *Fundamentals of Embryology* by B. M. Patten; *A Textbook of Histology* by J. L. Bremer and H. L. Weatherford. The Williams and Wilkins Co.: *Human Embryology* by W. J. Hamilton, J. D. Boyd and H. W. Mossman; *Medical Embryology* by Jan Langman. The Ronald Press Co.: *Human Developmental Anatomy* by J. Davies. F. A. Davis Co.: *A Textbook of Human Embryology* by R. G. Harrison. John Wiley & Sons, Ltd.: *The Essentials of Human Embryology* by G. S. Dodds; *Vertebrate Embryology* by W. Shumway. The Macmillan Co.: *Fundamentals of Comparative Embryology of the Vertebrates* by A. F. Huetner. Henry Holt and Co.: *Principles of Development* by P. Weiss. Lea and Febiger: *A Textbook of Histology* by J. C. Finerty and E. V. Cowdry. J. B. Lippincott Co.: *Histology* by A. W. Ham. Pitman Medical Publishing Co., Ltd. and J. B. Lippincott Co.: *Basic Human Embryology* by P. L. Williams and C. P. Wendell-Smith.

In most cases an illustration was first prepared by myself, then redrawn later by Mr. Frank Price. I am deeply indebted to him for his great contribution to the book. Last, but not least, I wish to extend my sincere thanks and special appreciation to Mr. Owen R. Evans, Managing Director of William Heinemann Medical Books Limited, for his kind, patient, hard work in getting this book published.

August, 1968

H.W.

Further Reading:

Arey, L. B. (1965) *Developmental Anatomy* (Philadelphia and London: W. B. Saunders)

Balinsky, B. I. (1960) *An Introduction to Embryology* (Philadelphia and London: W. B. Saunders)

Patten, B. M. (1953) *Human Embryology* (New York: McGraw-Hill)

Hamilton, W. J., Boyd, J. D., and Mossman, H. W. (1962) *Human Embryology* (Baltimore: The Williams and Wilkins Co.)

Langman, J. (1963) *Medical Embryology* (Baltimore: The Williams and Wilkins Co.)

Davies, J. (1963) *Human Developmental Anatomy* (New York: The Ronald Press Co.)

Weiss, P. (1939) *Principles of Development* (New York: Henry Holt)

Williams, P. L. and Wendell-Smith, C. P. (1966) *Basic Human Embryology* (London: Pitman Medical Publishing Co. and Philadelphia: J. B. Lippincott)

Willier, B. H., Weiss, P., and Hamburger, V. (1955) *Analysis of Development* (Philadelphia and London: W. B. Saunders)

Waddinton, C. H. (1956) *Principles of Embryology* (London and New York: The Macmillan Co.)

CONTENTS

PART I

GENERAL EMBRYOLOGY

CHAPTER 1

GERM CELLS

Heredity and environment

Every individual develops from a fertilized egg called the zygote. It contains genes contributed from both parents (Fig. 1–1), and it is these genes that determine the course of development and its outcome. For the complete realization of the hereditary role of the genes, however, the environment must provide the necessary and proper conditions; even though environment creates nothing, its influence upon development is clearly recognized (see Chapter 8). The action of genes sets the hereditary machine going, but it is the environmental factors which exercise effective control over this machinery in the production of an organism.

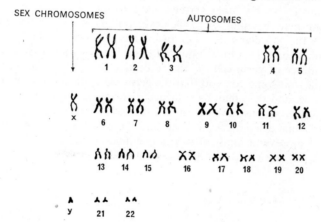

FIG. 1–1. Karyotype of chromosomes from a human male cell (numbering system based on Danver Convention).

Since an individual starts from a germ cell, and yet the fully formed body consists of both somatic and germinal tissues, a segregation between germ cells and somatic cells must take place sometime during the course of development. The significant thing is that the germ cells give rise to the somatic tissues, not the reverse. This is the thesis of Weismann's theory of continuity or immortality of germplasm. The somatic tissues live for one generation whilst the germ cells pass on from generation to generation in an unbroken line which has continued from the beginning of life. Figure 1–2 shows schematically three successive generations, in each of which the small inner circle represents the germ plasm. The arrows which point from the inner to the outer circle indicate the influence of the genes in determining the body form of an individual.

FIG. 1–2. Diagram illustrating the concept of continuity of germplasm. Three generations are shown; in each, the small circle represents germplasm, the large circle, the somatic tissue. Arrows point in the direction of determination, only from germ to soma, never the reverse.

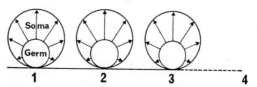

It should be noted that there are no arrows pointing in the opposite direction, denoting an inability of the somatic tissues to affect the germ plasm. It is a " one-way traffic ", so to speak.

The question naturally arises: At what stage in ontogeny does the separation of germ plasm and somatic tissues occur? In the parasitic roundworm, *Ascaris*, one of the 16 cells (blastomeres) becomes segregated out as the first germ cell at the end of the fourth cleavage division. In higher forms, it is much more difficult to ascertain when this separation occurs. However, it is safe to say that in the vertebrates this event takes place much later; thus the earliest traceable sex cells are found in young embryos. Whichever is the case, it remains true that any inheritable changes must be first present in the genes. In other words, only genes or chromosomes changed by mutation, or mishaps during disjunction of synaptic allelomorphic chromosomes can cause changes in the somatic tissues. That is the reason why acquired characters (which represent only somatic changes resulting from operation of environmental factors) are not inheritable. Lamarck's theory of inheritance of acquired characters has been proved false simply because, as far as we know, there is no mechanism whereby changes in the soma can induce changes in the germ plasm.

Origin of germ cells

From observations and careful experiments it is now established that in amphibians, birds, rats, mice and humans (probably other vertebrates, too) the earliest germ cells arise from yolk sac endoderm. From there they journey to the developing gonad via either the dorsal mesentery (a, in Fig. 1–3) or by the vascular route, i.e., inside blood vessels (b, in Fig. 1–3). These germ cells are the primordial sex cells which, upon entering the gonadal blastema of either sex, will constitute the only source of germ cells of the respective sex. This statement is not challenged in the case of the male, but some contend that the germinal epithelium of the ovary is potentially capable of forming ova, and thus may be regarded as being a secondary source of germ cells in the female. This contention has never been satisfactorily proved, however. On the contrary, recent lines of experimental evidence seem to support the view that the germinal epithelium of the ovary, whilst originating several kinds of ovarian cellular elements in addition to the granulosa cells (p. 136), is probably not capable of giving rise to new egg cells.

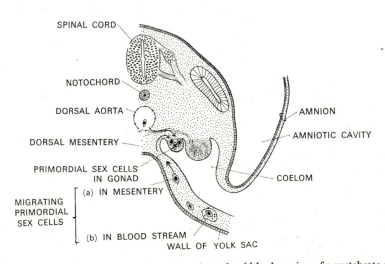

FIG. 1–3. Schematic representation of a section through mid-body region of a vertebrate embryo illustrating the origin of primordial germ (sex) cells and their migration to the developing gonad via two routes: (a) through mesenteries and (b) through the blood stream.

Destiny of the primordial sex cells (cf. p. 129)

The activity of the primordial sex cells after their arrival in the gonad differs somewhat in the two sexes, although in both male and female these cells are the only precursors of definitive gametes. In a developing testis, the number of these cells increases tremendously by active proliferation (Fig. 1–4) and they become incorporated as spermatogonia into the developing seminiferous tubules. In the ovary, primary sex cords (homologous to the testis cords, the fore-runners of seminiferous tubules) are also formed; some of the primordial sex cells become incorporated into these cords which are also known as medullary cords, because they are present in the medulla of the ovary. The remaining primordial sex cells find their way into the developing cortex of the ovary, where they come to lie scattered among other cells. It is this latter source that will later participate in follicular development. The medullary cords, on the other hand, degenerate almost completely. Any remnants of them become dormant, but under certain conditions they may be reactivated. In fact, both natural and experimental cases of hypertrophy

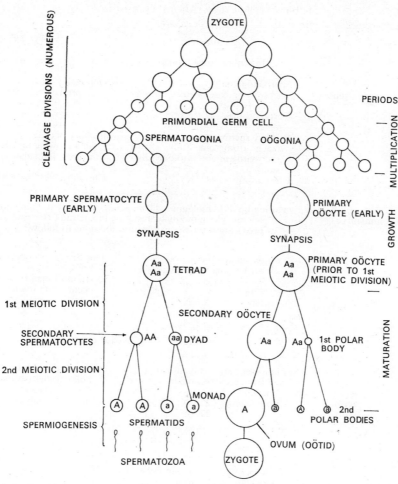

FIG. 1–4. Graphic representation of the history of the gametes, from zygote to zygote, in the two sexes. (The many mitotic divisions undergone by the primordial germ cells before they become spermatogonia or oogonia are not shown in the diagram.) The two possible divisions of the " tetrads " are represented: the first meiotic division being a reductional division in the male line; an equational division in the female line.

of medullary cords are known to occur; in birds, for instance, removal of the left functional ovary invariably causes the right rudimentary ovary to develop into an ovo-testis. In extreme cases (which are rare) the hypertrophied medullary cords may even produce spermatozoa, indicating strongly that the original primordial sex cells residing in these cords could be stimulated to spermatogenic activity. In the present example this stimulation is brought about by removal of the female sex hormone, which normally inhibits the medullary (male) component of the right ovary. This example demonstrates quite conclusively that the vertebrate ovary may contain a residual male component that often retains some dormant primordial sex cells.

THE MATURATION OF GERM CELLS

The main events whereby the spermatogonia and oögonia are transformed into their respective mature gametes, spermatozoa and ova, are summarized in Table 1–1, and also shown schemati-

Table 1–1. MATURATION OF GERM CELLS

Period	Sex:	Male	Female
	Site:	In seminiferous tubules	In ovarian cortex
Multiplication (by mitosis; many generations)		Spermatogonia (resting on basement membrane) Chromosomes: 44+XY	Oögonia (in primary follicle with one layer of follicular cells) Chromosomes: 44+XX
Growth		Primary spermatocytes (each from one fully grown spermatogonium without division) Chromosomes: 44+XY	Primary oöcytes (in a growing follicle with multi-layered follicular cells and an antrum) Chromosomes: 44+XX
Synapsis (no cell division involved)		Pairing-up of homologous chromosomes; after that, each chromosome of a pair splits longitudinally, resulting in a tetrad (from each synaptic pair) as preparation for the maturation divisions to follow	
Maturation (Meiosis)	First division	Two secondary spermatocytes (from 1 primary spermatocyte) Chromosomes: 22+X / 22+Y	One Secondary oöcyte and 1 polar body (first) (In most mammals, this division occurs after ovulation) Chromosomes: 22+X / 22+X
		Chromosome in each cell is a dyad.	
	Second division	Four spermatids (functional) (2 from each secondary spermatocyte) Chromosomes: 22+X; 22+X / 22+Y; 22+Y	One oötid (mature ovum) and 3 polar bodies (secondary) (This division occurs in some mammals only after fertilization)
		Chromsome in each cell is a monad.	
Spermiogenesis (no cell division involved)		Each spermatid enters a process of morphological transformation into a definitive spermatozoon, characterized by a tail and a head containing the chromosomes (Fig. 1–9).	

cally in Fig. 1–4. This process does not begin until puberty when the necessary hormones produced by the anterior pituitary become available (see Chapters 7, 13 and 17). For spermatogenesis FSH and LH (ICSH) are required. For oögenesis, both FSH and ovarian oestrogen (female sex hormone) are indispensable.

One significant feature occurring during the maturation of germ cells is the reduction of chromosomes from the diploid (2N) to the haploid (N) condition. (In man, N is 23, of which 22 are autosomes and one is a sex chromosome, either an X or a Y). All somatic cells and germ cells up to the time of the first maturation (meiotic) division contain 2N (46) chromosomes. One complete set (N) of these chromosomes has come from each of the two parents; this is the foundation of biparental inheritance. It follows that functional spermatozoa and eggs must contain only one complete haploid set of chromosomes in order that at the time of fertilization the diploid chromosome number specific of the species is restored. The mechanism, provided by nature to achieve this important end, consists of pairing (synapsis) of homologous chromosomes in the primary spermatocytes and oöcytes followed immediately by two meiotic divisions. As a result, a future germ cell receives one chromosome of each synaptic pair; whether it receives the paternal or maternal chromosome is entirely a matter of chance. And since this fifty-fifty chance applies independently to each homologous pair of chromosomes the higher the number of chromosomes a species has, greater will be the variability in the chromosomal makeup of the resulting spermatozoa or eggs (see p. 6). As will be shown later this is also the basis of the mechanism for sex determination.

Mitosis vs. Meiosis (Fig. 1–5)

Mitosis is the regular process of cell division whereby the two resulting daughter cells each receive an exact copy of the chromosomes present in the cell before division starts. The mechanism making this possible is that during late prophase each chromosome splits longitudinally into two chromatids which arrange themselves on the equatorial plate of the spindle at metaphase; the two identical chromatids then separate, one going to each of the daughter cells. Meiosis is a special or modified kind of cell division designed for reducing the diploid chromosome number of the species (2N) to N, the haploid state with equal precision. Meiosis differs from mitosis in a number of ways. The primary spermatocytes and primary oöcytes about to enter the first meiotic division undergo a series of changes during the prophase. These changes involve only the nuclear material, converting it from the diffuse state of chromatin to that of definitive chromosomes. Four such stages are illustrated in Fig. 1–5 (Meiosis: prophase 1, 2, 3, and 4). In stage 1, (leptotene) the chromosomes are elongate and relaxed; in stage 2, (zygotene) the homologous chromosomes come together in pairs (synapsis; see Fig. 1–4); in stage 3, (pachytene) the paired chromosomes become further thickened; and in stage 4, (diplotene) the synaptic pairs become " tetrads ". That is, each chromosome of a synaptic pair duplicates itself so that each synaptic pair becomes a composite of 4 chromatids, known as a tetrad. These latter now enter the metaphase of the first meiotic division. During the anaphase of the first meiotic division a phenomenon known as disjunction occurs to each of the tetrads, separating them into " dyads ".; thus the secondary spermatids and secondary oöcytes have their chromosomes in the state of dyads. Since in most cases the second meiotic division follows immediately upon the first, the " dyads " become separated into " monads " without repeating the chromosomal changes just described for the prophase preceding the first meiotic division. The products of the second meiotic division, spermatids and oötids (mature ova), have their chromosomes in the state of monads and the chromosome number is reduced from the diploid (2N) to the haploid (N) condition.

Significance of " synapsis " and " tetrad " formation

The pairing of homologous chromosomes during synapsis is a chemical phenomenon; it is attributed to a high chemical affinity existing between similar chromosomes, one coming from each parent. " Dissimilar " chromosomes do not undergo synapsis. It is thus a precise mech-

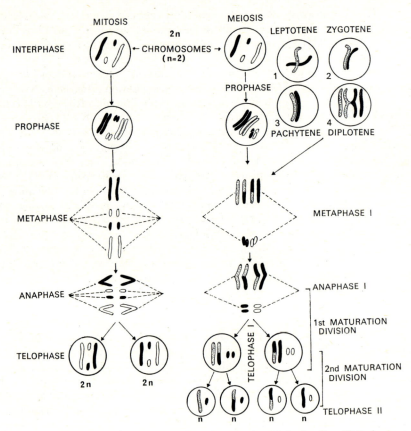

Fig. 1–5. A comparative diagram of mitosis and meiosis in cells having four (2N) chromosomes (solid from one parent, blank from the other). Only one pair of the two homologous (allelomorphic) chromosomes is shown for the stages of prophase in the first meiotic division. Notice that one pair of chromosomes in meiotic division has undergone crossing-over.

anism for ensuring that the resulting germ cells each have a complete haploid set of chromosomes, characteristic of the species. By this mechanism each germ cell receives one member of every synaptic pair formed during the zygotene stage of prophase of the primary spermatocytes and primary oöcytes. The purpose of tetrad formation occurring during the diplotene stage is to set the stage for the two meiotic divisions which follow in quick succession. Taking one synaptic chromosome-pair into consideration, the two meiotic divisions can be graphically represented as in the following diagram.

It is evident that a tetrad could divide according to either possibility 1, (in which case the first meiotic division is a reductional division) or possibility 2, (equational division). They will be then followed, respectively, with an equational division and reductional division. But in both instances (occurring with equal chance) the end results of the two maturation divisions are the same, namely four spermatids each with the haploid number of chromosomes. It is important to bear in mind that these two possibilities regarding the order of the two meiotic divisions apply to each and every tetrad at random and completely independently of one another. This is the basis for Mendel's Law of Independent Assortment; it explains the origin of tremendous variability in the chromosomal make-up of the mature germ cells in each sex. The possible number of gametes obtainable can be calculated by the formula 2^n, where n represents the haploid

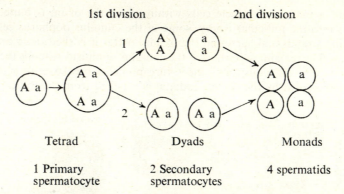

1st division   2nd division

Tetrad   Dyads   Monads

1 Primary   2 Secondary   4 spermatids
  spermatocyte   spermatocytes

chromosome number of the species, (e.g., 23 in man). The variability is further multiplied by random union of the two gametes at time of fertilization to 4^n.

One realizes, of course, that in spite of the precise nature of this mechanism things still could go wrong, especially during disjunction, thereby resulting in many kinds of chromosomal aberrations such as loss or gain of a whole chromosome, inversion or translocation of parts (Fig. 8–11). In particular, crossing over of genetic material at pachytene results in much variability. Many abnormalities of development are attributable to chromosomal aberrations (Chapter 8).

Differences in the gametes of the two sexes

Certain differences in the gametes produced by the two sexes should be noted. Most conspicuous is the fact that whereas four functional spermatozoa result from one primary spermatocyte, only one functional ovum is obtained from a primary oöcyte together with three polar bodies. The latter invariably disintegrate; often the first polar body fails to enter a second division. Another difference between the gametes is one of size. It is estimated that in the human, an oögonium in a primary follicle may measure 0·02 mm. in diameter. By the time it reaches maturity in a Graafian follicle ready to ovulate it has a diameter of approximately 0·14 mm. This presents a sharp contrast to the spermatozoa, which are much smaller cells. This difference in size has functional significance. The egg cell, during the period of growth, accumulates a large number of food granules (yolk) in its cytoplasm, and being large, it is an immotile cell. The spermatozoa, on the other hand, are adapted for great mobility (see Fig. 1–9).

Follicle Development (Fig. 1–6)

This phenomenon has no parallel in the male. Unlike the maturing male germ cells, which require no protection, the growing ovum on its way to maturity incorporates around itself a large number of non-germinal cells to form a follicle. These follicular cells are derived exclusively from the germinal epithelium (see Chapter 13). At first, an oögonium in the cortex of the ovary becomes surrounded with a single layer of follicle cells. As the oögonium increases in size the follicle cells become several layers thick. These are known as, respectively, primary (Fig. 1–6A, B, C) and growing (Fig. 1–6D) follicles. It has been estimated that 40,000 to 300,000 such primary follicles are present at birth. After puberty there comes a time when some of these primary follicles begin to develop further. Due to the secretory activity of the follicle cells, a fluid-filled space appears between the follicle cells. This space is called an antrum, and it marks the beginning of the maturation stage of the follicle; the germ cell within it is a primary oöcyte (Fig. 1–6D). The follicle continues to grow until it attains a tremendous size, all the time being pushed toward the periphery of the ovary. In the meantime, the follicular cells immediately surrounding the maturing ovum secrete a substance, chemically identified as glyco-protein, which forms a distinct layer, the zona pellucida, next to the vitelline membrane of the egg. At this stage the follicle cells are differentiated into the stratum granulosum which lines most of the follicle, and the cumulus oöphorus, a mound of follicle cells within which the ovum is buried. As the ovum gradually projects into the follicular cavity, some of the cumulus oöphorus cells arrange themselves into radiating strands and surround the ovum. After it is shed these cells will constitute the corona radiata. The remaining portion of the cumulus oöphorus sustains the ovum by linking it to the granulosa cells and constitutes the future point of breakage at ovulation, when the liberated ovum, surrounded by the corona radiata, is expelled from the follicle (Fig. 1–6G).

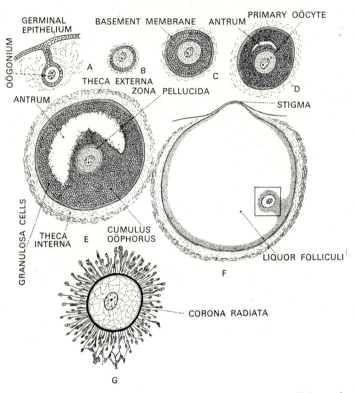

FIG. 1–6. Stages in the development of the human ovum and ovarian follicle: A, beginning of follicle formation as an oögonium becomes surrounded by follicular cells of ovigerous tube; B, primordial monolaminar follicle; C, growing (multilaminar) follicle with beginning of basement membrane formation; D, follicle with an antrum; E, maturing follicle with zona pellucida fully developed and a theca of connective tissue differentiating outside it; F, maturing (Graafian) follicle ready to rupture at a point known as the stigma; G, enlarged view of the ovum from stage F surrounded by the zona pellucida and cells of the corona radiata.

The process just described is completed approximately every four weeks and is under the control of hormones (Fig. 1–7). Within each menstrual cycle many oögonia start to differentiate, but only one reaches maturity; the others which fail to ovulate, become atretic (Fig. 1–7) and disintegrate. The process of degeneration may set in during any stage of growth or maturation. These events of follicular development and maturation of the ovum, together with ovulation, are summarized in Fig. 1–7 (Nos. 1 to 7). Subsequent changes in the ruptured follicle are shown in numbers 8, 9 and 10 of Fig. 1–7. The remains of the follicle grow into a fully formed and functional corpus luteum. In the event of fertilization followed by successful implantation of the embryo this persists for several months, otherwise atrophy results in the formation of a corpus albicans (No. 10, Fig. 1–7) after a fortnight or so. The stages of follicle maturation take place one after another with precision in close relation to the menstrual cycle and the changes in the uterine endometrium under the control of hormones (see Chapter 7).

Follicles containing 2 to 3 primary oöcytes have been reported. However, they probably do not constitute a source of twins or triplets as it is known that these abnormal follicles usually degenerate long before they ever reach maturity. Similarly, abnormal pre-implantation ova with multinucleated blastomeres are known. The cases studied show various degrees of cellular degeneration and pyknosis in the blastomeres, which suggests that they could not have continued to develop for very long.

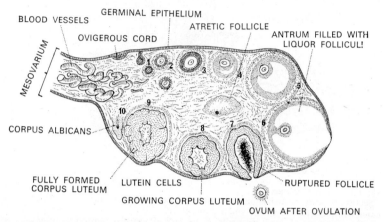

FIG. 1–7. Diagram of mammalian ovary showing the life cycle of one egg and its follicle (1–6, before ovulation; 7–10, after ovulation): 1, ovigerous tube; 2, primary follicle with one layer of follicular cells; 3, growing follicle with two layers of follicular cells; 4, growing follicle with an antrum; 5, a follicle approaching maturity; 6, mature follicle; 7, ruptured follicle with blood clot; 8, young corpus luteum; 9, fully formed corpus luteum (of menstruation or pregnancy—see p. 70); 10, corpus albicans. The egg cell in 1, 2, 3 is an oögonium; in 4, 5, 6, a primary oöcyte.

Spermatogenesis (Fig. 1–8)

The maturation of spermatozoa from spermatogonia takes place inside each seminiferous tubule; the process starts at puberty. The spermatogonia are located next to the basement membrane and may be one or several layers thick. Slender, somewhat oblong cells are located between the spermatogonia at fairly regular distances; these are the Sertoli cells (sustentacular cells). Mature spermatids may be attached to the apical portion of these cells which suggests that the function of the Sertoli cells is support and nutrition of the spermatids. The primary and secondary spermatocytes, many of which are in meiotic division, are located progressively toward the lumen of the tubule. The former are generally larger cells than either the secondary spermatocytes or the spermatogonia. Approaching the lumen much smaller spermatids are found, and filling the lumen are maturing spermatozoa in various stages of spermiogenesis (Fig. 1–9). It must be stressed, however, that spermatogenesis does not occur simultaneously in all the seminiferous tubules. The process in each tube is cyclical and waves of activity alternate with periods of rest. Thus, seldom does one find all the stages from spermatogonia to spermatozoa present at one time in any one section of seminiferous tubules.* A spermatogonium takes, on the average, 64 days to reach the final stage of mature spermatozoa.

* This suggests that mature sperms are produced cyclically (spermatogenic cycle). Recent experiments on the seminiferous tubules in mammals have disclosed evidence that the control mechanism of this phenomenon lies with the Sertoli cells. The mechanism works in the following manner: a residual body is shed by each maturing spermatid (see Fig. 1–9); the discarded residual bodies are phagocytosed by the Sertoli cells. This act of phagocytosis probably triggers the Sertoli cells to secrete a steroid hormone, and a new cycle is thus initiated.

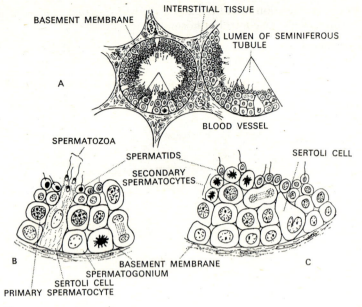

FIG. 1–8. Human spermatogenesis:
  A. Section of testis showing outlines and portions of six seminiferous tubules surrounding one complete tubule with cellular contents
  B. and C. Sections of small segments of the wall of active seminiferous tubules as indicated in A, showing the position and morphology of the male germ cells at successive stages of growth and maturation.

The differences in the maturation process of the two sexes are summarized below:

Male	Female
Spermatogonia: Dormant until puberty, then proliferate throughout reproductive life; tremendous number produced (millions of spermatozoa contained in a single ejaculation).	**Oögonia:** Full complement present at birth located in the cortex; probably no new ones added after birth; some growth in size (preliminary maturation) occurs.
Primary spermatocytes: No pause; maturation divisions ensue almost immediately.	**Primary oöcytes:** Produced only after action of FSH on the primary follicles. Second maturation division usually delayed until after ovulation.

Products of Meiosis

Four functional spermatozoa from 1 primary spermatocyte.	One mature ovum, plus polar bodies (2 to 3, depending on whether 2nd polar bodies are produced in the second maturation division)
Spermiogenesis (Fig. 1–9): Unique process transforming the four spermatids (from each primary spermatocyte) into fully mature spermatozoa.	
	Follicular atresia: Unique process in which some follicles become involuted during each maturation cycle, leaving only one to reach maturity.
Spermatogenesis in general: Maturation process is continuous once started.	**Oögenesis in general:** Maturation process is cyclical, leading to ovulation of a mature ovum once in every four weeks.

Spermiogenesis

Spermiogenesis is the process whereby spermatids are transformed into mature spermatozoa. The different stages involved in this process can be followed in Fig. 1–9. The nucleus of the spermatid, containing the genetic material, is condensed into the head of the spermatozoon; the Golgi body secretes the acrosome or head cap through an intermediate stage, the acrosomal granule; the centriole is transformed into the axial filament or flagellum; and the mitochondria become aggregated into the middle piece (body and neck) of the spermatozoon. All the remaining cytoplasm not utilized in this process is finally cast off (Fig. 1–9). With the electron microscope the 9 + 2 configuration of the fibrils can be seen to be present throughout the middle piece and axial filament (G2, G3, Fig. 1–9); this is the characteristic pattern of all motile cilia. There is some evidence that the head cap may secrete a substance, which in some way facilitates fertilization (see p. 15).

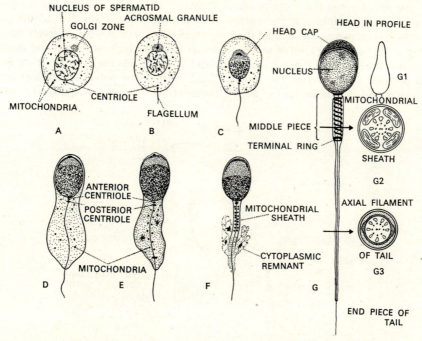

Fig. 1–9. Stages in the maturation of spermatids into definitive spermatozoa, the process known as spermiogenesis.

Abnormal human spermatozoa

Morphologically abnormal sperms are rather common. They comprise a great variety: dwarfs, giants, double-head, double-tail, double neck and body, abnormal tail, abnormal alignment of head and body, and so on. It has been suggested though that a person's fertility may not be adversely affected if the anomalous spermatozoa do not exceed 10 % of the total number in the ejaculate.

CHAPTER 2

FERTILIZATION AND SEX DETERMINATION

Sperm transport

Mature sperms are stored in the epididymis. They are non-motile in this environment, which is rich in metabolites of these cells. When they are expelled from the epididymis two kinds of secretions are added along the route of sperm transport (Fig. 2–1, also see Fig. 13–6). The first is contributed by the ampulla of the ductus deferens, the seminal vesicle and the prostate; in this fluid, which is known as the seminal fluid or semen, the spermatozoa are freely suspended and become motile. The second kind of secretion comes from the bulbo-urethral and urethral glands (Fig. 2–1); it is the so-called " pre-ejaculation fluid ", which fills the entire urethra and precedes the actual seminal fluid. When the seminal fluid reaches the pelvic (posterior) urethra, it is forcefully ejaculated by contraction of the bulbo-cavernosus (bulbo-spongiosus) muscle.

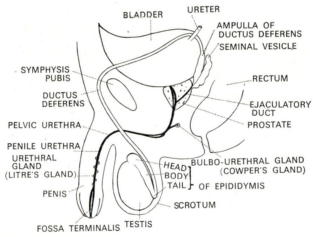

Fig. 2–1. Male organs of reproduction (showing the passages for sperm transport) in sagittal section.

The secretions of the accessory sex glands are alkaline and serve to neutralize the immediate neighbourhood of the spermatozoa, thereby making them motile, and they also neutralize the acidity of the male urethra and vagina.

An ejaculate averages from 3–5 ml. with a sperm density of 60 to 200 million per ml. About 75–80% of the sperms have normal morphology (Fig. 1–9) and motility. Their speed of movement is in the range of 2–3 mm. per minute, depending on the surrounding pH, averaging 0·5 mm./min. in the acidic vagina but becoming much faster during the ascending journey in the uterine cavity because of the alkalinity of the uterine fluid.

The seminal fluid contains fructose, which is metabolized by an enzyme contained in the mitochondrial sheath of the sperm's middle piece (Fig. 1–9); the energy thus released is utilized by the active spermatozoa. The movement of sperms through the uterine cavity towards the tube, against the general direction of the fluid currents, is credited mostly to their own power. It has also been suggested that the current created by some of the ciliated epithelial cells lining the tube and mild peristaltic movements of the uterine wall assist in their movement.

Present evidence shows that the movement of the spermatozoa after they enter the cervix is governed by a chemotactic factor attributable to the ovum. If there is no egg in the uterine tube, they move aimlessly and at random (Fig. 2–3A); but if an ovum is present, even quite a distance away, they move in the direction of the egg (Fig. 2–3B). Such an attraction by the egg indicates strongly that some substance must have been released by the egg cell for the specific purpose of attracting the spermatozoa into the uterine tube, which they reach within a few hours. From there they migrate towards the upper third of the tube where the ovum is and where fertilization is to take place.

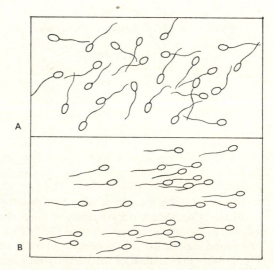

FIG. 2–3. Drawing of human spermatozoa showing the effect of the ovum on their orientation:
A. Randomly oriented when no ovum is present in the vicinity;
B. Definitely oriented with their heads towards the location of the ovum.

The viability of the sperm in the human female genital tract is estimated at no more than two days, although they may remain motile for a much longer time. There is evidence that fertilizing power is lost before motility and that a motile sperm may not be capable of fertilizing an ovum. Artificial insemination, now widely practised in animal breeding, has shown that sperm viability can be prolonged by low temperatures, e.g., freezing with a protective medium such as glycerol.

Sterility is more often the fault of the male than female. In all, four factors, acting either singly or in combination, may be responsible: (a) sperm ejaculate may have a volume below 2 ml. and a density under 20,000,000/ml.; (b) sperm motility may be low, with more than 40% non-motile spermatozoa and a speed below 1·5 mm. per minute; (c) sperm morphology may be unusual, with for example less than 60% with normal morphology (p. 11); and (d) there may be an insufficient hyaluronidase concentration in the semen.

Female factors conducive to sterility: (a) Acidity of vaginal fluid (with a pH lower than 3·0) caused by the bacterium, *Lactobacillum*, which converts glycogen into lactic acid; (b) blockage of the passage from the fallopian tube to the uterus; (c) anovulatory menstrual cycles; (d) a lethal factor present in the vagina that kills all spermatozoa. This last is a recent finding; the chemical responsible for the phenomenon is under intensive investigation in an attempt to elucidate its nature. Its potential value in contraceptive medicine is obvious.

Ovum transport

The mucous membrane of the uterine tube is thrown into folds, by means of which the lumen of the tube is divided and subdivided into numerous intercommunicating spaces. The folds are especially highly developed at the ampullary end, continuing onto the peritoneal end of the tube as finger-like projections, the fimbriae (Fig. 2–2). The movements of these fimbriae ensure that an ovum finds its way after ovulation into the uterine tube. Following its entrance (virtually being swept in!), the ovum stays in the upper third of the tube where it remains, waiting to be fertilized. Its viability does not extend beyond two days and if not fertilized within that time, it dies and is carried down into the uterus, where it quickly disintegrates.

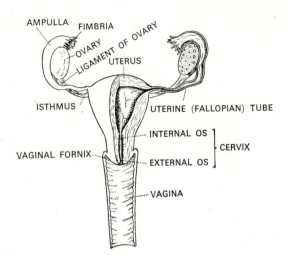

FIG. 2–2. Female organs of reproduction, anterior view (part in section). The ovaries have been displaced for purposes of illustration.

The ovum, which is surrounded by a multi-layered cellular corona radiata (Fig. 2–4A), is in most cases a secondary oöcyte ready to enter the second meiotic division. The first polar body can usually be seen enclosed between the vitelline membrane and the zona pellucida (Fig. 2–4B). The second meiotic division is completed while the ovum lies in the tube, just prior to fertilization (Fig. 2–5A). Penetration of the sperm serves as a stimulus to complete the division.

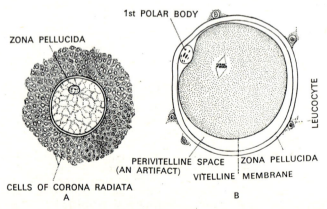

FIG. 2–4. A. Drawing of a photomicrograph of a human ovum immediately after ovulation. It is surrounded by a thick multi-layer corona radiata immediately outside the zona pellucida;
B. Drawing of a section of a human ovum showing the second maturation (meiotic) division spindle and a dividing polar body. The wide perivitelline space separating the vitelline membrane of the ovum from the zona pellucida is an artifact.

FERTILIZATION

The first sperm, after coming into contact with the egg, adheres to and penetrates it. (The entire cell, including the tail, enters the egg cytoplasm (Fig. 2–5B)). This penetration which may be regarded as specific as an antigen-antibody reaction, involves a reciprocal action on the part of both gametes. The peripheral part of the acrosome (Fig. 1–9) dissolves to release a lysin, hyaluronidase, which acts to disperse the cells of corona radiata. The remaining central portion of the acrosome is transformed into an elongate acrosomal filament. With the aid of this filament, the sperm pushes through the zona pellucida, its pathway being already cleared by the action of the sperm lysin. The egg immediately responds to the acrosomal filament by lifting a " fertilization cone " from the surface of the vitelline membrane at the point of contact with the spermhead. The cell membrane of this cone fuses with that of the spermatozoon so effecting entry of the sperm into the egg and the cone, then retracts to carry the sperm deep into the interior of the egg cytoplasm.

The formation of the fertilization cone is a sign of activation. Two changes follow in rapid succession: (a) a change in the peripheral cytoplasm of the egg results in the formation of a " fertilization membrane ". The latter, which spreads like a wave from the point of penetration over the whole surface of the egg, is a mechanism to prevent polyspermy by blocking the entry to further spermatozoa; (b) chemical substances are given off by the egg to slow down all remaining spermatozoa, causing them to lose their directive activity. (Spermatozoa arriving at the site, however, all contribute significantly toward dissolution of the cells of corona radiata).

Syngamy—union of pronuclei

The sperm nucleus immediately moves toward the egg nucleus (Fig. 2–5B). The two which

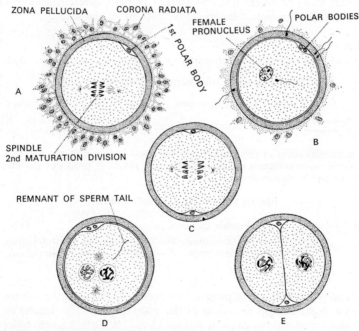

FIG. 2–5. Schematic drawing of fertilization and syngamy in the human:
A. Nucleus of primary oöcyte in anaphase (first polar body shown);
B. After entry of the sperm, with heads of four other spermatozoa immobilised in the zona pellucida (first and second polar bodies shown);
C. Anaphase of first cleavage division following syngamy;
D. Telophase of first cleavage division;
E. First two blastomeres at end of first cleavage division.

are now known as pronuclei, resolve their chromosomes into complete haploid (N) sets, and organize them on the spindle for the metaphase of the first cleavage division (early anaphase of this stage is shown in Fig. 2–5c). The centrosomes for the first cleavage division are supplied by the spermatozoon (Fig. 2–5D, E).

Results of fertilization

Three things are accomplished by the act of fertilization. These are: (1) Activation of the egg. Normally, the sperm provides this stimulus; it can, however, be replaced by other agents, both physical and chemical, as in cases of artificial parthenogenesis (p. 78). (2) Restoration of 2N (diploid) chromosome number for the species. (3) Chromosomal sex determination.

Experiments have shown that initiation of development requires a minimum of three conditions. They are: (a) a non-specific stimulus to bring about activation of the egg (b) at least a haploid set of chromosomes of either maternal or paternal origin (c) some egg cytoplasm, which can never be substituted by any part of the spermatozoon.

SEX DETERMINATION

In each species one pair of chromosomes, the sex chromosomes, is set aside for the purpose of sex determination, the remainder being known as the autosomes (Fig. 1–1). The two sex chromosomes, one arising from each parent, are homologous and they make a synaptic pair during meiosis. They can be present in either the homozygous or the heterozygous condition. It is obvious that the heterozygous individual produces two kinds of gametes in equal numbers while the homozygous individual produces just one kind of gamete. Herein lies the key to the mechanism of sex determination, namely " heterogamy " of one of the sexes.

Normal mechanism (Fig. 2–6)

Sex is determined by either male heterogamy or female heterogamy as follows:

Male heterogamy (this occurs in insects and man):

Male gametes	Female gametes	Off-spring
N autosomes + X	N autosomes + X	2N autosomes + XX (female)
N autosomes + Y		2N autosomes + XY (male)

(Note: A slight modification of this pattern is where XO is found in place of XY, i.e., in the male, the X chromosome is not paired, and as a result, it produces gametes either with or without the X chromosome.)

Female heterogamy (occurs in birds):

Male gametes	Female gametes	Off-spring
N autosomes + W	N autosomes + W	2N autosomes + WW (male)
	N autosomes + Z	2N autosomes + WZ (female)

Sex-ratio

The 1 : 1 sex ratio is not realized as precisely as expected. Among the human population the latest figure shows a slight margin in favour of the male sex, 48·47% females to 51·53% males. This difference is significant, but its cause is not yet clear. What is known, however, is that it is not due to differential deaths in the uterus.

Deviations from the normal mechanism

Generally speaking, the presence of the X chromosomes results in femaleness and that of the Y chromosome and autosomes in maleness. However, in some species the Y chromosome

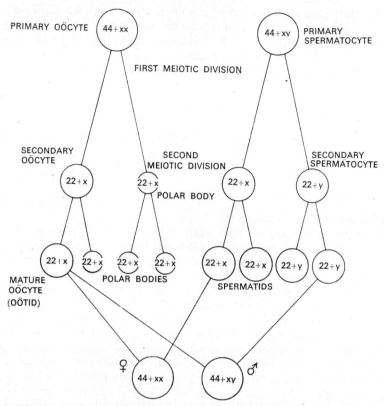

FIG. 2–6. Diagrammatic representation of the mechanism of sex determination in human (female at left; male, at right). The significance of this mechanism lies in the reduction of the number of chromosomes characteristic of the species from diploid (2N) to haploid (N) by means of the meiotic divisions.

apparently carries no male-determiners at all. This has been found to be true in the fruit fly, *Drosophila melanogaster*. It was noted that occasionally flies with more male characteristics than normal males or more female characteristics than normal females appeared in a population. In order to explain this satisfactorily Bridges proposed his "Theory of Genic Balance". *Drosophila* has 4 pairs of chromosomes (N = 4; A = 3). Of these, 3 pairs are autosomes (A) and 1 pair are sex chromosomes. A normal female fly has this formula: 2A + XX. But sometimes "non-disjunction" happens, i.e., chromosomes of synaptic pairs fail to separate during meiosis (p. 88). Should this occur, a viable egg with 2A + XX is produced (the polar bodies not getting any chromosome at all). When this egg is fertilized by a normal sperm, the resulting zygote gives rise to a "triploid" female as follows:

$$\left.\begin{array}{l} 2A + XX \text{ (egg)} \\ A + X \text{ (sperm)} \end{array}\right\} \longrightarrow 3A + 3X \text{ (triploid female)}$$

This triploid female is viable and produces four classes of eggs. The latter, when fertilized, produces six varieties of zygotes (genotypes) differing in their "sex status", thus:

Zygotes		Eggs from triploid female		Zygotes
2A + 2X		A + 2X		2A + 3X
3A + X	A + Y	2A + X	A + X	3A + 2X
3A + 2X	(sperm)	2A + 2X	(sperm)	3A + 3X
2A + X		A + X		2A + 2X

If we classify the above zygotes on the basis of the ratio X/A (not counting the Y chromosome), they would constitute a series ranging from the value 1·5 to 0·33 in the order of decreasing femaleness and increasing maleness. Such an interpretation based on actual observations gives considerable support to the theory of genic balance. It means that in *Drosophila* the Y chromosome plays no role in sex determination. The six genotypes demonstrating this are summarized as follows:

Zygotes	Frequency	X/A	Sex of the individual
2A + 3X	1/8	1·5	Superfemale
3A + 3X	1/8	1·0	Triploid female
2A + 2X	2/8	1·0	Normal female
3A + 2X	2/8	0·67	Intersex
2A + X	1/8	0·5	Normal male
3A + X	1/8	0·33	Supermale

Sex-chromosome aberrations in the human

Great progress has been made in recent years in the diagnosis of clinical cases of sex dimorphism and abnormalities. This progress is attributable largely to the discovery (by Barr in 1956) of a distinctive chromocentre (basophilic and Feulgen-positive), the sex chromatin, found in the interphase nuceli in most female (not male) cells in man and some other mammals; the chromatin is usually seen lying close to or directly against the nuclear membrane (Fig. 2–7). At present the origin of sex chromatin is not yet clearly understood; it is regarded by many as an XX chromosome derivative, therefore not present in either XO or XY sex-chromosomal patterns.

With this technique, cases were discovered in which a subject with a predominantly female appearance may exhibit male sex-chromatin pattern, and vice versa, indicating strongly that the sex chromosomes of these individuals were not normal. Careful cytological studies soon revealed that they were the results of aberrance of the Y chromosome. Since the loss or gain of the Y chromosome grossly affects the sex of the individual, the Y chromosome in the human (contrary to that in *Drosophila*) carries maleness determiners. Also, these cases are associated with another phenomenon called " Mosaicism ", which is thought to be caused by nondisjunction of the sex chromosomes during mitotic cleavage divisions. The two most common examples of these aberrations of sex chromosomes are given below:

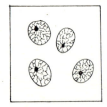 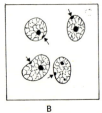

A   B

Fig. 2–7. Drawing of the nuclei of heart mesenchyme cells showing the sex chromatin pattern; (A) represents the male and (B) the female. The arrows point to the sex chromatin

1. Turner's syndrome — gonadal dysgenesis. The individual has principally female characteristics, but with a male (negative) sex-chromatin pattern, and a " streak " ovary, i.e., consisting mostly of connective tissue. The sex chromosome complement is either XO (a Y having been lost from XY) or XX/XO mosaicism; such an individual apparently starts out as a male (XY), but turns in the direction of femaleness after losing the Y chromosome. This proves that XO and XY complexes are not equivalent in the genetic sex-determining mechanism.
2. Kleinefelter's syndrome — seminiferous tubule dysgenesis. The individual is phenotypically a male, but with small testes and fibrosis and hyalinization of the seminiferous tubules and no spermatogenesis; there is a female sex-chromatin pattern. The sex

chromosome complement is either XXY (a Y being added to XX) or XX/XXY mosaicism; it is a case of one Y chromosome overriding the effect of the two X chromosomes, again demonstrating the male-determining property of the Y chromosome. Incidentally, a fair percentage of the individuals exhibiting these syndromes are mongoloid, or mentally underdeveloped or retarded.

Sex-linked inheritance

The X chromosome carries certain genes for somatic characteristics in addition to determiners for femaleness. These genes are, of course, transmitted according to Mendelian laws, but their phenotypical expression in the two sexes depends on whether or not the gene in question is dominant or recessive. The best known examples of sex-linked maladies in man are colour-blindness and haemophilia. In both, the gene involved is recessive, hence the mechanism of transmission is identical. The genotypes and phenotypes of colourblindness are given below so that the results of any marriage between a man and woman with known genotypes can be worked out without difficulty.

The gene for colourblindness is represented by $\overline{X}$

Genotypes	Phenotypes
XY	Normal man
XX	Normal woman
$\overline{X}$Y	Colourblind man
$\overline{X}$X	a " carrier " for colourblindness; herself not colourblind
$\overline{X}\,\overline{X}$	Colourblind woman

Note: It takes only one $\overline{X}$ chromosome to make a man colourblind, and that $\overline{X}$ can only come from the mother. A woman, on the other hand, requires homozygosity of $\overline{X}$ in order to exhibit colourblindness. However, a woman heterozygous with respect to the colourblind gene can nevertheless give that $\overline{X}$ gene to either her sons or daughters. For this reason, she is known as a " carrier ".

CHAPTER 3

CLEAVAGE, GASTRULATION AND MESODERM FORMATION

This chapter presents a comparative review of early vertebrate development. *Amphioxus*, frog, chick and mammals are chosen to represent the different patterns of cleavage, gastrulation and mesoderm formation. Lengthy descriptions of developmental processes and the mechanisms involved are avoided; instead, key information is condensed and summarized in tables and illustrated by drawings in order to help an understanding of the basic facts in development. It is believed that these basic facts are of value to a study of comparable stages in human development.

CLEAVAGE

Eggs are classified on the basis of the amount of yolk they contain and how it is distributed in the egg (Table 3–3). The yolk or deutoplasm represents an inert material in the egg cytoplasm. Because it offers resistance to cell division, the inert yolk affects both the form (pattern) and rate of cleavage divisions, as well as the degree of completeness of a cell division. Some of these influences are clearly seen in the following rules of cleavage, which were formulated by early embryologists from very careful observations.

Rules of cleavage
1. Cells tend to divide into two equal parts.
2. Each new plane of division tends to intersect the preceding plane at right angles. (Rules 1 and 2, by Sach.)
3. The typical position of the nucleus (and mitotic figure) tends to lie in the centre of its sphere of influence, i.e., the protoplasmic mass.
4. The axis of the spindle typically lies along the longer axis of the protoplasmic mass; division cuts this axis transversely. (Rules 3 and 4, by Hertwig.)
5. The rate of cleavage is inversely proportional to the amount of yolk present (by Balfour).

It must be remembered that the two factors which cause these differences are (*a*) the amount of yolk and (*b*) the way in which it is distributed. But, despite the differences, cleavage consists of a rapid series of mitotic divisions almost immediately following fertilization, the end product being a spherical hollow structure known as a blastula (Table 3–1).

The significant thing about this blastula, regardless of the size of blastomeres or whether or not a segmentation cavity is present, is that the several hundred cells which compose it constitute all the material that is necessary to develop into a complete organism. Cleavage is, therefore, primarily a device for providing the prospective embryo with a sizeable stock of building material, even though the cells in a blastula look much alike and are yet morphologically undifferentiated.

Although the first few cleavage planes may vary in different animals, they are, nevertheless, fundamentally similar. Let us take *Amphioxus* as a typical example (Fig. 3–1). The first plane divides the zygote from pole to pole into 2 equal blastomeres. The 2nd cleavage plane is also meridional, bisecting the 2 cells into four as in quartering an apple. The 3rd division is latitudinal (parallel to equatorial plate), resulting in 8 blastomeres, 4 at each of the two poles. The blasto-

Table 3–1. A Comparison of Blastulae

Feature:	Blastomeres		Segmentation cavity (blastocoele)		
Animal	Layer of cells	Size of cells	shape	position	origin
Amphioxus (Fig. 3–2)	Most typical: a single layer of blastoderm (Fig. 3–2B)	almost equal, only slightly smaller at the animal pole	Spherical	Central and closed	Typical true blastocoele
Frog (Fig. 3–3)	Several layers (Fig. 3–3F)	Considerable difference in size of micromeres and macromeres	Semi-spherical with a flat bottom	Eccentric in apical hemisphere; displaced toward animal pole; closed (Fig. 3–3F)	Same as in *Amphioxus*
Chick (Fig. 3–4)	A small cap of cells (like a disc) on top of yolk	about equal	A flat cleft	underneath the blastoderm	Not derived from segmentation activity;* formed by withdrawal of blastoderm from yolk
Mammal (Fig. 4–3A)	Blastocyst (preceded by a solid morula) as an aberrant (atypical) blastula	Inner cell mass (equivalent to blastoderm in chick); Trophoblast, (comparable to periblast in chick)			Equivalent to lecithocoele in chick

* The rapid cleavage planes never extend to the edge of the blastoderm disc, hence the marginal cells are connected with a ring of unsegmented protoplasm, periblast. Tangential divisions keep adding new cells to the central region of the blastoderm, but not all these are complete cell divisions. As a result, the periblast soon becomes a multinuclear syncytium, which retains its connection with the yolk at the margin and with the central cells of the blastoderm. It forms the germ wall.

The blastoderm overlying the original lecithocoele is area pellucida (no yolk); the marginal ring added from the germ wall is area opaca. The exterior margin of the germ wall advances out over the yolk to form the wall of the yolk sac.

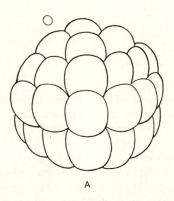

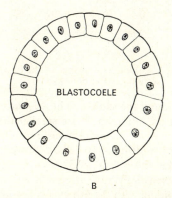

BLASTOCOELE

A   B

FIG. 3–2. Cleavage of *Amphioxus*; A, 32-cell stage; B, section of blastula.

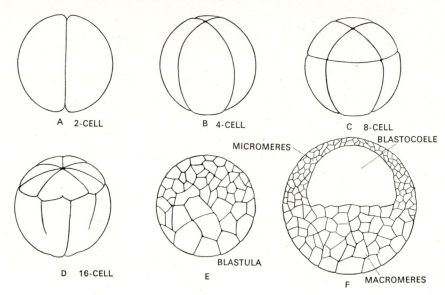

FIG. 3–3. Outline drawings of cleavage in the frog.

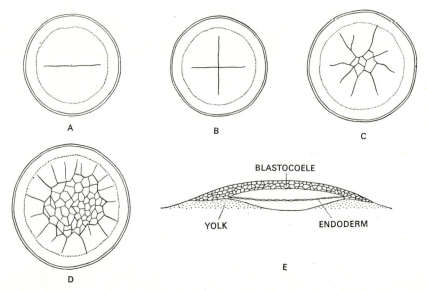

FIG. 3–4. Outline drawings of the discoidal cleavage of the chick, A–D, in surface view. E in section. (After Ballisky.)

meres are about the same size in *Amphioxus*, but often (in eggs with an increased amount of yolk) the cells at the animal pole are smaller than those at the vegetal pole. The 4th and 5th cleavages consist each of two simultaneous division planes: the 4th of 2 meridional ones at right angles to each other (resulting in 16 cells) followed by the 5th, two latitudinal ones, thereby converting the 16-cell stage into a total of 32 blastomeres. From there on, divisions are no longer precise, but become increasingly more irregular with regard to timing and degree of completeness of divisions. Also, beginning with the 6th cleavage four division planes will occur more or less simultaneously, all of which are meridional. Likewise, the next (7th) cleavage will consist of four latitudinal division planes taking place about the same time. The number of division planes will double but alternate from meridional and latitudinal in this manner. They cannot be followed as easily as the early cleavages. As cleavage advances, the resulting blastomeres become smaller and smaller, and they soon become arranged spherically to enclose a segmentation cavity (blastocoele) in typical cases (Fig. 3–2). The blastomeres may form a layer several cells thick (Table 3–1).

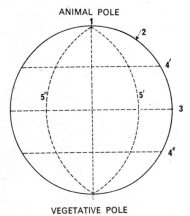

FIG. 3–1. Diagram to show the first five cleavage division planes in an isolecithal egg such as that of *Amphioxus*.

GASTRULATION

Up to the time prior to gastrulation there has been no growth in mass. The blastomeres, except for differences in size, are essentially indistinguishable and the cavity they enclose, the blastocoele, does not communicate with the exterior.

Table 3–2. A COMPARISON OF THE METHODS OF GASTRULA FORMATION.

Amphioxus (Fig. 3–5A, B, C)	Frog (Fig. 3–6A–F; J–L)	Chick (Fig. 3–7A, D)	Mammal (Fig. 4–5A)
(a) Invagination: Macromeres form the primary endoderm, lining the gastrocoele or archenteron assisted by: (b) Epiboly (arrows, Fig. 3–5A): Local growth of blastopore, the dorsal lip; the cells formed at this point segregate into ectoderm and endoderm. The endoderm formed this way is secondary endoderm, the increased extent of gastrocoele is the deutenteron. The opening of gastrocoele (blastopore) grows smaller as epiboly continues. The phenomenon is called concrescence. (Fig. 3–5B, C)	(a) Epiboly: Most of the endoderm formed is secondary endoderm (arrows, Fig. 3–6B): (b) Invagination: Only by small cells derived from the macromeres. Hence, the anterior portion of the gastrocoele is an archenteron. Yolk plug gets smaller and smaller as concrescence of the blastopore progresses. (Fig. 3–6J)	Practically entirely by epiboly (Fig. 3–4E); enoderm is completely secondary and the gastrocoele, a deutenteron with a floor of undivided yolk. Epiboly may be assisted by some delamination. A gastrular lip is formed at the posterior-most end of the blastoderm (Fig. 3–7A). The margin begins to thicken and inward migration of cells starts to form the lower germ layer (secondary endoderm) as an involution of the blastoderm. The egg is laid at an early stage of gastrulation (Further development is suspended unless incubated).	Predominantly by delamination from the ventral cells of the inner cell mass to become the endoderm layer.

Just as division is the one characteristic feature of cleavage, so the key feature of gastrulation is the movement of cells (Fig. 8–3); as a result of this process cells are translocated as they become differentiated. During gastrulation there will be growth and differentiation (p. 80) accompanying the processes of cell division and localization.

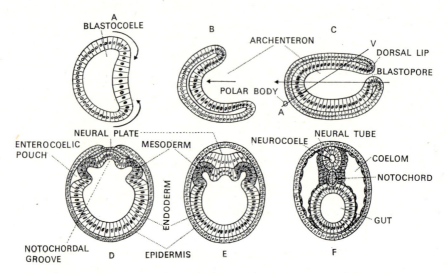

FIG. 3–5. Gastrulation (A, B, C) and mesoderm formation (D, E. F) in *Amphioxus*.
  A. Sagittal sections of early gastrulation (arrows indicate directions of epiboly and involution);
  B. More advanced stage of gastrulation (the arrow indicates the direction of invagination);
  C. Late gastrulation (the arrow indicates the antero-posterior axis and the line AV marks the original animal-vegetal poles);
  D. to F. Transverse sections of postgastrular stages, showing the formation of the neural tube, somites and notochord.

MESODERM FORMATION

In *Amphioxus*. Cells destined to form the mesoderm are carried in with the endoderm, to separate out later as enterocoelic pouches and notochordal groove by a process of folding. Each of them separates off from the remainder in the form of a vesicle; the one in the centre becoming the notochord, the two lateral ones, somites (Fig. 3–5D–F).

In the Frog. The endoderm and mesoderm separate as they are formed at the lip of the blastopore. The process is advanced in time until it is almost synchronous with gastrulation. A second plane of delamination appears at the dorsal lip of the blastopore, with the result that cells formed by epiboly become segregated into 3 layers, ectoderm above, mesoderm between, and endoderm below. The dorsal mesoderm separates into 3 cephalocaudal strips, of which the median one gives rise to notochord whilst the lateral ones grow forward and downward as mesothelial sheets. To the latter are added: mesodermal mass delaminated *in situ* from the primary endoderm and from the secondary endoderm formed at the lateral and ventral lips of the blastopore (Fig. 3–6G–I).

In the Chick (Fig. 3–7E–H). In the chick endoderm is formed at the first appearance of the dorsal lip. Mesoderm is formed from the primitive streak (Fig. 3–7C, D), an axial thickening of the ectoderm in the posterior two-thirds of the area pellucida formed after 16 hours of incubation. The primitive streak has the following components comparable to parts of the blastopore:

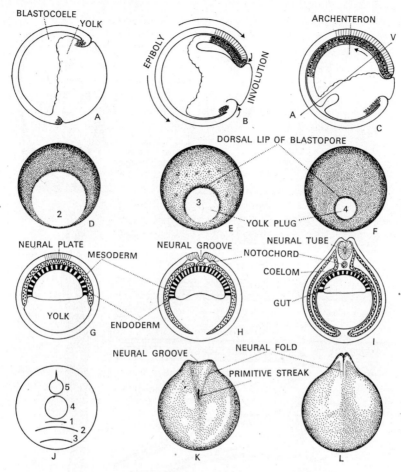

FIG. 3–6. Gastrulation and mesoderm formation in the frog.

A. Section of early gastrulation, the arrow indicating involution at the dorsal lip; a large yolk plug is present.

B. Later stage of gastrulation showing ectoderm of the neural plate (lined) chordamesoderm (small solid dots) and endoderm (small circles), the latter two are segregated as cells formed by epiboly turn inward at the blastopore lips; the yolk plug is decreasing in size (the arrows indicate epiboly and involution).

C. A still later stage of gastrulation, showing further advanced involution (arrow) and the future antero-posterior (primary) axis of the animal (the line AV).

D, E, and F. External posterior views of stages approximately corresponding to A, B, C, respectively, showing progressive reduction of the yolk plug due to closing of the blastopore (numbers 2, 3, 4 correspond to those of J).

G, H. and I. Transverse sections of frog embryos showing successive stages in the formation of mesoderm, notochord and neural tube (ectoderm, lightly lined; mesoderm, dotted; endoderm, heavily lined).

J. Diagram, (dorso-posterior view) to show the successive positions of the blastoporal lip as gastrulation proceeds from 1 to 5 (4 and 5 also indicating size of yolk plug).

K. Early neurula stage. L. neural fold stage.

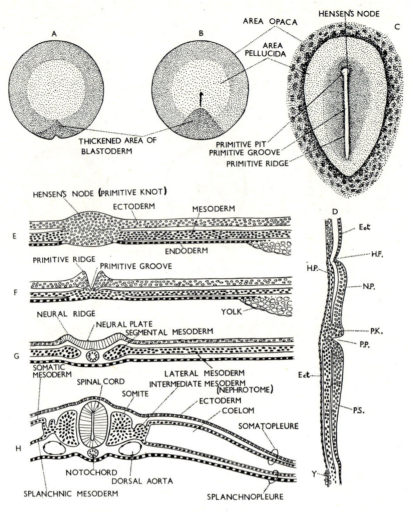

FIG. 3–7. Gastrulation and mesoderm formation in the chick.
A. 3–4 hour incubation;   B. 5–6 hour incubation;
C. Primitive streak stage (about 17 hours);
D. Sagittal section through the head process and head fold (20 hours);
E. Transverse section through the primitive knot (Hensen's node);
F. Transverse section through central portion of the primitive streak;
G. Transverse section through the neural plate (23 hours);
H. Transverse section through the neural folds (36 hours).

(a) primitive groove (homologous with the blastopore, but modified);
(b) primitive folds (ridges) — (homologous with gastrular lips);
(c) primitive knot (Hensen's node), from which cells migrate forward to become the head process; this is the forerunner of the notochord.
(d) primitive pit. From the sides and posterior end of the streak mesothelial mesoderm grows out to form a shield-shaped middle layer interrupted only by the streak itself and the notochord in front. Thus, the primitive streak corresponds to the gastrular lip in amphibians.

In Mammals. Mesoderm is formed essentially as in the chick, i.e., by means of a primitive streak (Figs. 4–10; 4–13).

Table 3–3. A SUMMARY OF EARLY DEVELOPMENT IN *Amphioxus*, FROG, CHICK AND MAN

Animal	Egg	Cleavage	Method of gastrulation	Mesoderm formation	Neural tube formation
Amphioxus	Isolecithal; holoblastic	Equal and total	Invagination of macromeres and some epiboly at blastopore	From secondary endoderm into 2 enterocoelic pouches and a central notochordal groove ⎱ overlapping ⟷	Immediately following the establishment of axial structure: notochord (chordamesoderm) and mesothelia
Frog	Lecithal (moderately telolecithal); holoblastic	Unequal; partial	Epiboly and Invagination	Precocious (simultaneous with gastrulation): (a) from involuted cells at dorsal lip 3 layers delaminated: middle mesoderm immediately dividing into 3 cephalic strips (b) Delamination from secondary endoderm formed at lateral and ventral lips of blastopore	Same in all Vertebrates (see p. 213)
Chick	Macrolecithal (highly telolecithal); meroblastic	Discoidal	Epiboly and Delamination	From the primitive streak by active cell movement of two lateral halves of blastoderm toward the centre	
Man (mammals in general)	Isolecithal	Atypical morula and blastocyst	Delamination	Essentially the same as in chick, i.e., from the primitive streak	

CHAPTER 4

IMPLANTATION AND EARLY DEVELOPMENT

Cleavage, morula and blastocyst formation

The human zygote spends its first three days journeying down the uterine tube (Fig. 4–2); during this time it undergoes cleavage. By the time it reaches the isthmus it consists of 8 blasto-meres (comparable to Fig. 4–1E). The first two blastomeres may not, however, divide at the same time, thereby resulting in an intermediate 3-cell stage (Fig. 4–1B) intervening between the first two cleavage divisions. For the same reason, there may be a 6-cell stage (Fig. 4–1D). Shortly after arriving in the uterine cavity the zygote has become a morula (Fig. 4–1F) which is a solid cluster of 16–32 cells without a central segmentation cavity. It does not therefore strictly corres-pond to a blastula, see p. 21; (it is an atypical blastula).

During the next 2 to 3 days the ovum remains unattached and is nourished by a glycogen-rich secretion (uterine milk) from the uterine glands. In preparation for implantation, the zona pellucida disintegrates and the morula differentiates into a blastocyst. The latter is a hollowed-out, ball-like structure, formed by delamination of a layer of cells from the main group of cells. The delaminated cells arrange themselves into a spherical membrane, the trophoblast, which

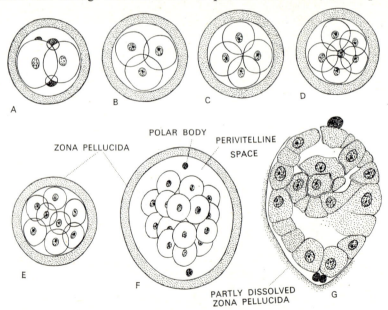

Fig. 4–1. Drawings of the cleavage stages of the macaque monkey (A to E).
  A. 2–cell stage;   B, 3–cell stage;   C. 4–cell stage;
  D. 6–cell stage;   E. 8–cell stage.
  F. Drawing from a photomicrograph of a living morula of macaque monkey, containing 16 cells.
  G. Drawing from a photomicrograph of a section through a 58–cell human blastocyst removed from the uterine cavity. (After Hamilton, Boyd and Mossman, after Lewis and Hartman and Hertig and Rock.)

encloses a central cavity, the blastocoele (Fig. 4–3A). The trophoblast so formed is attached to the remaining cell mass, now known as the inner cell mass. The cells of the inner cell mass, some-times called the embryoblasts, will give rise to the future foetus, while the trophoblast and all its derivatives form only extra-embryonic tissues, which do not contribute materially to the embryo proper but form the forerunner of the chorion, destined to be the foetal component of the placenta.

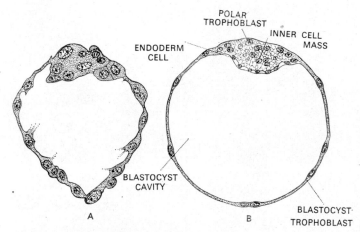

FIG. 4–3. A. Drawing from a photomicrograph of a section of a human blastocyst (about 107 cells). (After Hamilton, Boyd and Mossman.)
B. Drawing of a 9-day zona macaque monkey blastocyst which has lost the zona pellucida and is ready to be implanted. (After Hamilton, Boyd and Mossman.)

Implantation

Implantation takes place while the ovum is at the blastocyst stage of development, around the 7th day following fertilization (Fig. 4–2). The phenomenon is believed to require reciprocal action on the part of both maternal and foetal tissues. That of the former is represented by a "sensitization" of the endometrial stroma cells, and is known as the "decidual reaction". Contact may be made at any point on the surface of the blastocyst, but adhesion results only from cells directly overlying the inner cell mass (Fig. 4–3B). This implies that the foetal cells must be " properly " prepared for implantation. After an initial attachment is made in this way, the area of adhesion rapidly spreads.

Abnormal implantation sites and resultant ectopic pregnancies.

An egg infrequently goes astray and lands at places other than the normal implantation site. Such an egg, if fertilized, will be implanted as long as there is peritoneum present. Six ectopic implantation sites are known: (1) the abdominal cavity, particularly the recto-uterine cavity; (2) the ampullary region of the uterine tube; (3) inside the uterine tube itself; (4) inside the uterus, but in abnormal places; (5) in the region of the internal os (see Fig. 2–2); and most rarely (6) inside the ovary itself. Pregnancy at these sites (with the exception of no. 4) never reaches completion, but invariably leads sooner or later to the death of the embryo and haemorrhage of the mother; there may even be other complications. In category no. 4, the most frequent (and normal) site of implanta-tion is the posterior or anterior wall of the uterus; then in descending order of frequency, on the sides, near the internal os, and finally at the fundus. Of these abnormal sites, that which is the most serious and of greatest clinical significance is the internal os site, on account of the fact that the placenta blocks the opening to the vagina and antepartum haemorrhage results. This condition is known as " placenta praevia ".

One interesting feature about ectopic pregnancies is that even in those cases where the embryo is far removed from the endometrium, the latter nevertheless responds as if normal implantation had

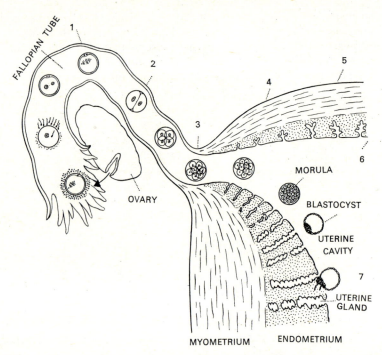

FIG. 4–2. Diagrammatic representation of the process of ovulation, fertilization, cleavage, and implantation of the blastocyst. Numbers 1 to 7 indicate days counting from the time of fertilization. (After Dickinson.)

taken place. There have been rare cases in which spurious labour, followed by extrusion of decidua, actually took place. These instances emphasize strongly the general mechanism of hormonal actions.

Events immediately following implantation

Following implantation, development proceeds in the inner cell mass and in the trophoblast. From the former a layer of small polyhedral cells is delaminated ventrally to become the endoderm (Figs. 4–3B; 4–4C and 4–5A). Almost simultaneously with this, the amnion is formed. Unlike reptiles and birds (p. 62), the human amnion takes its origin from those cells of the inner cell mass immediately underneath the polar trophoblast, (Fig. 4–3B) which are consequently called the amnioblasts; these cells are soon separated from the remainder of the inner cell mass by the formation of a cavity, the amniotic cavity. This is the product of coalescence of numerous tiny spaces created as a result of secretory activity of the amnioblasts. The amniotic cells thus delaminated and now lining themselves up in a single layer above the cavity, nevertheless remain connected peripherally to the inner cell mass (Fig. 4–5A). Subsequently, the rest of the inner cell mass flattens out and organizes itself into a layer of columnar cells which form the primitive ectoderm. Up to this time the embyro is a bilaminar disc, consisting of two loosely packed germ layers, one (the ectoderm) sitting on the top of the other (the endoderm).

At the same time the implanting trophoblast cells (Fig. 4–4A) (originally polar trophoblast, Fig. 4–3B) burrow deeper into the endometrium. At this spot the trophoblast cells have already differentiated into an outer layer of syncytiotrophoblast and an inner cellular layer, the cytotrophoblast (the black and light zones respectively in Fig. 4–5A; the syncytial layer is shown dark in Fig. 4–4A). The initial activity during implantation and subsequent further extension and enlargement of this area are due to the invasive action of the syncytiotrophoblast. The differentiation of the trophoblast into two layers spreads from the implantation site to the entire prospective chorionic vesicle.

The early activity of the syncytiotrophoblast to secure a foothold for the embryo is by way of erosion of maternal tissue at points of contact. The implanted blastocyst may be likened to a parasite invading its host, the activity of the syncytiotrophoblast being not unlike the cells of a malignant tumour in many respects (see p. 60). The moving front of the syncytiotrophoblast spreads deeper and wider as it keeps digging into the endometrium; stroma cells in its path break down and blood vessels rupture. In this way the sprawling trophoblastic syncytium gives rise to numerous irregular spaces of various sizes separated by syncytiotrophoblastic strands or irregular trabeculae (Fig. 4–5B); these spaces are the trophoblastic lacunae. The merging of these lacunae with the ruptured sinusoids and capillaries of the endometrium (Fig. 4–5B) results in the formation of many blood-filled spaces, which constitute the forerunners of intervillous spaces. The embryo is completely buried in the mucosa by the 11th day; during this time it has been nourished by a composite cellular material known as " histiotrophe " or " embryotrophe ", which consists of a cellular debris mixed with blood, i.e., the products of its own erosion of the endometrium.

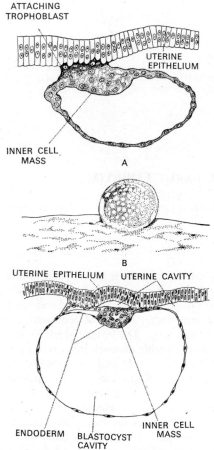

FIG. 4–4. A. An early stage of attachment of the trophoblast of a macaque monkey. (After Wislocki and Streeter.)
B. Drawing (from a photomicrograph) of an external view of the side of the above blastocyst. (After Heuser and Streeter.)
C. A slightly later stage of attachment of the blastocyst than shown in B. (After Heuser and Streeter.)

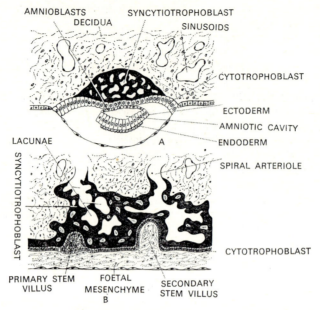

FIG. 4–5. A. Drawing of a section of 7½-day human embryo, to show the early development of placenta. (Modified from Davies.)

B. A later stage in placenta development showing (a) the formation of lacunae within the syncytiotrophoblast and rupture of the decidual capillaries (b) the formation of primary stem villi; and (c) the formation of secondary stem villi. (Modified from Davies.)

FURTHER DEVELOPMENT OF THE EARLY EMBRYO

Further development of the human embryo will be studied in four successive stages: approximately 9, 12, 14 and 21 days of age.

9-day human embryo (Fig. 4–6)

This embryo, which closely resembles that described by Miller in 1913, is about 1½ days later than that which has just been described. This later embryo has an amnion with a well defined amniotic cavity and consists of two germ layers, the ectoderm (high columnar cells) and endoderm (small polyhedral cells). It has an embryonic vesicle (0·4 mm) larger than that represented in Fig. 4–5A and also a much larger trophoblast (0·9 mm. in diameter). The latter (which by now has spread almost all around the embryonic vesicle, enclosing a sizable exocoelomic cavity) consists of an extensive outer layer, the syncytiotrophoblast (black, Fig. 4–6) and an inner layer of cytotrophoblast (stippled, Fig. 4–6). Many irregular spaces, trophoblastic lacunae, are enclosed in the syncytiotrophoblast. The trophoderm has developed further and a layer of mesothelial cells has delaminated from the surface of the cytotrophoblast. This is Heuser's membrane, which is the forerunner of extra-embryonic mesoderm. It rapidly lines the entire exo-coelomic cavity (primitive yolk sac) as well as covering the embryonic disc. The point of entry of the trophoblast into the endometrium is closed by a fibrin coagulum. There is, as yet, no definitive yolk sac in the embryo or chorionic villi on the trophoderm.

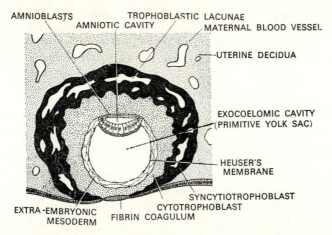

FIG. 4–6. Drawing of a section of a 9-day human blastocyst.

12-day human embryo (Fig. 4–7)

The embryo proper has advanced relatively little, except for a change in the orientation of the ectodermal and amniotic cells (cf. Fig. 4–6; Fig. 4–7). The trophoderm has, however, further differentiated in many respects. The trophoblastic lacunae have increased in number and extent, but more importantly, some of them lying close to the border have established open connections with the maternal sinusoids. The trophoblast at the abembryonic pole is still poorly differentiated. Due to the continual delamination of cells from the cytotrophoblast, the extra-embryonic meso-derm has increased considerably in extent, and contains many spaces between the anastomosing strands of mesenchymal cells. When these spaces coalesce they will form the extra-embryonic coelom (Fig. 4–9). Because of the rapid growth of this extra-embryonic mesoderm, Heuser's membrane has remained as a thin layer, lining the inner surface of the extra-embryonic mesoderm. Some endodermal cells have begun to spread over the inner surface of the receding Heuser's membrane. The extra-embryonic mesoderm has thus differentiated into outer somatopleuric and an inner splanchnopleuric layers.

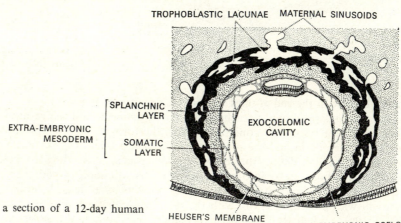

FIG. 4–7. Drawing of a section of a 12-day human blastocyst.

14–16 day human embryo (Peter's embryo) (Fig. 4–8)

At this stage the trophoderm has reached 1·1 mm. in diameter. The two most important features of difference are the formation of a definitive (secondary) yolk sac by cells delaminated from the endodermal layer and the beginning of villi formation. The trophoblastic lacunae have now extended from the embryonic to the abembryonic pole, encircling the entire chorionic vesicle and a uteroplacental circulation begins for the first time by virtue of an increasing number of intervillous spaces. The villi at this stage of development are primary stem villi (Fig. 4–19A), which, as yet, lack a core of any kind. The somatic layer of extra-embryonic mesoderm has differentiated into an outer dense and an inner loose portion. Blood vessels will arise from the former and so the developing villi will be provided with a vascularized core.

The spaces developing within the extra embryonic mesenchyme have by now coalesced to form a large confluent space, known as the extra-embryonic coelom, whilst the original exo-coelomic cavity (primitive yolk sac) has atrophied, forming a remnant (exo-coelomic cyst), which will soon disappear altogether.

The beginning of the formation of a body stalk is indicated and the amniotic cavity has flattened somewhat, accompanied by thinning down of its roof cells. The embryonic disc, thus rather flattened, is now ready for the formation of the primitive streak (Fig. 4–10A).

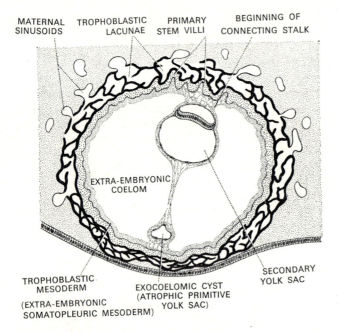

MATERNAL SINUSOIDS   TROPHOBLASTIC LACUNAE   PRIMARY STEM VILLI   BEGINNING OF CONNECTING STALK

EXTRA-EMBRYONIC COELOM

TROPHOBLASTIC MESODERM (EXTRA-EMBRYONIC SOMATOPLEURIC MESODERM)

EXOCOELOMIC CYST (ATROPHIC PRIMITIVE YOLK SAC)

SECONDARY YOLK SAC

FIG. 4–8. Drawing of a section of 13–15 day human blastocyst.

Human embryo at the end of third week (Spee's embryo) (Fig. 4–9)

The trophoderm disc has reached 8·0 mm. in diameter and the germ disc advanced from the bilaminar to the trilaminar condition. With the formation of the primitive streak, both intra-embryonic mesoderm and the notochord will soon appear (Fig. 4–10B). The establishment of these axial structures defines the embryo's primary axis. Extending from the posterior end of the embryo is the body stalk, into which an allantois will soon extend. The loose portion of the extra-embryonic mesoderm has disappeared, while its inner dense layer has provided the primary stem villi with a core; the villi with this yet unvascularized core are known as secondary villi (Fig. 4–19B). When this mesoderm becomes vascularized, the secondary villi become transformed into the functional stage, definitive or tertiary villi (Fig. 4–19C). This event coincides with the beginning of a vitelline circulation, when blood vessels are formed in the extra-embryonic splanchnic mesoderm of the yolk sac. These features mark the end of the early period of development.

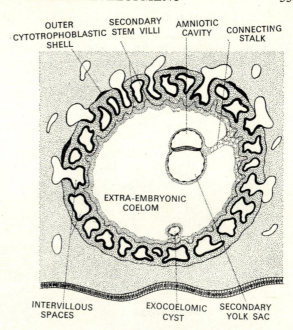

OUTER
CYTOTROPHOBLASTIC   SECONDARY   AMNIOTIC   CONNECTING
SHELL   STEM VILLI   CAVITY   STALK

EXTRA-EMBRYONIC
COELOM

FIG. 4–9. Drawing of a section of a 21-day human
embryo. (Modified from Langman.)

INTERVILLOUS   EXOCOELOMIC   SECONDARY
SPACES   CYST   YOLK SAC

Abnormal human blastocysts

Hertig, Rock and Adams in 1956 reported their study on 26 implanted blastocysts ranging from
$7\frac{1}{2}$–17 days of age, all recovered from patients of normal fertility. Of these, 35% were normal
blastocysts showing a varying degree of trophoblastic hypoplasia, some with a disoriented germ disc,
and two completely devoid of an embryoblast.

It is doubtful if any of these would have resulted in pregnancy; most of them probably would
have been aborted with the following menstrual flow. This is because of the inability of their
defective trophoblast to produce enough hormone to sustain the corpus luteum (p. 70). On the
other hand, cases of pathological overactivity of the trophoblast are also known. Sometimes the
persisting chorionic sac of an abnormal embryo becomes a cluster of fluid-filled vesicles known as a
hydatidiform mole. It is a benign tumour, and may attain a considerable size. Yet in other cases
(rare), the chorionic trophoblast turns into a malignant tumour known as a chorio-epithelioma.

Formation of the primitive streak

The third week of development constitutes a significant landmark. On or about the 15th
day, the ectodermal cells in the caudal half of the germ disc begin to round up; they proliferate
at a terrific rate and the resulting cells all migrate toward the midline. This fast " dumping " of
new cells along the embryo's primary axis gives rise to a median longitudinal prominence, the
primitive streak (Fig. 4–10). It is characterized by a narrow groove, the primitive groove, flanked
on both sides with slightly elevated edges, the primitive ridges (Fig. 4–10A). The cells thus aggregated at the streak belong potentially to all three germ layers (i.e. they are pleuripotent); those
that are destined to become mesoderm migrate forward from Hensen's node (see below), as the
notochordal process (or head process), and laterally between the ectoderm and endoderm as
definitive mesoderm (Fig. 4–10B). This latter is intra-embryonic mesoderm and is the last
germ layer to be formed. It eventually becomes continuous with the extra-embryonic mesoderm,
which covers the amnion and yolk sac.

The primitive streak bulges slightly into the amniotic cavity (Fig. 4–10C), and the embryonic
disc gradually elongates and assumes the form of an inverted pear-shaped disc. Its broad
cephalic end comes as a result of rapid expansion of new ectodermal cells from the streak
anteriorly, while new cells are also added to its caudal end (Fig. 4–10A). Thus, the primitive

streak is to be regarded not as an end in itself, but rather as a mechanism to attain an end, namely the formation of mesoderm and notochord. It persists until the end of the somite stage after which it retrogresses rapidly. The mesoderm derived from its terminal (caudal) portion contributes to some of the external genitalia (p. 137).

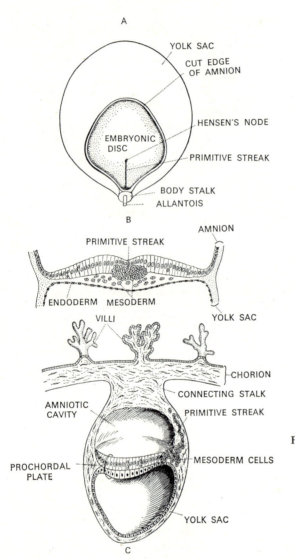

FIG. 4–10. A. Drawing of the dorsal aspect of a 16-day pre-somite embryo.
B. Transverse section through the region of the primitive streak, showing mesoderm cells being formed and invaginated from the primitive streak.
C. Schematic drawing of a mid-longitudinal section of such an embryo as that shown in A and B. (After Hamilton, Boyd and Mossman.)

Formation of the notochord

At the same time as the intra-embryonic mesoderm is formed, a further marked thickening of ectoderm appears at the extreme cephalic end of the primitive streak. This thickening constitutes Hensen's node. Rapid inward movement of surface cells in the node creates a pit, known as the blastopore (Fig. 4–11, 13). (On this basis, it is generally believed that the primitive streak is homologous with the blastopore of amphibians.) A cord of mesodermal cells then migrates forward from Hensen's node to become the primordium of the notochord, known at this stage as the notochordal or head process (Fig. 4–11). The invagination of the blastopore continues and extends into the notochordal process as a canal known initially as the notochordal canal and later as the neurenteric canal (Fig. 4–13).

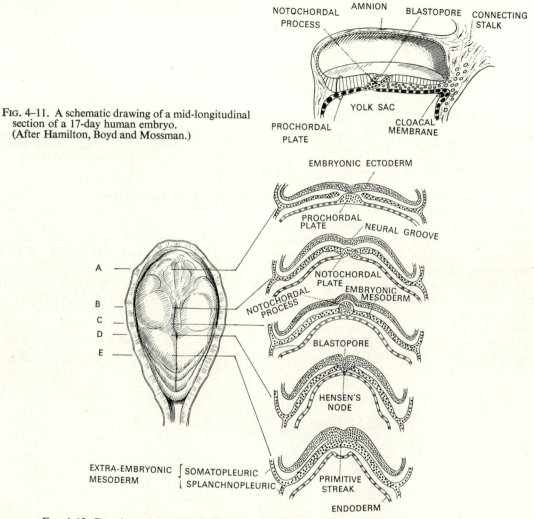

FIG. 4–11. A schematic drawing of a mid-longitudinal section of a 17-day human embryo. (After Hamilton, Boyd and Mossman.)

FIG. 4–12. Drawing of the dorsal aspect of an 18-day pre-somite embryo, with transverse sections of it at five levels (A to E) as indicated. (After Hamilton, Boyd and Mossman.)

As development proceeds, the notochordal process fuses with, and becomes intercalated in, the embryonic endoderm (Fig. 4–13; 12B); subsequently, an opening appears in the floor of the notochordal canal, bringing it into communication with the yolk sac cavity (Fig. 4–13). The situation thus creates a temporary communication between the amniotic cavity and the yolk sac cavity (Fig. 4–13). About this time, two significant events occur at opposite ends of the embryo. Immediately cephalic to the notochord on the one hand, and right behind the primitive streak on the other, the endoderm and ectoderm cells meet and fuse to form a bilaminar membrane. They are called respectively, the prochordal plate, (the forerunner of the buccopharyngeal membrane) and the cloacal membrane, (the forerunner of urogenital and anal membranes

(Fig. 4–13)).   At the same time, the posterior end of the yolk sac gives rise to a small diverticulum, which constitutes the allantois, and extends into the lengthening body stalk.   The body stalk, as a link between the placenta and embryo will be, in time, transformed into the umbilical cord.

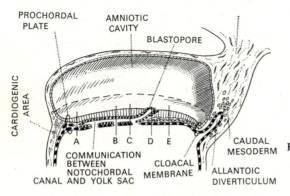

FIG. 4–13. Drawing of a sagittal section of the same embryo as in Figure 4–12.   The sectional levels used in the latter are indicated. (After Hamilton, Boyd and Mossman.)

In a 19-day pre-somite embryo (Fig. 4–14) the body folds have begun to undercut the embryo, bending it ventrally (this is more pronounced at the cephalic end), (Fig. 4–14B) with the result that the developing embryo takes on a marked dorsal convexity.   The embryo overhangs the extra-embryonic layers, displaying a tendency to lift itself above them.   Under this general influence a body stalk is further developed and the lateral and ventral body walls of the embryo are also established.   The portion of the yolk sac lying beneath the head becomes a closed foregut, lined by endoderm all around except caudally where it communicates with the mid-gut through the anterior intestinal portal.   Similarly at the posterior end, a hind-gut makes its appearance. The remaining mid-gut is open and has no floor (Fig. 4–15B).   Meanwhile, the ectodermal cells laying directly above the notochord thicken greatly and constitute a neural plate.   Blood island formation has begun in the splanchnopleuric mesoderm of the yolk sac and a primordium of the heart has appeared (Fig. 4–14B).

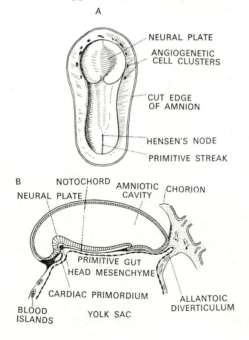

FIG. 4–14. A. Drawing of the dorsal view of a later pre-somite embryo about (19 days) showing the angiogenetic. cell clusters in front and on each side at the cephalic end. (After Langman.) B. Drawing of a sagittal section of an embryo of approximately of the same age as in A (possibly slightly older).   (After Patten.)

Only one day later (20-day embryo) three mesodermal somites have formed (Fig. 4–15A), and the neural plate has further developed by sending up two lateral folds (neural folds) which demarcate a resultant neural groove between them. The somites represent segregated blocks of paraxial mesoderm, arranged with one pair per segment. The first pair arises just behind the tip of notochord; from this point, new somites are added caudally in sequence at an approximate rate of four pairs per day until, by the end of the first month, 39–40 such pairs are present.

Coinciding with further undercutting of the embryo by the body folds, both the fore-gut and hind-gut have lengthened considerably (Fig. 4–15B). A tubular heart enclosed in a primitive pericardial coelom is seen to have developed immediately below the fore-gut. Posteriorly, the allantois has extended still further into the body stalk.

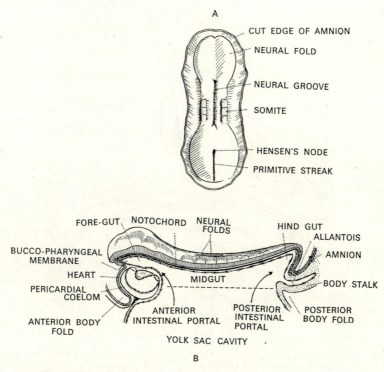

FIG. 4–15. A. Dorsal view of a 20-day human embryo.
B. Mid-longitudinal section of the above embryo.

In a 23-day embryo (Fig. 4–16) development has further advanced. Some of the features now present are best shown in transverse sections (Fig. 4–17). Up to this time the embryonic gut ends blindly at both ends, but by 23 days of development, an oral opening, the stomodaeum, and a cloacal opening, the proctodaeum, have appeared. In both instances the indented area comes as a result of a depression of the surface ectoderm followed by a sinking in of the latter to meet with the gut endoderm (Fig. 4–16B).

The neural tube is only partially closed by the dorso-medial fusion of the neural folds (approximately between levels C and E, Fig. 4–16A). The portions of the tube which remain open are represented by a large anterior neuropore and a sinus rhomboidalis at the caudal end (Figs. 4–16A; Fig. 4–17B, E).

The heart and pericardium are well established (Fig. 4–16B), with dorsal and ventral aortae already formed (Fig. 4–17A). Primordia of lung and liver are indicated (Fig. 4–15B). The process of formation of somites may be traced in Fig. 4–17 (B, C, D), in the last section of which the differentiation of epimere (somite), mesomere (intermediate mesoderm) and hypomere (lateral mesoderm) is clearly represented.   The caudal end of the primitive streak is still active in forming mesenchyme (Fig. 4–17E, F), and further narrowing down of the open mid-gut (Fig. 4–17E) has coincided with the furtherance of the under-cutting activity of the body folds.   As a result, both ends of the embryo have been lifted free from attachment to the underlying embryonic disc, thereby forming a subcephalic pocket (Fig. 4–17A) and a corresponding pocket at the caudal end (Fig. 4–16B).

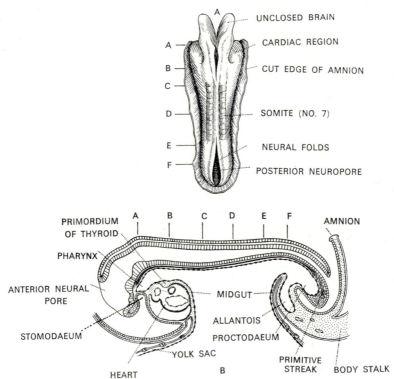

FIG. 4–16. A. Dorsal view of a 10-somite human embryo (approx. 25 days) on which are indicated six transverse levels (A to E) used in Figure 4–17.
B. Longitudinal section of an embryo of similar age to that above with corresponding six levels of transverse sections.

Further development of the trophoblast

The development of the trophoblast has been traced to the stage of the formation of primary and secondary stem villi (Fig. 4–19A, B), the formation of trophoblastic lacunae and the coalescence of the latter with ruptured endometrial sinusoids (Fig. 4–5B).   The next step in villi formation is the vascularization of the mesodermal core to convert the secondary stem villi into definitive or tertiary villi (Figs. 4–18A; 4–19C).   This process is accomplished by formation of blood vessels in the foetal trophoblastic mesenchyme (p. 145).   The deeply-penetrating mesenchymal cells are accompanied by a layer of cytotrophoblast.   At the tip of the villus, however, the cytotrophoblast proliferates so fast that it breaks through the overlying layer of syncytiotrophoblast (Fig. 4–18A).   These active cytotrophoblast cells constitute the cytotrophoblastic cell columns.   The confluence of the lacunae and the ruptured blood vessels form the intervillous spaces, which are virtually enclosed pools of maternal blood.

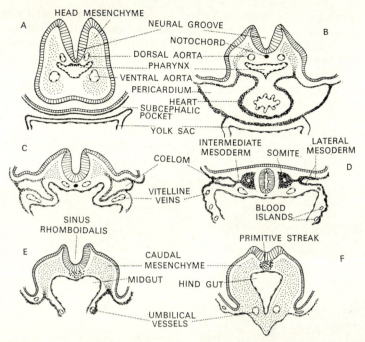

FIG. 4–17. The structure of human embryos (the same age as that in Figure 4–16) seen from transverse sections, the levels of which are indicated on Figure 4–16. (Bartelmez embryo.)

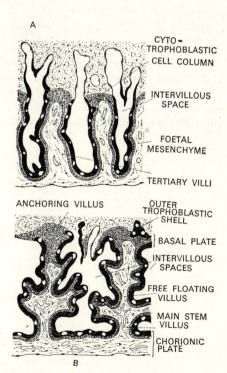

FIG. 4–18. A. A late stage in the formation of the chorionic villi.
B. A later stage in the development of the placenta.

The fully developed villus consists of a chorionic plate at its base (foetal side) and the basal plate at the maternal end. The latter plate becomes anchored in the decidua, hence the name " anchoring villus " which is sometimes used (Fig. 4–18B). In between these two ends, the villus undergoes repeated branching into countless smaller and smaller free floating villi (bush-like true villi), all of which regardless of size are provided with a vascularized core. The basal plate thus comprises three distinct components: (1) the cytotrophoblastic cell columns, (2) the outer trophoblastic shell (syncytiotrophoblast) and (3) the adjoining decidua basalis (Fig. 4–9; Fig. 4–18B). The function of this composite structure is to attach the foetal placenta firmly to the uterine wall. One characteristic of the basal plate is that it is pierced by maternal blood vessels, passing to and from the intervillous spaces (cf. Fig. 5–23A). It also constitutes the complex junctional zone of the definitive placenta (p. 59).

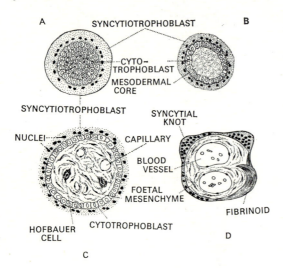

Fig. 4–19. Structure of human chorionic villi at four stages of development, as seen in transverse sections. A. Primary stem villi; B. Secondary stem villi; C. in the early weeks of pregnancy; D. at full term.

In late pregnancy the syncytiotrophoblastic layer gets thinner and becomes closely adherent to the foetal capillaries; in places it deforms into heaps, containing many nuclei, known as syncytial knots (Fig. 4–19D), which are believed to represent degenerated cells. The clinical significance of the syncitial knots, if any, is little understood except that it is known that they may sometimes get detached and subsequently find their way into the maternal circulation.

CHAPTER 5

THE DEVELOPMENT OF THE EMBYRO AND FOETUS

A. THE EMBRYONIC PERIOD (4th to 8th weeks)

The development of the human embryo during the period from $3\frac{1}{2}$ to 8 weeks of age will be studied by means of two approaches: (a) a listing (in summary form) of the major developmental events pertaining to each of the three germ layers, and (b) a presentation of six representative stages of development in this period (Figs. 5–3 to 5–8 inclusive) accompanied by a summary of comparative data (Table 5–1). The growth in length of the human embryo during this period based on the report of Streeter with Heuser and Corner in 1951, as presented by Davies (1963), is given in Fig. 5–1.

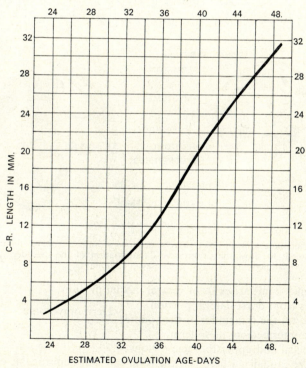

FIG. 5–1. Growth curve of human embryos up to the first 50 days of development. This is based on studies reported by Streeter with Heuser and Corner, 1951. (Modified from Davies.)

1. Differentiation of mesoderm (the derivatives of each component are listed)

Mesoderm
- Paraxial mesoderm (forerunner of somites)
- Intermediate mesoderm
- Lateral plate mesoderm
  - somatic or parietal layer
  - splanchnic or visceral layer

At the end of 3rd week the somites begin to give a segmental appearance to the body; first pair are located just caudal to the tip of notochord: 40 pairs are present at the end of first month. Differentiation of the somites (Fig. 5–2):

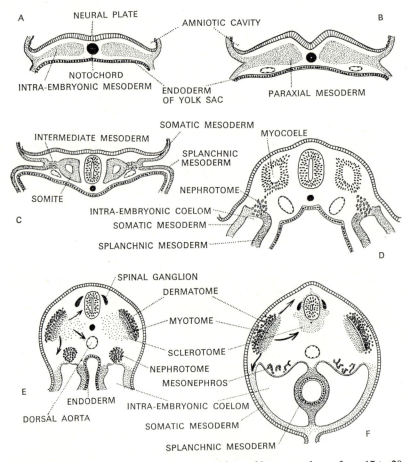

FIG. 5–2. Diagrammatic drawings of transverse sections of human embryos from 17 to 28 days of development to show the progressive differentiation of the mesoderm; A, 17 days; B, 19 days; C, 20 days; D, 21 days; E, 26 days; F, 28 days.

Sclerotome (mesenchymal) arises from ventral medial portion;
Dermatome arises from dorso-lateral portion
Myotome, constitutes the remainder of the somite } Dermomyotome
Differentiation of the intermediate mesoderm:
　Segmented in cervical and upper thoracic regions;
　Unsegmented more caudally, where it is the forerunner of nephrogenic cord.
Differentiation of the lateral plate mesoderm:
　Somatic layer, which is destined to form the mesothelial (serous) membranes of the peritoneal, pleural and pericardial cavities;
　Visceral layer is destined to form the smooth muscles and connective tissue coat of viscera.

2. Cardiovascular system (beginning at the middle of the 3rd week)
　(a) Angiogenetic cell clusters or blood islands appear.

(b) Bulging of embryonic disc upward into the amniotic cavity occurs.

(c) Cephalo-caudal folding of the body takes place, resulting in formation of the head and tail folds.

     (Note: Processes b and c, together with lengthening of the embryonic disc along the primary axis, constitute the basic developmental processes leading to the formation of the embryo) (see p. 38).

(d) Shifting of the angiogenetic clusters from their initial position in front of prochordal plate to more ventral aspects occurs.

(e) There is a gradual lifting of the germ disc from the yolk sac, producing the lateral body folds; at the same time angiogenetic cell clusters on each side approach each other ventrally in the midline.

(f) The angiogenetic cords fuse after acquiring a lumen, thereby establishing a single primitive endocardial tube suspended in the pericardial cavity; a conspicuous bulge, the pericardial swelling is thus produced.

(g) Formation of umbilical, vitelline and villous blood vessels takes place from the extra-embryonic mesoderm; these make connections with vessels of the embryo proper.

3. Pharyngeal (branchial) arches

somites (pairs) present		Arches
10		1st arch
14	{ Maxillary swelling { Mandibular swelling } 1st arch { 1st pharyngeal cleft	2nd arch (hyoid)
25		3rd arch

4. Endodermal germ layer

(a) Cephalocaudal folding produces the closed fore-gut.

(b) The closed fore-gut and open mid-gut both become lined with endodermal epithelium.

(c) The buccopharyngeal membrane ruptures at the end of the third week.

(d) The cloacal membrane becomes divided into the ventral urogenital and dorsal anal membranes.

(e) The open mid-gut is connected to the yolk sac by means of a broad stalk (vitello-intestinal duct), which continually narrows and lengthens; the yolk sac is never larger than 5 mm. in diameter and soon it is to be found alongside the allantois in the umbilical cord.

(f) The endoderm forms: (a) the epithelial lining of the respiratory tract, tympanic cavity and Eustachian tube, bladder and urethra (in part); (b) the parenchyma of tonsils, thyroid, parathyroids, thymus, liver and pancreas.

5. Ectodermal germ layer

(a) By the end of the 3rd week, the nervous system is an elongated slipper-shaped plate, the neural (medullary) plate, overlying the notochord and part of paraxial mesoderm.

(b) Fusion of neural folds begins in the region of the 4th somite, proceeding from there cephalically and caudally.

(c) Both anterior and posterior neuropores are present for a while. The former closes at a stage of 18–20 somites, the latter, at 25 somites.

(d) Otic placode differentiation is visible; from this an otic vesicle will be formed by invagination at end of 4th week.

(e) Optic vesicle has been formed.

TABLE 5–1. FEATURES OF SIX HUMAN EMBRYOS FROM 3½ TO 8 WEEKS OF DEVELOPMENT

FEATURES		3½-week	4-week	5-week	6-week	7-week	8-week (Transition between embryo and foetus)
Somites	No.	14	25	33	40	40	40
	Visibility	Externally distinct			decreasing external prominence	no longer visible externally	
Length (C.R.)		2·5 mm.	3·4 mm.	6·7 mm.	13·4 mm.	17·0 mm.	30·7 mm.
Brain	Neuropore	Present at both ends of neural tube	Anterior closed; posterior open	Both closed			
	Forebrain	indicated	projects markedly	Head bends ventrally	Marked head growth with decreased cervical flexure	Further increase in head size	Human appearance, for the first time
	Hindbrain			Rhombencephalon shows thin roof plate, bends ventrally	Cerebral vesicle indicated		
Brain Flexures				Cervical and Pontine flexures present			
Sense Organs	Eye			Optic vesicle showing pigment in retina and lens	Optic cup and lens	Eyes open; with lids developed	Eyes still open; will soon be closed by special ridges
	Ear	Otic placode present	Otic placode depressed	Otic vesicle present	External ear indicated	External ear and auditory meatus established	More distinctly developed
	Nose			Olfactory pit present			Nostrils sealed up
Pharyngeal arches and grooves		Maxillary and mandibular processes of 1st arch bounding stomodaeum	1st and 2nd, plus 3rd beginning to appear	2nd arch (hyoid) overlapping posterior ones with cervical sinus		A mouth with lips; tongue; and 20 milk-tooth buds	
Body curvature		Head and tail folds barely indicated					
Tail			Appearing	Well developed	Still present	Receding	Has disappeared
Head, trunk, neck				Head, trunk well marked; no neck yet		Neck established for the first time	Neck well established
Heart		As an elevated region below mandibular process	Prominent pericardial swelling; heart 9 times adult by proportion	Swelling still noticeable		Externally no longer visible	
Forelimb				As paddle-shaped buds;	Hands showing outlines of digits	Hands showing separated digits	Assuming embryonic position with radius and tibia directed cranially; fingers and toes well developed
Hind limb				Smaller than forelimb buds	Vague divisions of thigh, leg and foot	Digits of foot still closed	
Gut			Stomodaeum separated from foregut by bucco-pharyngeal membrane				
Liver					Bulging	A bulbous liver	
Yolk sac, Vitello-intestinal duct and Umbilical cord		As wide as midgut	Constricted				Umbilical cord further reduced; begin attachment to ventral abdominal wall
Cartilage and bone				First appearance of cartilage			First appearance of bone

Critical Period for limb development

Period of Sensitivity to harmful influence in environment e.g., thalidomide

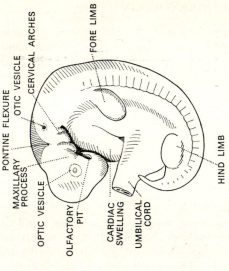

ANTERIOR NEUROPORE
1st PHARYNGEAL GROOVE
1st PHARYNGEAL ARCH
CUT EDGE OF AMNION
OTIC PLACODE
2nd PHARYNGEAL GROOVE
2nd PHARYNGEAL ARCH
1st SOMITE
CARDIAC SWELLING
CUT EDGE OF YOLK SAC
14th SOMITE
POSTERIOR NEUROPORE

FIG. 5-3. Schematic drawing (lateral view of left side) of a 14-somite embryo aged approx. 25 days.

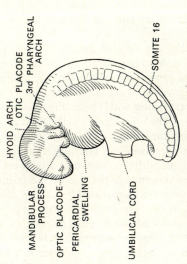

HYOID ARCH
OTIC PLACODE
3rd PHARYNGEAL ARCH
MANDIBULAR PROCESS
OPTIC PLACODE
PERICARDIAL SWELLING
UMBILICAL CORD
SOMITE 16

FIG. 5-4. Schematic drawing of the left side of a 25-somite human embryo aged approx. 4 weeks.

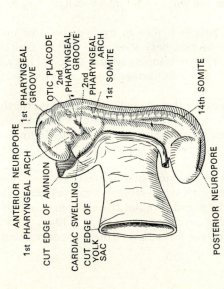

PONTINE FLEXURE
OTIC VESICLE
CERVICAL ARCHES
FORE LIMB
MAXILLARY PROCESS
OPTIC VESICLE
OLFACTORY PIT
CARDIAC SWELLING
UMBILICAL CORD
HIND LIMB

FIG. 5-5. Schematic drawing of a human embryo aged approx. 5 weeks

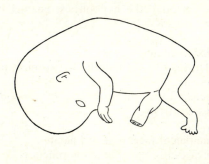

NASO-LACRIMAL FURROW
MID BRAIN
OPTIC CUP
EXTERNAL AUDITORY MEATUS
CERVICAL FLEXURE
HAND
CEREBRAL VESICLE
LEG

FIG. 5-6. Left side view of a 6-week human embryo, CR length = 13 mm.

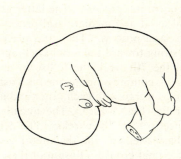

FIG. 5-7. Left side view of a 7-week human, embryo, CR length = 17 mm.

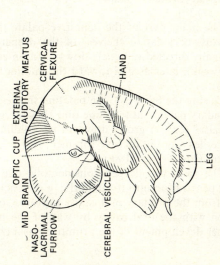

FIG. 5-8. Left side view of a 8-week human embryo, CR length = 30 mm.

(*f*) The ectoderm is destined to form the central nervous system, peripheral nervous system, sensory epithelium of sense organs, epidermis and its derivatives (hair, nail, subcutaneous glands), the hypophysis, enamel organs of teeth, and epithelial linings of some other organs.

6. External appearance

During the 2nd month the two most important factors to account for foetal external appearances are (*a*) the formation of the face, ear, nose and eyes; (*b*) the formation of the limbs, especially their aquisition of a 90° torsion with the result that the elbows point dorsally and the knees, ventrally.

Formation of face, nose and palate

The centre of facial development is a shallow ectodermal depression, the stomodaeum. This is soon bounded by a series of rounded elevations (processes or swellings) consisting of proliferations of head and/or branchial mesenchyme. Various muscles, bones and blood vessels differentiate from the mesenchymal cores of the branchial arches whilst their epithelial covering and lining give rise to other structures (see Chapters 17 and 21). The completion of these transformations results in the appearance of a neck (Fig. 5–7) which is a characteristic of the Amniotes. An elongation of this region involving vessels, nerves, muscles and the digestive and respiratory organs will take place later.

At $4\frac{1}{2}$ weeks, there are a pair of mandibular swellings, a pair of maxillary swellings and a median frontal process. The latter is composed of three definitive components, the frontonasal, lateral nasal and medial nasal processes (Fig. 5–9), the latter two arising slightly later than the frontonasal process. The nasal placodes mark the beginning of the nose. The maxillary swellings swing toward the nasal swellings without, however, fusing with them (Fig. 5–10).

In the 7th week the following events take place. The maxillary swellings keep growing medially, compressing the medial nasal swellings toward the middle line. As a result, the nasal swellings merge with each other and also with the maxillary swellings laterally, thus forming the upper lip (Fig. 5–10c). The maxillary swellings and mandibular swellings fuse over a short distance to form the cheeks. The degree of this fusion determines the size of the mouth. The maxillary swellings and the lateral nasal swellings are originally separated by a deep groove, the nasolacrimal groove. Fusion of these swellings results in the formation of a portion of the nasolacrimal duct underneath (p. 248). During the formation of the middle portion of the nose through merging of the medial nasal swelling, the following structures are formed: (*a*) the philtrum of the upper lip, (*b*) a maxillary component carrying four incisor teeth, and (*c*) the triangular primary palate. These three together are known as the intermaxillary segment (Fig. 5–12c).

The main part of the definitive palate (secondary palate) is formed by two shelf-like outgrowths, or palatine shelves, of the deeper parts of the maxillary swellings. These shelves, originally directed obliquely downward on either side of the developing tongue (Fig. 5–11, I AB) (6th week), later ascend toward the midline as the tongue moves further downward (Fig. 5–11, II AB).

During the 8th week, the palatine shelves approach each other medially and fuse to form the secondary palate; at the same time they merge anteriorly with the primary palate. Concurrently, the nasal septum grows down in the midline and joins the cephalic part of the newly-formed palate, leaving the incisive foramen as a middle landmark between the primary and secondary palates (Fig. 5–11, III AB).

The nasal pits deepen considerably, due to growth of the surrounding nasal swellings and their penetration into the underlying mesenchyme. The oronasal membrane which separates the pits from the primary oral cavity ruptures so placing the primitive nasal chambers in communication with the oral cavity by way of the newly formed primitive nares (Fig. 5–12AB). With further development of the primitive nasal chambers and the formation of the secondary palate,

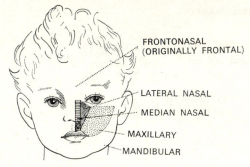

Fig. 5–9. Schematic representation of the human face showing the contributions of four components (differentially hatched areas) to the definitive face.

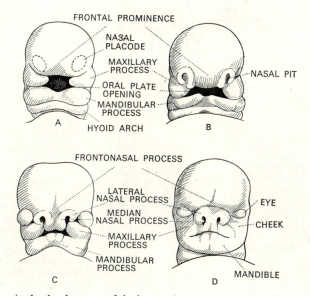

Fig. 5–10. Steps in the development of the human face shown from frontal aspect; A, 6 mm.; B, 10 mm.; C, 15 mm.; D, 20 mm. approximately.

Table 5–2. Summary of the Development of Facial Components

Embryonic part (Processes)	Fleshy derivatives
Frontonasal (originally frontal) . .	Forehead
Mandibular	Lower lip and gum; Lower cheek
Maxillary	Most of upper lip and gum; Upper cheek
Lateral nasal	Alae of nose, side and wing
Medial nasal	Middle portion of nose and nasal septum; Philtrum of upper lip and gum; Maxilla, carrying 4 incisor teeth; Primary palate

Note: The nasal septum is believed by some to be formed from the frontal process. The alternative view of Veau and Streeter holds that in man there is no separate frontonasal process.

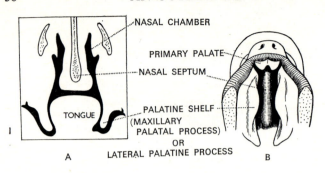

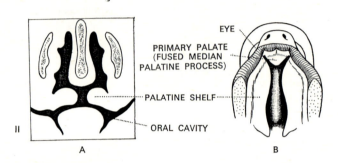

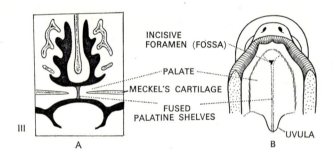

FIG. 5–11. Schematic drawings to show stages in the development of the human palate and nasal septum. Approximate ages are as follows: I, 6½-weeks II, 7½-weeks III, 10-weeks (frontal sections are shown at A, and a ventral view view of the palatine shelves after removal of the lower jaw and tongue at B).

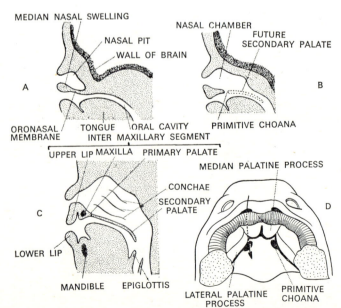

FIG. 5–12. Development of the nasal chambers and related structures as shown in medial sections through the face in 6-week (A), 7-week (B) and 9-week (C) embryos. (D) Developing palate viewed from the oral side of an 8-week embryo. (Modified from Langman, Hamilton, Boyd and Mossman, and Arey.)

the nares shift their original positions more posteriorly to a junction between the nasal cavity and pharynx (Fig. 5–12D).

Malformations of the human face (Fig. 5–13)

A. *Agnathia* (absence of lower jaw).

B. *Oblique facial cleft joining a median cleft of the lip.* The condition is due to incomplete union between the maxillary process and the adjacent nasal processes.

C. *Unilateral cleft* (or hare) *lip.*

D. *Bilateral cleft lip.* Conditions C and D are usually limited to the fleshy part of the lip only, but may also involve the bony upper jaws as well (cf. Fig. 5–14D). The condition is caused by faulty spreading of mesenchyme into the normally merging maxillary and medial nasal processes. Sometimes, cleft lip is combined with cleft palate (see below).

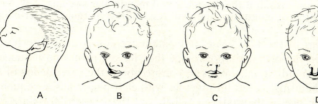

FIG. 5–13. Malformations of the human face. (After Arey.)

A. Agnathia (no jaws).
B. Oblique facial cleft joining a median cleft of the lip.
C. " Hare " lip or unilateral cleft lip.
D. Bilateral cleft lip.

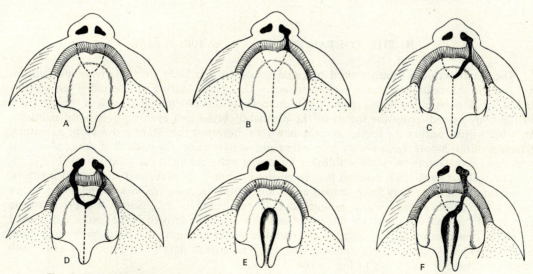

FIG. 5–14. Malformations of the human palate, lip or both (ventral view of the palate, gum, lip and nose). (After Langman.)

A. Normal condition.   B. Unilateral cleft lip extending into the nose.
C. Unilateral cleft involving lip and jaw, and extending to the incisive foramen.
D. Bilateral cleft involving lip and jaw.   E. Isolated cleft palate.
F. Cleft palate combined with unilateral anterior cleft.

Malformations of the human palate (Fig. 5–14)

I. Cleft lip and cleft palate

A. *Clefts lying anterior to the incisive foramen.* (1) Lateral cleft lip (Fig. 5–14B, Fig. 5–13C);

(2) Cleft upper jaw. (Fig. 5–14c); (3) Cleft between primary and secondary palates (Fig. 5–14d). Cause: failure of proper mesodermal penetration into the grooves between medial nasal and maxillary swellings.
  B. *Clefts lying posterior to the incisive foramen.* (1) cleft (secondary) palate (Fig. 5–14e); (2) cleft uvula (Fig. 5–14f). Cause: failure of the palatine shelves to fuse.
  C. Combinations of A and B in various degrees.
 II. Median cleft lip (rare). The cause is incomplete merging of the two medial nasal swellings in the midline. It is usually accompanied by a deep groove between the right and left sides of the nose.
III. Oblique facial cleft. This is due to failure of the maxillary process to merge with its corresponding lateral nasal swelling, with the result that the nasolacrimal duct is exposed on the surface (Fig. 5–13b).
 IV. Macrostomia and microstomia.
  (*a*) Macrostomia will result if the maxillary and mandibular swellings fail to merge;
  (*b*) Microstomia (small mouth opening) will result if this merging is over-done, or excessive.

The above anomalies of the face, nose and palate are compatible with life, but because of their damaging effect on the personal appearance they have a profound influence, both psychological and social, on the individual. We know more about their frequency of occurrence than about their causal mechanisms. Cleft lip together with cleft palate has a frequency of 1 per 1000 births with a preponderance in the male; it is believed that these defects are genetically transmitted. Little correlation between the two defects has been ascertained. Cleft palate occurs at a rate of 1 per 2500 births and is not related to the maternal age. Modern research indicates strongly that some of these anomalies may be corrected by surgical and other means if done early. Certain teratogenic agents such as cortisone, hypervitaminosis A, and pteroylglutamic acid deficiency have been found to be effective in causing cleft palate in mice and rats; it is doubtful however, whether these results apply to the human.

B. THE FOETAL PERIOD (3rd to 10th months)

The foetal period is characterized by rapid growth of the body with relatively insignificant advances in differentiation of the various tissues. The growth during this period is not proportional for all parts of the body. In fact, the character of this differential growth of various parts of the body extends from the foetus to the postnatal period and even right on until maturity. In other words, neither the foetus, nor the newborn, nor even the infant is a man in miniature. Changes of this nature, i.e., in body proportion and size are under the control of genic, hormonal and nutritional factors (possibly with other factors as well), acting at the proper time.

The young foetus (2–3 months) has an enormous head, no neck, and small hind quarters. The infant is still relatively large-headed and short-limbed in comparison with the individual in early adolescence, a stage which is marked by long slender limbs. Some of these changing features of the body with time are illustrated in Fig. 5–15. The growth of the foetus is expressed in either crown-rump (C.R.) length or crown-heel (C.H.) length, the latter measuring from vertex of skull to heel (i.e., the standing height). The growth data for the human foetus, both length and weight, are shown in Fig. 5–16.

The 3rd month is marked by (1) changes which make the face more human-looking; the eyes come to lie more ventrally and the ears more to the sides; (2) the limbs reaching their full relative length in comparison to the rest of the body; and (3) development of the external genitalia.

During the 4th and 5th months, concluding the first half of intra-uterine life, body length reaches approximately half of the total length of the new-born infant. Also, foetal movements begin to be felt. The embryo has a human appearance; the eyes are still closed, but the nose, lips and ears look human. Head, neck and spine of the foetus curve to conform to the circular uterine cavity. The umbilical cord loops between the arms and down past its leg.

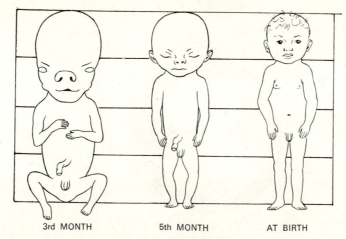

3rd MONTH   5th MONTH   AT BIRTH

FIG. 5–15. Schematic drawing to show the changing proportions of the size of the head with respect to the rest of the body in foetuses of 3 months, 5 months, and at birth.

During the second half of the intra-uterine life, the weight of the foetus increases considerably and, during the last 2½ months, this increase amounts to 50% of its full-term weight. Another noteworthy change is that the foetus obtains a well-rounded contour due to deposition of subcutaneous fat during this period.

At term, the foetus is about 50 cm. long and weighs over 3000 gm. Its skull still has the largest circumference of all bony parts, and the testicles of a male foetus should have descended into the scrotum.

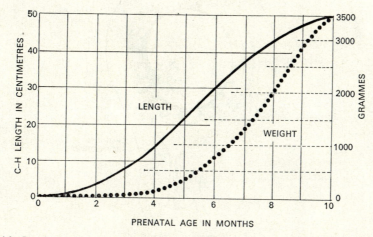

FIG. 5–16. Graphs representing increase in length (solid line) and increase in weight (broken line) of human embryos during prenatal months. (After Williams and Wendell-Smith.)

PLACENTATION

Origin and development of placenta

The placenta is a complex organ formed of intricately woven maternal and foetal tissues. Its origin goes back to the time of implantation when an initial contact is made between the tropho-

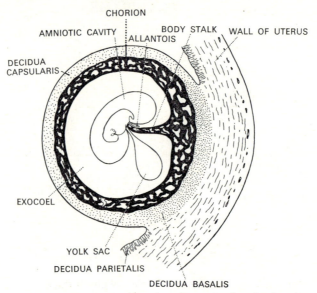

Fig. 5–17. Diagrammatic drawings of a 4-week embryo showing the foetal membranes, the extent of chorion development and its relationship with maternal (decidual) structures.

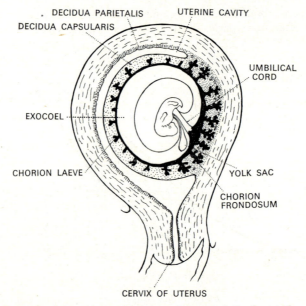

FIG. 5–18. The uterus and the embryo with its membranes and chorion at about the middle of the second month.

blast and the uterine mucosa. Thereafter, due mostly to the incessant activity of the trophoblast, a chorion characterized by the presence of villi, is formed. At first, formation of the latter structure is confined to the embryonic pole of the chorionic vesicle; gradually the formation of villi spreads to the abembryonic side (Figs. 4–6 and 7) so that, by the third week, the chorion is of about equal thickness all around the vesicle (Fig. 4–9). From the 4th week onwards, the chorionic villi on the abembryonic surface start to atrophy whilst those on the embryonic side continue to

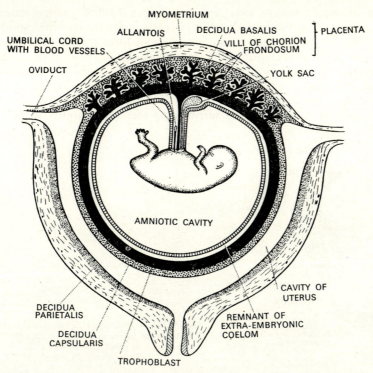

FIG. 5–19. Sectional view of a human uterus showing the foetal membranes and their relationship to the uterus and embryo (approximately 3 months).

grow and differentiate with increased vigour (Fig. 5–17). By the 6th week, as the chorionic vesicle slowly bulges into the uterine cavity, it can be differentiated into two regions. That part which is firmly attached to the uterine wall bears extensive villi and is known as the chorion frondosum, whilst that part bulged into the uterine cavity is the chorion laeve (Fig. 5–18) which shows only scanty, degenerating villi. The process of degeneration proceeds until, 2–3 weeks later, the chorion laeve will have lost all its villi and presents a smooth surface (Fig. 5–19). By then, the chorion frondosum has developed into the functional foetal component of the placenta. As such, it is intimately and immediately apposed to a well circumscribed area of the endometrium, the decidua basalis (Fig. 5–19). The definitive placenta therefore comprises two components: the foetal chorion frondosum and the maternal decidua basalis.

Along with this development of the chorion and with continuing enlargement of the embryonic vesicle, which keeps pushing the abembryonic side out into the uterine cavity, the decidua (uterine mucosa of pregnancy) has been differentiated into three portions: (1) The decidua basalis, as just described, is that part involved in the formation of the placenta. (2) Continuous with the decidua basalis, and expanding beyond the limit of the latter onto the surface of the chorionic vesicle, is a relatively thin decidual tissue, the decidua capsularis. (This layer, subject to continuing growth pressure originated from the foetus, gets thinner with time.) These two portions of decidua are more or less directly concerned with the foetus. (3) The remaining portion, which lines the remainder of the uterine cavity, and is not directly involved with the embryo, is known as the decidua parietalis (Figs. 5–17, 18, and 19).

Changes in the structure of decidual membranes

These changes occur as a consequence of " growth pressure " exerted by the ever enlarging foetus on the chorionic vesicle. The first change occurring between the 5th and 6th week is a fusion between the amnion and chorion (laeve), resulting in the elimination of the extra-embryonic coelom. Next, as the chorionic vesicle comes in contact with the decidua capsularis, these also fuse, thereby eliminating the narrow chorionic cavity (a space formed after the atrophy of the chorion laeve, part of which is contributed from its coalesced lacunae). This happens around the end of 2nd month. Still later, with continuing growth, the surface epithelium of the decidua capsularis comes into contact with the decidua parietalis and fuses with it (Fig. 5–21), so obliterating the uterine cavity; this happens about the end of the 3rd month. After that, the only space separating the growing foetus from the surrounding foetal membranes is the amniotic cavity

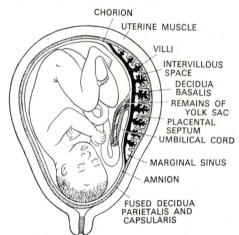

CHORION
UTERINE MUSCLE
VILLI
INTERVILLOUS SPACE
DECIDUA BASALIS
REMAINS OF YOLK SAC
PLACENTAL SEPTUM
UMBILICAL CORD
MARGINAL SINUS
AMNION
FUSED DECIDUA PARIETALIS AND CAPSULARIS

FIG. 5–20. Diagrammatic longitudinal section of the uterus, illustrating the relationship of an advanced foetus to the placenta and other membranes.

and its fluid. It may be noted that this final change coincides with the degeneration of the cytotrophoblastic covering of the villi, leaving the syncytiotrophoblast alone surviving for the remainder of gestation (Figs. 5–19, 20).

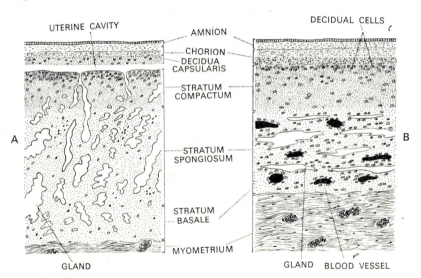

UTERINE CAVITY
AMNION
DECIDUAL CELLS
CHORION
DECIDUA CAPSULARIS
STRATUM COMPACTUM
A   B
STRATUM SPONGIOSUM
STRATUM BASALE
MYOMETRIUM
GLAND
GLAND   BLOOD VESSEL

FIG. 5–21. Vertical sections through the decidua parietalis of a gravid human uterus.

A. In the third month, showing intact decidua capsularis;
B. At 7-months, after the atrophy of the decidua capsularis and fusion of the chorion and decidua parietalis has obliterated the uterine cavity. Note the flattening of the uterine glands and the thinning of the mucosa as a result of the fusion.

The structure of the placenta

The basic structure of the chorionic villi and their relationship with adjoining decidual tissues has been discussed (Fig. 4–18AB). At full term the placenta is a disc-like structure containing a completely closed compartment, which is incompletely divided into some 20 cotyledons by septa. That is to say, the intervillous space is correspondingly divided into cotyledonous bays which are filled with maternal blood. Bathed in the latter are the profusely branching villi. The septa grow down from the basal plate (without, however, touching the chorionic plate); they are composed mainly of decidua cells mixed with some cytotrophoblast (prolongations of the cytotrophoblastic cell column) and covered with syncytiotrophoblast (Fig. 4–18). The septa are considered as derivatives of the junctional zone (p. 59).

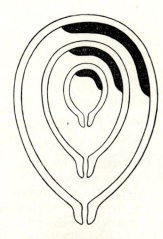

FIG. 5–22. Schematic representation to show the relative sizes of the human placenta at 75, 163 and 261 days of gestation.

The placenta grows in extent with progressing pregnancy until at full term (Fig. 5–25) it has a diameter of 15–20 cm., a total effective surface area estimated at 7 to 14 square meters, and it weighs 500 g. and is 3 cm. thick. It has been estimated that the total length of the villi placed end to end would be some 30 miles. At 3 weeks the placenta covers $\frac{1}{5}$ of the uterine surface; this increases to $\frac{1}{3}$ at 8 weeks and by the end of the 5th month half of the entire uterine surface is covered by placental tissue (Fig. 5–22).

Blood flow and the " placental barrier "

The maternal blood flows into the intervillous spaces from the terminal portions of the coiled (spiral) arteries of the endometrium (Fig. 4–18) and returns by the uterine veins. Both the arteries and veins pierce the basal plate to reach the cotyledonous bays (Fig. 5–23A). This blood is never at any time in contact with the foetal blood, the two being separated by a number of cellular membranes, collectively known as the " placental barrier " (see below). Embedded in the mesenchymal core of the villi are branches of the foetal umbilical arteries and veins of the allantoic circulation. This arrangement of the maternal and foetal blood vessels makes possible the transfer of a great variety of substances across the " barrier ", to and from the mother. The primary mechanism of this transfer is diffusion, with the placental barrier acting as a unique semipermeable membrane. Maternal blood entering the cotyledons is forced toward the chorionic plate and is then turned back, with a slowed down rate of flow, towards the basal plate. The flow of foetal blood inside the villi is in the reverse direction, initially towards the basal plate, and then turned backwards in the direction of the foetus. Such a countercurrent flow of blood in the placenta constitutes a mechanism permitting the most efficient exchange of gases and other dissolved materials between the maternal and foetal circulations (Fig. 5–23B).

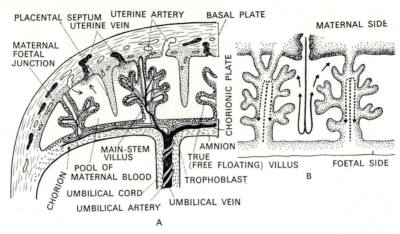

Fig. 5–23. A. Diagrammatic section through a human placenta showing two cotyledons separated by septa. A primary stem villus and free floating villi branching from it are shown in one of the cotyledons. Uterine arteries (spiral) and veins entering and leaving the intervillous spaces are indicated with arrows. (Modified from Harrison.)

B. Diagrams to show the principle of counter current flow of blood in the human placenta.

The coiled arteries are unique in that they respond to pregnancy by reactions which are believed to be conducive to the formation of an efficient placental circulation. There is an increase in both diameter and muscularity of these vessels and, more significantly, their lumen becomes narrower at the points at which they pierce the basal plate; this serves as a means to enhance local blood pressure and blood volume entering the intervillous spaces. The decreased lumen may be correlated with the fact that the spiral arteries open into the intervillous spaces through gaps in the cytotrophoblastic shells.

In the early stages, the blood filling the lacunae in the syncytiotrophoblast is stagnant. Later, when the intervillous spaces are established through the confluence of the lacunae and ruptured sinusoids and capillaries, a slow circulation is generated in the blood. It is only when the large coiled arteries begin to open into the intervillous space through irregular gaps in the trophoblastic shell (p. 73) that the final pattern of placental circulation commences. Since specific paths of blood flow to and from the intervillous spaces have not been demonstrated, some mixing of the entering and departing blood during their passage through the narrow entrances and exits seems unavoidable.

It is estimated that the placenta has a total capacity of 500 ml. of which 350 ml. is foetal villi, and 150 ml. intervillous spaces occupied by maternal blood. The blood circulates at a rate of 500 ml. per minute (i.e., complete replacement occurs 2–3 times in one minute).

The human placental barrier consists of 7 membranes (including basement membranes) prior to mid-pregnancy (cf. Table 6–2). These are: (1) syncytiotrophoblast (2) cytotrophoblast (3) cytotrophoblast basement membrane (4) foetal mesenchyme (villous core) (5) basement membrane of the villous core (6) basement membrane of foetal capillaries (7) endothelium of foetal capillaries. After midpregnancy, due to atrophy of the cytotrophoblast, Nos. 2 and 3 listed above are eliminated. This reduction, though generally believed to be a step towards increasing the efficiency of active transfer by the placenta, may not be of significance.

Significance of the junctional zone

This is where the invasion by foetal tissues terminates and where some mixing of cellular elements belonging to the mother and foetus has occurred. For instance, there are patches of very large cells (giant cells) of uncertain origin; they could possibly be either decidual cells or syncytiotrophoblast, or both. Some of these cells are seen to be surrounded by mucopolysaccharides, substances which are known to resist the action of proteolytic enzymes, a finding which may be of significance in understanding the mechanism of cessation of the trophoblastic invasion.

The cytotrophoblast that persists from the original cytotrophoblastic cell columns (Fig. 4–5B) and remains in this zone may continue to produce some chorionic gonadotrophins until the end of pregnancy. The junctional zone is suspected of being the site for transport of substances of high molecular weight, such as proteins, from the decidua to foetus. Finally, it is at this site that separation occurs at parturition.

Functions of the placenta

The human placenta is a dynamic organ; it performs the functions of the yolk sac, chorion and allantois in the lower Amniotes (reptiles and birds). In this respect the placenta performs the physiological exchanges involved in obtaining nutrients, oxygen, and water from the mother and, in return, passing back CO_2 and nitrogenous waste products. In this exchange (p. 58; Fig. 5–23) the placental barrier acts as a semi-permeable membrane, permitting passage of substances with a low molecular weight such as gases, simple ions, amino-acids, urea, uric acid, creatin, creatinine, and monosaccharides. The function of the placenta as an important endocrine organ has been treated elsewhere (pp. 69–72; Table 7–2), hormones being transported both ways across the placenta by diffusion.

The transport of more complex substances of a high molecular weight (e.g., certain proteins, antibodies) is not completely understood.* In such cases it is assumed that the mechanism is one of " facilitated diffusion " or " active transport ", which means that the permeability of a particular substance is not governed by laws of diffusion applicable to the composite placental membrane as a whole, but rather that the permeability of one or more of the barrier membranes operates in a specific way. Under this category, the mother's antibodies against immunizable diseases pass freely to the foetus, thereby providing it with acquired immunity against any disease for at least 5–6 months after birth or until such time the baby commences to manufacture its own antibodies. The RH (Rhesus) factor is an example of reversed passage of antibodies. The antigens of a Rh+ve baby pass to the mother and the antibodies produced by the latter pass back to the foetus, causing haemolysis of the foetal blood. Just how the foetal antigen reaches the intervillous space is unknown. It has been suggested that the transfer may have resulted from detachment of minute fragments of the chorionic villi or from minute villous haemorrhages.

The placenta is also an effective barrier against many pathogenic micro-organisms. So far, only two exceptions to this rule are definitely known; (a) the spirochaete causing syphilis can be transmitted from mother to baby (b) the virus of German measles, rubella, if contracted by the mother during the first 3 months of pregnancy, can lead to a variety of congenital anomalies in the baby, affecting especially the heart and sense organs (pp. 86,169).

Age changes in the placenta

The placenta reaches its functional peak slightly after mid-pregnancy, after which time a number of structural changes have been observed and generally confirmed as manifestations of aging. Among these, the most widely occurring is the production of fibrinoid (an amorphous material) which is deposited at the junctional zone. The fibrinoid is most likely secreted by the trophoblastic shell and the syncytium outside it, and aggregates on the surface of villi as so-called " knots ", and in the basal and chorionic plates. There is also an increase in the fibrous tissue content in the cores of villi and a thickening of the basement membrane of both trophoblast and

---

* Recent *in vitro* studies using dialyzable maternal sera indicated that human foetal membranes are able to select protein molecules for passage not only according to size, but also on the basis of their chemical nature.

foetal capillaries. Finally, obliterative changes occur in the peripheral vessels of the branching villous system. Despite these age changes, however, positive evidence of a decline in the efficiency of the placenta is lacking (Fig. 4–19D).

Some unanswered questions about the placenta and trophoblast

The early trophoblast, especially the syncytiotrophoblast is a remarkably invasive tissue. The outcome of its activity following implantation and during placentation poses two relevant questions: (1) How does the mother tolerate this invasive " foreign matter " (the foetus) for such a long time against the principle of the immunological defence system of the body. If that secret can be cracked, advances in organ transplantation will certainly be made. (2) What is the mechanism whereby the invasive behaviour of the trophoblast is stopped in time? Assuming, for a moment, that the syncytiotrophoblast behaves like a cancer cell, an answer to this question is likely to provide crucial information for cancer therapy. The implication is that the decidual cells of the pregnant endometrium somehow hold a weapon to check and stop invasion of the trophoblast. It seems that here lies an area involving enzyme and anti-enzyme chemistry which is most worthy of attention.

Conversely the syncytiotrophoblast has great potential as a possible cancer-killer. It has been shown that these cells, if transplanted elsewhere in the body will retain their inherent potency and invade and ingest whatever cells they come into contact with. It may be that they could do likewise to malignant cancer cells; but if so, under what new conditions?

Stages of nutrition of the embryo and foetus

1. Egg cytoplasm. The ovum is " on its own ", drawing upon a limited reserve of food material in its cytoplasm (possibly supplemented by secretions of the uterine tube).
2. Uterine " milk ". The cleaving zygote, up to the time of implantation, feeds on the secretion from uterine glands, mostly glycogen.
3. Histiotrophe. (embryotrophe). The blastocyst feeds on a mixture of cellular debris consisting of broken-down glandular, decidual and endothelial cells, which have resulted from the erosion of the endometrium during the implantation process.
4. A transitional haemotrophic nutrition. The embryo during the early phase of placentation, gets its nutrition haemotrophically. During this time its chorion vascularized with allantoic vessels is apposed to the wall of the implantation cavity (consisting of exposed decidual cells, eroded uterine glands and blood vessels). The implantation cavity and eroded glands are filled with extravasated blood.
5. Placental nutrition. The embryo enters upon its final phase of nutrition after structural completion and initiation of function of the placenta. This phase lasts throughout the remainder of the gestation period.

Umbilical cord and after-birth (Figs. 5–24 and 25)

During development the growing embryo tends to free itself from attachment to the trophoblast wall and finally is freely suspended in a completely fluid medium within its own amnion by means of the umbilical cord. This structure is traceable back to its forerunner (the body stalk (p. 34)) and it constitutes the only linkage between the mother and foetus. Both the allantois and yolk sac (with stalk) extend into it. It also houses the umbilical vessels, a pair of arteries and one vein, which represent the original vessels of the allantois. All these structures are embedded in a specialized stroma known as " Wharton's Jelly " (Fig. 5–24A). The cord is bounded by the inner lining of the amnion as its epithelial covering (a single ectodermal layer of cells). When fully formed it attains a length of 2·0 feet and is about $\frac{1}{2}$ inch in diameter; it is twisted and contains about 40 turns.

At birth, the amnion breaks and its fluid bursts out before the baby is expelled followed after some further minutes by a compound structure, the after-birth (Fig. 5–25), which consists of the umbilical cord and the attached placenta. The detachment of the latter from the uterus tears away the decidua parietalis from almost the whole inner surface of the uterus, and causes extensive bleeding. The after-birth is about 7 inches in diameter and its weight is approximately $\frac{1}{7}$ of that of the foetus. Its structural relationship with the umbilical cord and placenta is indicated as follows:

Afterbirth
- Umbilical cord*
  - Amnion (fused to decidua parietalis)
  - Allantoic stalk
  - Yolk sac stalk
  - Blood vessels
- Placenta
  - Maternal
    - Decidua parietalis (in shreds)
    - Remnants of decidua capsularis (if any left)
    - Decidua basalis
  - Foetal
    - Chorion frondosum } Placenta proper
    - Chorion laeve

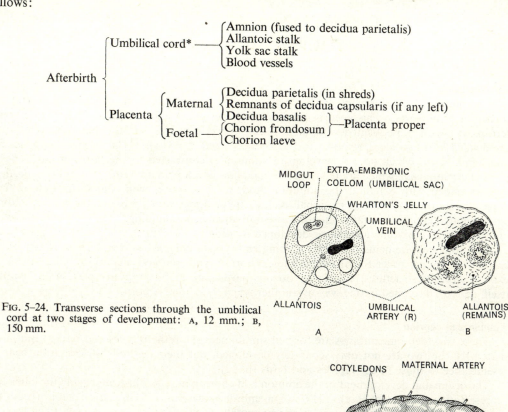

MIDGUT LOOP
EXTRA-EMBRYONIC COELOM (UMBILICAL SAC)
WHARTON'S JELLY
UMBILICAL VEIN
ALLANTOIS
UMBILICAL ARTERY (R)
ALLANTOIS (REMAINS)

A   B

FIG. 5–24. Transverse sections through the umbilical cord at two stages of development: A, 12 mm.; B, 150 mm.

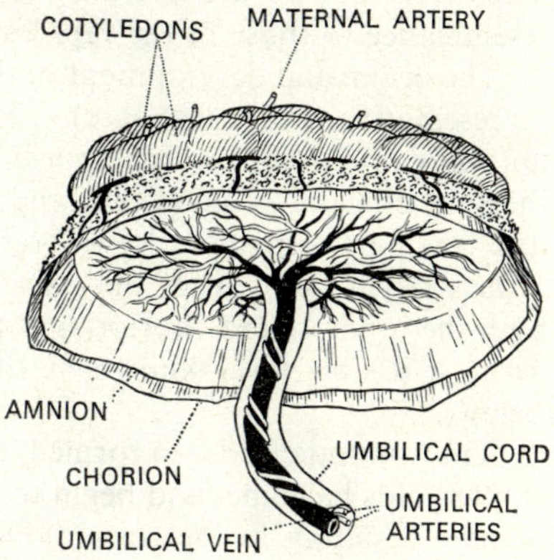

COTYLEDONS   MATERNAL ARTERY
AMNION
CHORION
UMBILICAL VEIN
UMBILICAL CORD
UMBILICAL ARTERIES

FIG. 5–25. Normal placenta and associated area of the chorion at full term.

* May show recognizable degenerate vitelline veins (a pair).

CHAPTER 6

FOETAL MEMBRANES

Introduction

For successful development of the foetus it must be cushioned against environmental disturbances of all sorts. This need is automatically met in aquatic animals, which have external fertilization with subsequent development taking place in water. On this basis the vertebrates are divided into two major groups: the Anamniotes and Amniotes. The former comprises fish and amphibians, which do not develop an amnion as contrasted to the latter group (reptiles, birds and mammals), which lay their eggs on land and develop an amnion. The embryo needs to be surrounded with a liquid, the amniotic fluid, for protection from shocks as well as from adhesion to either egg shell or maternal tissues. It is a device which provides the delicate embryo with a limited aquatic habitat in an otherwise non-aquatic surrounding. The amnion is therefore an early extra-embryonic membrane developed in all land vertebrates.

The other requirements of the developing embryo should also be met. These functions are carried out by the other foetal membranes: chorion, yolk sac and allantois. All of them are extra-embryonic structures, since they do not participate in forming any part of the embryo itself, and are discarded in one way or another when the young is born.

Amnion and chorion

These two foetal membranes are formed simultaneously in the reptiles and birds. But in the mammals, the two are not only separately developed, but their methods of formation bear no resemblance to those of the reptiles and birds (p. 32).

The origin and development of the amnion and chorion may be illustrated using the chick as a representative (Fig. 6–1a, b, c). The two membranes arise as a double-layered fold (head and tail folds of amnion) which appear at approximately 40 hours of incubation (a). Each layer of the fold consists of ectoderm and extra-embryonic mesoderm. The latter, by then, has split into two parts separated by the resulting cavity, the extra-embryonic coelom. The outer layer of mesoderm forms, with the ectoderm, a double-layer known as the somatopleure, from which both the amnion and chorion are derived. The inner layer of mesoderm forms, with the endoderm, a double layer known as the splanchnopleure from which the allantois is derived (see below).

The amniotic folds, so formed, arch upward above and over the embryo. In a 5-day embryo (b) the folds have met and begin to fuse, ectoderm with ectoderm and mesoderm with mesoderm, thereby resulting in the formation of an inner sac, the amnion, and an outer membrane, the chorion. The amnion, like the fold itself, consists of an inner layer of ectoderm and an outer layer of somatic mesoderm (c). It is filled with amniotic fluid, but the membrane is not vascularized at any time. It is in this fluid that the embryo completes its development. The chorion also consists of two layers, mesoderm within and ectoderm without. The space enclosed between the amnion and chorion is the extra-embryonic coelom, now greatly enlarged. In the mammals the amnion is formed rather hurriedly in a slurred-over manner by rearrangement of cells delaminated from the inner cell mass (p. 30) shortly after the formation of the blastocyst. Significantly, however, despite its different origin it has the same basic structure and function as the amnion in lower vertebrates. The human amnion further expands, eventually completely filling the extra-embryonic coelom, its wall being closely applied to the umbilical cord. In man and other mammals the chorion, too, is formed by a delamination process (p. 30) and because it is destined to be the foetal component of the placenta is one of the most important of the foetal membranes. It proceeds to form villi very early in development (p. 31).

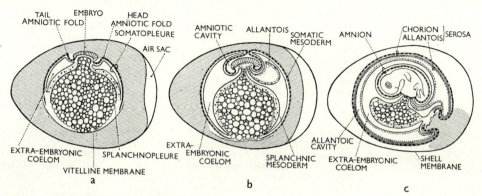

FIG. 6–1. Stages in the development of extra-embryonic membranes in the chick; A, 40 hours; B, 5 days; C, 10 days (egg shell not shown). (After Hamilton, Boyd and Mossman.)

Allantois

The method of formation of this foetal membrane is the same in all Amniotes. It arises as a double-layered (endoderm covered with splanchnic mesoderm) diverticulum from the posterior wall of the yolk sac. Subsequent development, however, differs in the chick and in man. In the former it extends into the extra-embryonic coelom (Fig. 6–1b) and eventually completely occupies it as seen in a 9-day embryo (Fig. 6–1c). As its outer wall comes into contact with the chorion, the two form a closely associated structure, composed of four layers of tissue. This compound structure is known as the serosa (c) and consists of the ectodermal and mesodermal layers of the chorion and the mesodermal and endodermal layers of the allantois. In consequence it is also sometimes called the chorio-allantoic membrane. It is highly vascularized, and by virtue of its outermost position, is the embryo's organ of respiration and excretion. In man, the allantois is formed the same way, but soon it turns into a rudimentary structure, retaining a tubular lumen, inside the body stalk. Its vessels, however, become the important umbilical vessels linking the embryo with the placenta.

Yolk sac

In those amniotes which have macrolecithal eggs the first foetal membrane to appear is the yolk sac. It is also a double-layered membrane, formed by primitive endoderm extending over the yolk mass and topped by a layer of splanchnic mesoderm. In these animals the yolk sac serves as the foetal organ of nutrition by virtue of its highly developed vitelline circulation. In man (as well as in most other mammals with isolecithal eggs) the yolk sac arises by delamination (p. 33), remains vascularized for a short while and acts as a haemopoietic organ (p. 146), but subsequently regresses to the point of leaving only a remnant inside the umbilical cord. It is thus largely a vestigial foetal membrane whose function is taken over by the placenta (p. 59). A summary of these features is presented in Table 6–1.

Placenta

The placenta is a structure evolved for the condition of viviparity, that is, where the embryos develop within the body of the mother. It is an unique " intermediary " organ between the foetus and the mother, performing the functions of all the foetal membranes put together. This is

TABLE 6–1. A COMPARISON OF FOETAL MEMBRANES OF BIRDS AND MAMMALS

Membrane	Manner of formation		Structure when fully developed		Vascularization	Functions	
	Birds	Mammals	Birds	Mammals			
Amnion	By folds of somatopleure	From cells delaminated from ectoderm in inner cell mass, enclosing a cavity	Ectoderm (inside) somatic mesoderm (outside)	Same	Same in both groups: not vascularized	Same in both groups: to equalize pressure; to prevent adhesion	
Chorion	Formed simultaneously with amnion	From cells delaminated from inner cell mass; consisting of 2 layers	Somatic mesoderm (inside) ectoderm (outside)	Same basic structure, but forms chorionic villi in close collaboration with extra-embryonic mesoderm	Richly vascularized in both groups	Birds: Joining allantois as respiratory and excretory organ	Mammals: Specialize in villi formation for: respiration, excretion & nutrition
Yolk Sac	That part of primary gut not included within body when embryo is folded off	Originates from cells delaminated from entoderm, enclosing a cavity	Entoderm (inside) splanchnic mesoderm (outside)	Same	In birds: important vitelline circulation In mammals: transitional vitelline	Nutrition	Vestigial; not functional
Allantois	Same in both groups: a diverticulum protruding from hind gut		Same as yolk sac	Same	In birds: important allantoic circulation In mammals: vessels of umbilical cord	See chorion	Vestigial; not functional
Placenta	None	See text					

accomplished by bringing the maternal and foetal circulations together to such a close proximity short only of a direct connection between them. In a limited sense the foetus may be compared to an additional part of the mother's body that needs to be nourished. The contrast arises, however, from the fact that the foetus has its own circulatory system under development and that no part of the foetus proper may be vascularized by the maternal blood vessels. The working of such a joint enterprise must depend, it seems, on the successful establishment of a functional relationship between certain highly specialized tissues of the foetus and mother (see p. 57).

Transitional stages

The first step toward placenta-formation is the acquisition by the chorion of the property to form villi (Fig. 6–2A). These are finger-like projections with a vascularized core that come into direct contact with maternal tissue. Phylogenetically speaking, these are at first formed sparsely all over the chorion; later they are concentrated in a smaller area of the chorion, but are more profusely developed.

In an early (primitive) placenta, the contact between the chorion and foetus is provided by the allantois.   A beginning in this direction is seen in Fig. 6–2A; marked progress in the same direction, in Fig. 6–2B, so that a tendency toward increased union or fusion between the allantois, chorion and uterine lining is clearly apparent.   This means that in some of the lower mammals the placenta is of the allantoic type.   (The yolk sac is never in any way involved.   Its role as a foetal membrane steadily decreases as one progresses phylogenetically).

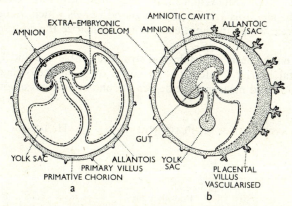

FIG. 6–2. Two stages in the evolution of foetal membranes of mammals;
    a. early stage (slightly more advanced than in Fig. 6–1b);
    b. a later stage, the beginnings of an allantoic placenta, with the foetal basis fully established.

Allantoic placentae

As indicated above, in this type of placenta the chorion brings the allantois into close relation with the uterine wall.   The degree of closeness of this relationship varies however.   In cases where the union is relatively loose, no maternal tissue is torn and shed at the time of parturition, and the placenta is known as a non-deciduate allantoic placenta.   The ungulates as a group have this type of placenta (Fig. 6–3).   On the other hand, if the union is made intimate by means of deep-burrowing villi, then parturition results in deciduation of maternal tissue.   This condition is represented by the dog (Fig. 6–4) and other carnivores and is known as a deciduate allantoic placenta.   As clearly indicated in both these figures, the placentae incorporate a large functional allantois.

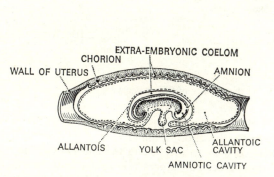

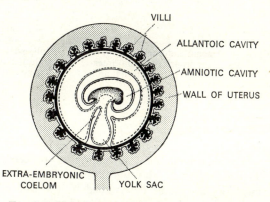

FIG. 6–3. The placenta of the pig; this is an example of an allantoic placenta of the non-deciduate type.

FIG. 6–4. The placenta of the dog; this is an example of an allantoic placenta of the deciduate type.

c

Non-allantoic placentae

In the course of evolution the role played by the allantois in placenta formation continually decreases until, in some of the highest mammals, the placenta has become of a non-allantoic type. The human placenta and those of the rodents are examples of this type. In these placentae the chorion takes over the function of the foetal component of the placenta while the allantoic sac regresses to a mere vestige. But even in such cases it must be pointed out that the degenerative process involves only the allantois as a sac, not its blood vessels which become the all important umbilical arteries and vein which, without exception, vascularize the chorionic villi.

Placental classification on the basis of histological structure (Table 6–2 and Fig. 6–5)

The term " placental barrier " refers to the layers of tissue (cells) actually separating the maternal and foetal blood and measures the degree of contact or gross union existing at the zone

TABLE 6–2.   CLASSIFICATION OF PLACENTAE BASED ON HISTOLOGICAL STRUCTURE

Type	Barriers	Examples

Epithelial-chorial (No union)	Foetal
	  Endothelium
	  Stroma } Villi
	  Trophoblasts
	Maternal (Endometrium)
	  Endothelium of mucosa capillaries
	  Stroma
	  Epithelium
		Horse
		Pig
		lemurs

Syndesmo-chorial (No union)	Foetal
	  Same as above
	Maternal
	  Stroma
	  Endothelium of capillaries
		Most ungulates

Endothelio-chorial (with foetal-maternal union)	Foetal
	  Syncytial chorionic epithelium
	  Stroma
	  Endothelium of capillaries
	Maternal
	  Endothelium of mucosa capillaries
		Carnivors

Haemo-chorial (with foetal-maternal union)	Foetal
	  Same as above
	Maternal
	  None, i.e., blood cells freely ooze
	  into intervillous spaces
		Man

Haemo-endothelial* (approaching actual intermingling of maternal and foetal blood)	Only barrier: Endothelium of foetal chorionic capillaries	Rat Guinea pig Rabbit

* Recent research has thrown doubt on the validity of this category.

of junction between the two components. Such a classification brings out a generally accepted significance, namely that evolution has proceeded in the direction of diminishing the " barrier ". This is fairly well (although not absolutely) correlated with an increase in the efficiency of permeability as can be determined by the rate of transfer of substances taking place inside the placenta to and from the two blood streams. For instance, it has been estimated that the human placenta (haemo-chorial) is 250 times more efficient in sodium transfer than the cow's placenta (syndesmochorial). In this classification (Table 6–2) only cellular layers are counted as contributing towards the placental barrier, the basement membrane is disregarded (cf. p. 58).

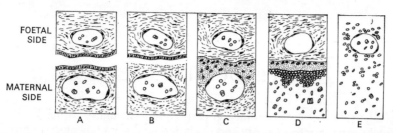

FIG. 6–5. Types of deciduate non-allantoic placentae, showing the progressive elimination of barriers between the maternal and foetal circulations (basement membranes are not taken into consideration).

A. Epithelio-chorial (some ungulates);   B. Syndesmo-chorial (ruminants);
C. Endothelio-chorial (carnivores);
D. Haemo-chorial (primates, including human);
E. Haemo-endothelial (rodents). This is the classical view; see footnote to Table 6–2.

CHAPTER 7

REPRODUCTIVE CYCLES

The reproductive cycle is a phenomenon pertaining particularly to the female. Its purpose is to bring one or more ova to maturity and ovulation, and simultaneously to prepare the uterus for implantation. The length of this cycle varies in different species:

Rat and mouse	5 days
Guinea pig	15 days
Sow, mare and cow	21 days
Monkey and human	28 days
Chimpanzee	37 days
Cat and dog	3–4 months

The cycle repeats itself unless fertilization takes place. If fertilization does occur, then the implanted embryo needs to be ensured of its continued successful development and provision must also be made for parturition. These events, closely coordinated between the ovary and the uterus, require the precisely timed action of a number of hormones. The secretions of three endocrine organs, working in a relay fashion, are involved in this control mechanism: the adenohypophysis (anterior pituitary), the ovary and the placenta (Fig. 7–1). The working of this rather complex system incorporates an indispensable feed-back mechanism (arrows, Fig. 7–1). Generally speaking, if hormone Y owes its production to hormone X, the accumulation of Y above a certain level inhibits X. For instance, the sex hormones (oestrogenic and androgenic) inhibit the follicle stimulating hormone of the adenohypophysis (FSH), as does chorionic gonadotrophin; see p. 72). Also, progesterone inhibits both luteinizing hormone (LH) and luteotrophic hormone (LTH) but stimulates FSH. Oestrogen stimulates LH. Modern oral contraceptives work on the principle of abolishing normal ovulation by supplying the patient with synthetic progesterone or a carefully worked-out combination of synthetic progesterone and oestrogen.

Sequence of hormonal actions concerned with reproduction

The development of the sex cells up to the stage of primary follicles (oögonia) formation is under the control of genes. After reaching puberty, a series of three gonadotrophic hormones of the anterior pituitary come into play. The first of these is follicle-stimulating hormone (FSH) which initiates the growth of a crop of young follicles. The second gonadotrophic hormone to act is luteinizing hormone (LH). Under its influence one of the growing follicles reaches maturity and ovulates. Other follicles become atretic and disintegrate (Fig. 1–7). In laboratory animals the theca interna cells of the atretic follicle may become scattered in the stroma as interstitial cells. Since LH is necessary for ovulation, it is sometimes called the ovulating hormone. Meanwhile, a steady increase in the concentration of oestrogens has been produced from the granulosa and theca internal cells of the growing follicles. At the same time as these events have been taking place in the ovary (follicular phase), oestrogens have also been acting on the uterine mucosa to repair the damage which occurred in the menses and to aid in the reconstruction of the endometrium (Figs. 7–2c; 7–3). Oestrogens increase the water content, vascularity, protein

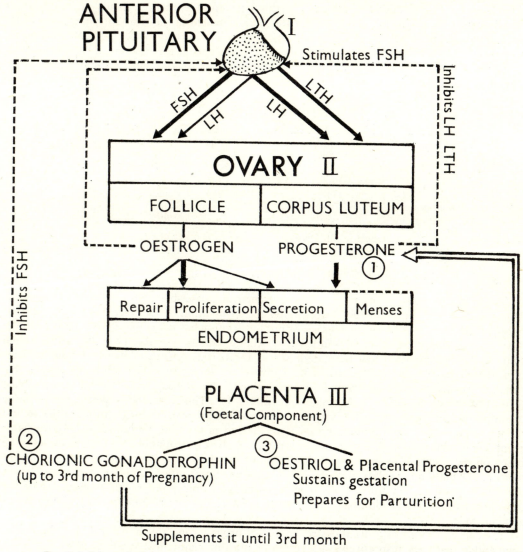

FIG. 7–1. Schematic representation to show how the sequence of hormonal actions concerned with reproduction act as a sort of " relay ", triggered by the anterior pituitary.

content and enzyme activity of the endometrium. In addition, they change the glandular epithelium from a cuboid to a columnar type and make the middle portion of these uterine glands tortuous and even stimulate them to secrete a serous secretion. These changes in the endometrium constitute the proliferative phase of the menstrual cycle (Table 7–1).

LH, which has been acting continuously on the follicle, finally converts the granulosa cells of the follicle after ovulation into a corpus luteum. When the latter is fully developed, the third gonadotrophic hormone, luteotropic hormone (LTH), stimulates the luteal cells of the corpus luteum to secrete the hormone, progesterone. This hormone, as the name implies, prepares the endometrium for implantation and the early part of gestation. Its secretion is responsible for the luteal phase of the ovary and the secretory phase of the endometrium (Fig. 7–2). The concentration of progesterone in the blood steadily increases as the corpus luteum increases in size

(Fig. 7–2A: *a, b*). Under the influence of this hormone the uterine glands gradually attain their maximal development; the bodies of the glands located in the stratum spongiosum of the endometrial stroma lengthen and their lumens become dilated (Fig. 7–2C). Accompanying the growth of the glands is an extensive growth of blood vessels in the now much thickened endometrium. The arteries consist of short ones in the stratum basale and long spiral ones in the remaining portion of the endometrium.

TABLE 7–1. PHASES IN OVARIAN AND UTERINE CYCLES

Hormone responsible		In Ovary					In Uterus	
		Days of the menstrual cycle						
Oestrogen	Follicular phase	1–4	.	.	.	.	. Menses	subject to variation
		4–6	.	.	.	.	. Repair	
		6–14	.	.	.	.	. Proliferative	
Progesterone	Luteal phase	14 (variable) .		.	.	.	Ovulation	
		14–28 (constant)* .		.	.	.	Secretory	

*That is, time from ovulation to onset of menstruation is always 14 days.

The events of the secretory phase of the endometrium, described above, proceed to about day 26 of the cycle, i.e. approximately 3 weeks after the termination of the preceding menses. What follows from here on depends on whether or not fertilization has taken place. If it has (assuming it to occur on day 16), and is followed by successful implantation on day 19 or 20, the functional state of the endometrium will be maintained as the corpus luteum of menstruation becomes transformed into a corpus luteum of pregnancy (Fig. 7–2B: *b*). The hormone responsible for this transfer is chorionic gonadotrophin, which is produced by the cellular trophoblast (cytotrophoblast) of the early chorionic villi (Fig. 7–1). This hormone is synthesized in large quantities beginning shortly after implantation, reaching its peak production during the second month of pregnancy, and terminating at about the end of the third month (Fig. 7–3), the latter event being correlated with the complete atrophy of the cytotrophoblast. Pregnancy tests are based on the assays of the activity of this hormone which is present in the urine of a pregnant woman. Ovulation in rabbits, mice or even frogs some hours after they have been injected with the urine constitutes a positive test. The chorionic gonadotrophin insures the security of the implanted embryo and in addition is antagonistic to FSH; thus, it prevents the ovary from starting another cycle.

The concentrations of ovarian oestrogen and of progesterone are shown in Fig. 7–2B, by the solid and dotted lines, respectively. Progesterone must be maintained at a reasonably high level if pregnancy is to be successfully sustained. In some mammals a functional corpus luteum is maintained in the ovary throughout gestation; its removal will terminate the pregnancy. In others, such as the human, surgical removal of the corpus luteum does not lead to abortion because from the third month onwards, the role of the ovarian corpus luteum is taken over by a new endocrine organ, the syncytiotrophoblast, which elaborates two hormones, a placental progesterone and an oestrogen, oestriol (Fig. 7–1; Table 7–2). The transfer of function from the corpus luteum of menstruation to the corpus luteum of pregnancy, and from the latter to the syncytiotrophoblast of the placenta (Fig. 7–1: ①, ② and ③), illustrates the working of a relay mechanism in the hormonal control of the reproductive cycle. A graphic representation of the amounts of these hormones produced during pregnancy (as determined by assays of their metabolic end products in the urine) is given in Fig. 7–3. The amounts of the pituitary gonadotropic hormones produced during a menstrual cycle, with their respective roles as described, are graphically presented in Fig. 7–2D.

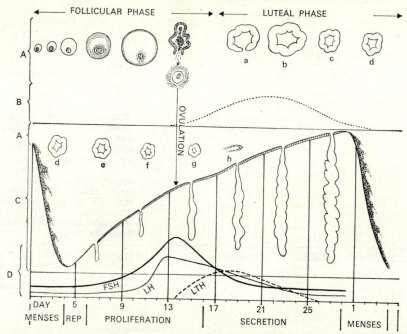

FIG. 7–2. Graphic representation of the events occurring during a menstrual cycle in the ovary (A) and uterus (C). The change in concentration of the hormones which are responsible for the different phases of the ovarian and uterine changes are also shown. Curve B represents the concentration of oestrogen and progesterone; curve D, concentrations of FSH, LH, and LTH. For a–h, inclusive, see text.

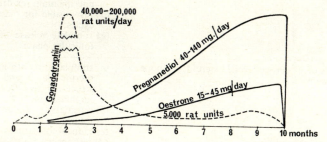

FIG. 7–3. Graphic representation of the amounts of placental hormones produced during pregnancy as determined by assays of their end-products in the urine. (After Arey.)

Should there be no fertilization, a decline in progesterone and oestrogen concentrations beginning about day 21 of the cycle brings on the regression of the corpus luteum. (A continuous supply of progesterone from a functional corpus luteum beyond day 28 is required to prevent degenerative changes occurring in the endometrium, and may also account for delayed and pseudo-menstrual cycles.) This, in turn, causes the onset of menstruation (Fig. 7–2c) and the cycle repeats itself. It is as if the endometrium, after being built up and fully prepared to receive the embryo, became suddenly frustrated! The atrophic changes undergone by the corpus luteum in such a case are portrayed by c to h inclusive in Fig. 7–2, A, c leading finally to a fibrous remnant, the corpus albicans (see Fig. 1–7).

Details of the microscopic appearance, drawn from histological sections, of the endometrium at six representative points of the menstrual cycle (days 7, 11, 23, 28, 2 and 5) are shown in

Endocrine organ	Cells producing the hormone(s)	Hormone	Chemical nature	Counter-part in male	Functions
Anterior Pituitary	Basophil cells	FSH	glyco-protein	same	(a) transforms solid follicles into vesicular ones; (b) stimulates secretion of female sex hormone, oestrogen; (c) promotes spermatogenesis
		LH	glyco-protein	same	(a) synergistic with FSH in completing follicular development, leading to ovulation; (b) stimulates oestrogen secretion from theca interna and granulosa cells; (c) transforms and develops a corpus luteum from the ovulated follicle, converting granulosa cells into luteal cells, and cells of theca interna into para-luteal cells; (d) stimulates secretion of male sex hormones by the testis
	Acidophil cells	LTH	protein	none	(a) synergistic with LH, causing the fully formed corpus luteum to secrete progesterone; (b) maintains the corpus luteum in functional state; (c) initiates milk secretion after parturition (see p. 75)
Ovary	Cells of theca interna, granulosa cells and possibly other ovarian stromal tissues	Oestrogens	steroid	male sex hormones	(a) responsible for the proliferative phase of the endometrium; its production constitutes the follicular phase of the ovary; (b) maintain general state of health of reproductive structures; (c) develop secondary sexual characteristics and maintain sex drive; (d) responsible for mammary and vaginal cycles; (e) stimulate release of LH during early follicular phase
	Luteal cells of corpus luteum	Progesterone	steroid	none	(a) stimulates growth and development of uterine glands and other endometrial structures involved in preparation for implantation; (b) sensitizes the endometrium for implantation; (c) induces formation of a placenta; (d) responsible for the secretory phase of endometrium and luteal phase of the ovary
Placenta (chorionic villi)	Cytotrophoblast (up to 3rd month)	Chorionic gonado-trophin	glyco-protein	none	(a) maintains the corpus luteum by transforming it from one of menstruation to that of pregnancy; (b) ensures the security of implanted embryo; (c) suppresses FSH, thereby stopping onset of another cycle Note: The presence of this hormone is assayed for in pregnancy tests.
	Syncytiotrophoblast (from 3rd month to end of pregnancy)	Oestriol (excreted as estrone)	steroid	none	(a) supplements ovarian oestrogen, keeping the level of female sex hormone high throughout pregnancy· (b) stimulates development of uterine muscles in preparation for parturition
		placental progesterone (excreted as pregnanediol)	steroid	none	(a) supplements ovarian progesterone (substitute for the corpus luteum in those species not requiring a functional corpus luteum in the latter part of pregnancy)

Fig. 7–4. On day 7, the damaged endometrium has entered a period of repair; on day 11, (about midway in the proliferative phase) the extent of growth of the stroma has increased and the stratum spongiosum and stratum compactum are clearly re-established; on day 23, at the height of the secretory phase, the glands are dilated and exhibit a typical " hacksaw " appearance, a sign of secretory activity. This secretion, consisting of mucin and glycogen and known as " uterine milk ", nourishes the embryo prior to implantation (see p. 60). By this time, the blood vessels have also reached a high degree of development; on day 28, the onset of menstruation, the endometrium shows oedema and blood has been extravasated under the epithelium; on day 2, about midway through the menstrual flow, advanced sloughing of endometrial tissues and blood vessels are evident; on day 5, menstruation terminates with only the basal layer of the endometrium (stratum basale) remaining. It is to be noted that the endometrium comprises three distinct layers: a dense upper stratum compactum, an extensive middle stratum spongiosum, which is loose and oedematous, and a thin stratum basale, which is dense and contains the bases of blood vessels and glands. The latter layer only remains at the end of the menstrual flow and from this regeneration and repair will begin. The strata compactum and spongiosum are known compositely as the functional layer, since both of them are involved in menstruation as well as in implantation.

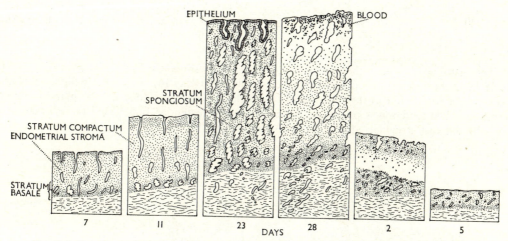

FIG. 7–4. Drawings of sections of the endometrium on days 2, 5, 7, 11, 23 and 28 of the menstrual cycle (the myometrium immediately beneath the endometrium is represented by horizontal wavy lines).

It is fairly certain that ovulation occurs at the midpoint of the cycle, i.e., on day 14, (the menses occupy the first four days of the cycle). The period from ovulation to the beginning of the next menses is constant at 14 days, but on the other hand, the length of period intervening between the end of the menses and the following ovulation is variable, being subject to such non-hormones factors as health, emotional state and so on. This variation probably accounts for the inaccuracy of the rhythm method of birth control (Table 7–1).

A structural interpretation of menstruation

The arteries of the endometrium are of a special coiled type (Fig. 7–5). As regressional changes begin in the endometrium just prior to the menses, these spiral arteries, with a slowed circulation, become constricted and somewhat buckled. They remain in this condition, causing a temporary blanching of the overlying endometrium. When this brief period of vasoconstriction ends, however, the vessels have already suffered enough damage to cause some blood to escape into the stroma, resulting in small pools of blood beneath the endometrial surface (cf. Fig. 7–4, day 28). These events are repeated, leading to a significant ischaemia in the endometrium, whereupon small pieces of tissue are detached. Bleeding then gradually spreads from the stroma onto the surface.

UTERINE GLAND:

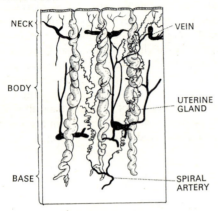

FIG. 7–5. Projection reconstruction of the glands and blood vessels of the endometrium on day 25 of the menstrual cycle.

The histology of the epithelium of a uterine gland is shown in Fig. 7–6. In A (day 10) the nuclei lie at the bases of the columnar epithelial cells; in B (day 16), drawn more highly magnified than in A, a slight shift in the position of the nuclei is seen; in C (day 25) the gland is actively secreting. The secretion is poured into the now much distended lumen and the epithelial cells are cuboidal with irregular edges (cf. the 23-day section, Fig. 7–4).

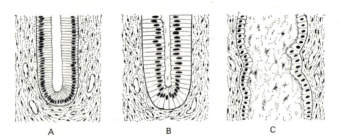

FIG. 7–6. High power drawing of the epithelium of a uterine gland on day 10 (A), day 16 (B) and day 25 (C) of the menstrual cycle.

A sex cycle comparable to the menstrual cycle does not exist in the human male; spermatogenetic activity is continuous from puberty until fairly advanced age, although it declines from middle age on. Successful spermatogenesis requires the synergistic action of FSH and LH (or ICSH, interstitial cell-stimulating-hormone, in the male). Since LH acts in the female as an ovulating hormone and in the male as a spermatogenetic hormone, it is often referred to as a gametokinetic hormone. So far as is known, there is no male counterpart of the hormone LTH.

In addition to the ovary and endometrium, both of which exhibit pronounced cyclic changes as just described, two other tissues also display cyclic phenomena under the influence of oestrogen. They are the mammary gland and the vaginal epithelium.

The mammary cycle

The pre-pubertal mammary gland is rudimentary with short sprout-like branches (Fig. 7–7A). Increasing amounts of oestrogen during the period of puberty enlarge the nipple and ducts, which grow and branch into a virginal or pre-pregnant state (Fig. 7–7B). During pregnancy there is remarkable growth of the ducts and secretory end-pieces (Fig. 7–7C). In this period possibly both oestrogen and progesterone act on the gland. This is certainly true for some species; but in the human, progesterone is not required, although it may very well act synergistically with oestrogen for the final stages of differentiation. In each menstrual cycle the breast becomes larger and firmer just prior to menstruation, when the oestrogens reach peak concentration. The actual initiation of milk secretion requires the specific action of LTH or prolactin as it is sometimes called (Fig. 7–7D), the secretion of which is inhibited prior to parturition by the placental oestrogen.

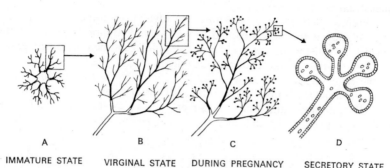

IMMATURE STATE   VIRGINAL STATE   DURING PREGNANCY   SECRETORY STATE

FIG. 7–7. Development of the mammary gland (after Arey):
A. Immature state; with rudimentary ducts.   B. Virgin state of the duct system;
C. Pregnant state, showing further branching of the ducts, plus budding of secretory end-pieces;
D. Initiation of milk secretion.

The two names for this hormone have developed because it acts on different tissues at different times. In both instances, it requires the prior action of another hormone, a phenomenon which is known as synergism, LTH must have the prior action of LH in initiating the corpus lutem to secrete progesterone; prolactin is effective only on the mammary gland that has been built up to a state capable of secretion by oestrogen. Similarly, as we have already seen, LH depends on the prior action of oestrogen to bring about ovulation.

The vaginal cycle

This is of little significance in humans. This cycle is also caused by the action of oestrogen and is very pronounced in rodents. The various cell types (characteristic of the different periods of the oestrous cycle) which are found in vaginal smears are as follows (Fig. 7–8A):

Stage	Duration	Cell types
Proestrus	1 day	Mostly epithelial cells; a few of them beginning to cornify;
Oestrus (heat)	1–2 days	Mostly cornified epithelial cells;
Dioestrus (interval)	2–3 days	Equal proportion of leucocytes and epithelial cells

Comparable stages in human vaginal epithelial smears are shown in Fig. 7–8B. The examination of a vaginal smear has become a standard laboratory practice for determining the condition of female rodents with respect to the oestrous cycle.

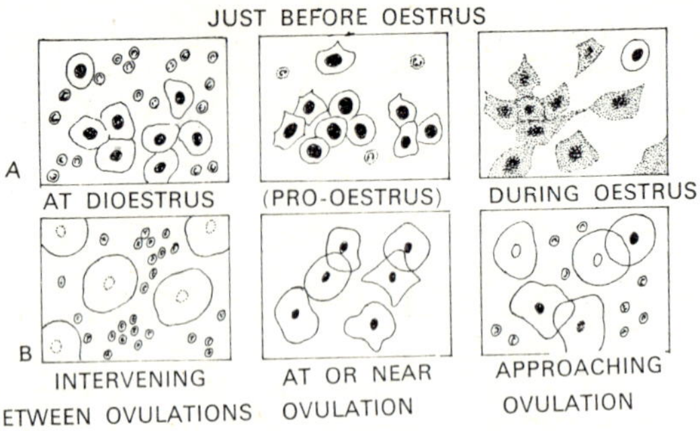

FIG. 7–8. A. Cellular types found in vaginal smears representing three stages of the oestrous cycle in rats. (After Arey.)
B. The vaginal cycle in the monkey (from left to right) shortly after cessation of menstruation; just prior to ovulation; shortly after ovulation.

Oestrous and menstrual cycles compared

The main differences between the two are: (1) Ovulation coincides with "heat" in the oestrous cycle; ovulation is not accompanied by any such comparable period in the menstrual cycle. (2) The menstrual cycle is characterized by the unique phenomenon of the menses, a bleeding resulting from the sloughing of the endometrial mucosa. (3) The time of ovulation occupies different loci in the two cycles. Ovulation is the terminal event in the oestrous cycle, ovulation taking place when the animal is in oestrus. In the menstrual cycle, ovulation occurs about mid-way in the cycle. Despite these differences, however, the two cycles are basically comparable in that their principal objective is to bring follicles to ovulation and the same hormonal mechanisms are involved in both.

CHAPTER 8

EXPERIMENTAL EMBRYOLOGY AND TERATOLOGY

The scope of descriptive embryology is limited to the study of normal developmental processes. Its sister discipline, experimental embryology, however, pursues a different objective, namely to analyze various phases and aspects of development in order to understand the multiple mechanisms by which a fertilized egg systematically changes into a complete organism. Obviously, development does not always proceed normally; numerous factors, intrinsic and extrinsic, can divert its course, thereby resulting in many kinds of anomalies involving either the whole organism (twinning), or parts of the body (malformations or deformities). The causes of developmental anomalies are not yet completely known, but great strides have been made in recent years towards the understanding, control, and rectification of developmental anomalies and malformations through advancement in experimental embryology, physiological genetics, cytochemical and chemical genetics, immunology, biochemistry, molecular biology and molecular pathology.

A number of basic techniques are at the disposal of the experimental embryologist, which he can use as tools for attaining his objectives. These are briefly as follows:

1. Defect experiments (effect of removal of a part from a whole).
2. Isolation experiments (growth and differentiation of an isolated part under artificial environmental conditions):
   (a) Explantation (tissue culture).
   (b) Interplantation (to some foreign site, e.g., anterior chamber of the eye).
3. Transplantation experiments (exchange of parts between two individuals):
   (a) Recombination:
       (1) autoplastic (on same individual)
       (2) homoplastic (between different individuals of the same species)
       (3) heteroplastic (between individuals from two closely related species)
       (4) xenoplastic (between individuals from two remotely related species, e.g., belonging to two genera)
   (b) Addition: (parabiosis) — combination of two whole individuals.
4. Segregation and Reaggregation experiments.
5. Tracer techniques using radio-active isotopes (in conjunction with radioautography).

The advantage of the experimental embryologist lies in his freedom to alter the environment (internal or external) in which a developmental process is taking place. For instance, he can add to the environment or subtract from it a single or multiple factors, in order to determine their specific effect. His success, however, often depends on whether or not a particular experimental design meets the requirement of a specific problem in mind.

Nature of development

Development is fundamentally an epigenetic process. It is a one-way process from zygote to the mature organism via a series of successive and interconnected events, each depending on the preceding ones. This continuous, progressive process, in general, goes from uniformity to diversity, from generality to specialization, from plasticity to rigidity, and from simplicity to complexity. The four characteristics of development are, therefore, progressiveness, discreteness, exclusiveness and genetic limitation. The entire course is controlled by multiple factors, chief among which are the genes. The action of genes and their interaction both between themselves and with their environment determine the final outcome.

Component processes of development

Growth, differentiation and organization are the three necessary components of development. Growth represents an increase both in number and size of cells and is the way to provide raw materials for differentiation. The latter is the process for creating and producing new cell types, which were not present before. Finally, the great diversity of parts produced by growth and differentiation are coordinated and brought under unified control through functional integration, so that they maintain specific mutual relationships and conform to specific patterns. This is organization, the final product of orderliness in development, which makes an organism what it is.

Basic conditions for initiation of development

From many experiments, as well as observations of nature, it has been established that initiation of development requires a minimum of three conditions. They are:

1. At least 1 N (haploid) chromosomes from either egg or sperm must be present.
2. A stimulus to activate the egg is necessary. This may be supplied by the sperm, or by various other agents, either physical or chemical (e.g., by pricking the egg with a needle, or by using an acid or a base). Instances of natural parthenogenesis and artificial parthenogenesis prove that the sperm is not indispensable.
3. Some cytoplasm of the egg is essential (this cannot be substituted by any part of the sperm cell).

Balance and cooperation between cytoplasmic and nuclear materials is vital to development. The cytoplasm of the egg (but not that of the sperm) contains indispensable specific developmental properties. The concept of " cytoplasmic inheritance ", originally stemming from these observations, is now well established, supported by demonstrable instances.

Multiplication vs. differentiation

Cells grow, divide, and differentiate with undisputable antagonism between mitotic activity and cellular differentiation. Rapidly dividing cells do not differentiate; in other words, a cell cannot divide and differentiate at the same time. A case in point is the cleaving egg. The zygote divides mitotically several times to produce a blastula which is scarcely larger than the zygote itself. This suggests at once that the resulting blastomeres have not undergone differentiation to any appreciable extent, and that cleavage is simply a means to make available a sufficiently large number of cells for subsequent differentiation.

When a cell enters into one of several lines of differentiation, it need not pursue this course in one uninterrupted stride; instead it may reach several intermediate levels of differentiation, at each of which progress can be temporarily suspended by an intervening period, to be followed again with mitotic activity. Many cells remain permanently arrested at early levels of differentiation (e.g., hepatic epithelium, and smooth muscle cells); only a certain proportion of them attain the highest possible degree of differentiation (e.g., neurons, erythrocytes, melanocytes, etc.).

At any level, including the highest, a cell is in a state of " plasticity " in which it is subject to the influence of environmental agents (e.g., hormones). The term " modulation " is applied by some to such cells whose morphology may thus alter, only to return to their original form the moment the causative agent is removed.

Finally, a fully differentiated cell is no longer capable of dividing, but is destined to die after serving its useful term. Aging, is at least in part, due to the loss of functional cells without replacement.

Some problems concerning cleavage

What relation exists, if any, between cleavage planes and the future symmetry of the embryo? The evidence at hand favours the interpretation that the egg, prior to segmentation, already displays a certain primary organization such as the possession of an animal and vegetal pole (primary axis), bilateral symmetry and certain centro-peripheral gradients. In most cases it is the bilaterally symmetrical organization of the egg cytoplasm that determines the cleavage planes, not the reverse. For example, the superficial grey crescent of a frog's egg (Fig. 8–1) invariably determines the first cleavage plane; it always bisects it so that the resulting two blastomeres each have an equal amount of the grey crescent material. In general, it may be said that the egg is precociously organized and that the cleavage pattern bears a definite relationship with this cytoplasmic organization.

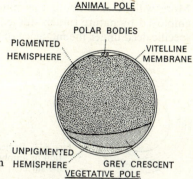

FIG. 8–1. Frog's egg after fertilization, showing the gray crescent. (The inner and outer layers of jelly surrounding the egg have been removed.) (After Shumway and Adams.)

Are the nuclei of blastomeres equivalent? If they are, then it would appear that differentiation depends on unequal divisions of the nucleus during cleavage. In newts, any nucleus at the 16-cell stage is interchangeable with others, and therefore is presumed to be equal in developmental potency (Fig. 8–2). It is now known, however, from experiments in which nuclei of chorda-mesoderm cells from late gastrulae are transferred to enucleated eggs, that such nuclei already have lost some of their intrinsic plasticity and the potency to direct normal embryonic development. In other words, the process of differentiation ultimately involves nuclear changes of a kind having to do with de-coding of genetic information.

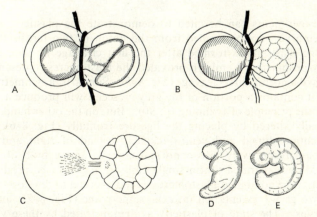

FIG. 8–2. Spemann's experiment for demonstrating equipotency of nucleus up to the 16-cell stage in amphibians. (After Balinsky.)

Significance of gastrulation

In contrast to cleavage, the primary function of which is to increase the number of cells, gastrulation is characterized by orderly (pre-destined) movements of aggregates (either sheets or layers) of cells so that a single germ layer is transformed into two germ layers (Fig. 8–3). In later gastrulae a third germ layer, the mesoderm, makes its appearance, and with the formation of a notochord, the primary axis of the embryo is established. The methods by which these developmental events are accomplished vary in different species. Regardless of the manner of formation, however, the significance of gastrulation lies in the establishment of a growth centre in the dorsal lip (amphibians) or primitive streak (birds and mammals). The latter is not just a focal point of cellular proliferation and movements, but it is endowed with the unique property of a primary organizer. It directs the chorda-mesoderm, a median strip of cells among the earliest involuted at the dorsal lip (or primitive steak), to induce the overlying ectoderm cells to form a neural tube. More will be said about this phenomenon of induction later. It is an effective mechanism employed by nature (much studied since the work of Spemann) whereby one tissue performs a specific deed under the influence of another in close contact. (see Chapter 3).

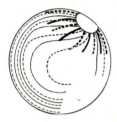

FIG. 8–3. Projection of the movements of parts of the maiginal zone during gastrulation in amphibians, seen in lateral view; the thick lines represent movements on the surface; the thin lines, movements of invaginated cells. (After Balinsky.)

The concept of potency

Potency is the total range of developmental possibilities a cell is capable of realizing under any condition, either normal or experimental. On this basis, blastulae and eggs may be divided into two groups: (1) *Mosaic*, those resulting from " determinate cleavage " (e.g., tunicates, molluscs, and annelids) and (2) *Regulative*, those resulting from " indeterminate cleavage " (e.g., vertebrates, including man). In the former, potency of a blastomere is equal to the fate it has received. For example, in *Dentalium* the removal of the polar lobe after the first cleavage division would result in a defective larva lacking an apical organ (Fig. 8–4). In the indeterminate type of cleavage, potency of individual blastomeres is much wider and less rigid. That is, they are plastic or undetermined.

Many classical experiments can be cited to demonstrate the plasticity in early amphibian embryos. A giant embryo may be formed from the union of two fertilized eggs; conversely, either one of the two blastomeres formed after the first cleavage division can develop into a smaller but perfectly proportioned embryo provided the blastomeres represent the right and left halves (i.e., products of a normal first cleavage (Fig. 8–5). Similarly, a symmetrical half amphibian blastula, as long as it contains a portion of the grey crescent, will produce a whole embryo. In fact, this constitutes the principle of twinning (p. 90). But, on the other hand, if the first cleavage plane is experimentally altered by placing the ligature frontally (Fig. 8–6), then the resulting blastomeres, representing dorsal and ventral halves (instead of right and left halves) when separated, will develop respectively into a normal embryo and a blob of unorganized tissue (Fig. 8–6). Mangold demonstrated that a single embryo may also be produced by fusing two 2-cell germs together. The combined blastomeres would proceed to develop into a single embryo provided that the two grey crescents fell into the same plane (Fig. 8–7); otherwise, the result would be two embryos. The state of plasticity as demonstrated by these various experiments lasts until the neural stage, at which time the potencies of the cells begin to be fixed.

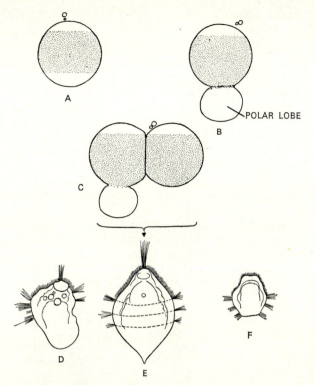

FIG. 8–4. Cleavage of the mollusc, *Dentalium* (A, B, C), larvae developing from a whole egg (E), larvae developing from separated blastomeres with the polar lobe (D), and without the polar lobe (F) (Modified from Balinsky.)

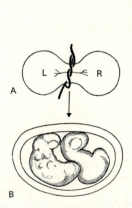

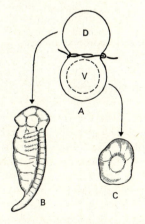

FIG. 8–5. Development potency of right and left half-blastomeres of newt egg.

FIG. 8–6. Development potency of dorsal and ventral half-blastomeres in newt.

FIG. 8–7. A 4-cell embryo arising from fusion of two 2-cell stages derived from two different species.

The mosaic and regulative types of development discussed above can be explained in terms of three factors, which interact with one another: (1) the time at which fertilization takes place, (2) the rate of cleavage and (3) the rate of segregation of cytoplasmic differences. One must bear in mind, however, that these factors may overlap and that their actions are relative to one another, hence a whole range of gradations between the extremes is possible. The relative influence of these factors on the determination of cleavage types is shown in Table 8–1.

TABLE 8–1.   FACTORS INFLUENCING CLEAVAGE TYPES (after Weiss)

Egg	Cleavage type	Time of fertilization	Rate of cleavage	Rate of segregation
Mosaic	determinate	relatively late	slow	rapid
Regulative	indeterminate	relatively early	fast	slow

Such an interpretation implies that there is a given degree of so-called "manifest organization" in the egg prior to segmentation. It folows-then, that cleavage is dependent upon pre-existing intrinsic differentiation of the germ. In amphibians presumptive organ regions of the blastulae are plastic i.e., when transplanted into new (strange) localities they develop in accordance with the requirements of their new site. This indicates that differentiation potency is greater than differentiation fate (Fig. 8–8).

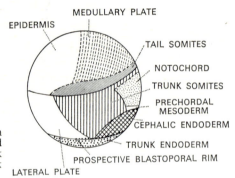

FIG. 8–8. Fate map of the early gastrula of an amphibian (axolotl), seen in lateral view; the positions of tissue destined to form medullary plate, tail somites, notochord, trunk somites, prechordal mesoderm, cephalic endoderm, and trunk endoderm are indicated. (After Balinsky.)

The problems of determination and differentiation

"Determination" is the result of loss of plasticity or regulative power. It is the fixation of fate by an irrevocable "assignment" for the future. Subsequent to gastrulation the embryo quickly becomes "mosaic", with well recognizable and established organ fields for the ear, nose, heart, limb, etc., each of which will be "self-differentiating (Fig. 8–9). "Determination" and "differentiation" are really inseparable processes, the latter actually being the result of the former. A part is said to be "determined" in fate when its component cells have become "intrinsically and irreversibly" different from other cells, and so it is a visible carrying-out of the assignment mentioned above. This represents an irreversible type of differentiation, which is most characteristic of the process of development and, no doubt, involves nuclear-cytoplasmic interplay, or more specifically DNA-RNA interaction.

Generally, three stages of differentiation are recognized, which are listed below in their chronological order:

1. Invisible differentiation — Chemical differences have occurred in cells without, however, giving any externally (morphologically) visible evidence of the change.

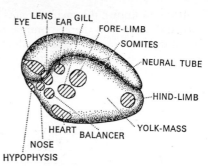

FIG. 8–9. Organ-fields of an amphibian embryo at the neurula
stage.

2. Histo-differentiation — Visible changes gradually appear, rendering tissues morphologically different from one another.
3. Auxano-differentiation — Organs are both morphologically and functionally established.

Induction

Induction is probably the most studied and experimentally analyzed mechanism of differentiation known, which was first investigated by Spemann and Mangold in 1924. In a classical experiment the dorsal lip of an amphibian gastrula was transplanted underneath the ventral lip of another embryo (in early gastrulation) (Fig. 8–10). In such a case the neighbouring host cells were induced by the graft to form a notochord, mesoderm and a neural tube (i.e., the axial structures) of a secondary embryo within the host embryo. Conversely, if the dorsal lip was removed from an embryo, development immediately ceased. Spemann called the formative influence exerted by the cells of the dorsal lip, induction, and the dorsal lip was referred to as an organizer or inductor. Since it is the first (earliest) induction, which establishes the axial structures of the embryo, the dorsal lip of the blastopore is popularly known as the primary organizer.

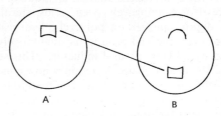

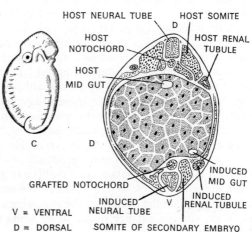

FIG. 8–10. An experiment by Spemann and Mangold showing induction of a secondary embryo in *Triturus* by means of a transplanted piece of blastopore from a donor (A) to a host (B). The induced secondary embryo, at the side of the host in a tail-bud stage (C) is shown in transverse section in D. D = dorsal; V = ventral.

It is now known that many organs in the body are formed by induction. During the course of normal development there are numerous instances in which two tissues come into contact so that one of them acts as an inductor which brings about specific changes in the other, resulting in the formation of a definitive structure or organ. The following chart summarizes the important and best known inductions in the chick. Note the tremendous inductive power residing with the mesoderm in particular:

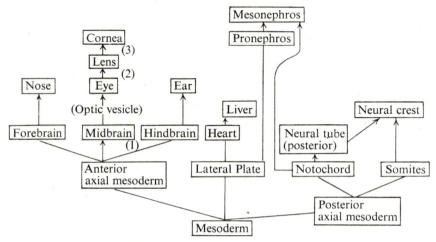

Organizers in the chick (modified from Weiss)
Arrows indicate induction;
(1), (2) and (3): Inductions, respectively, of the first, second and third orders.

It was soon discovered that dead inductors (killed in various ways) and various chemical substances (for example, glycogen, acids, sterol-like chemicals, methylene blue, cephalin, thiocyanate, digitin and certain polycyclic hydrocarbons) can induce competent tissues. In such cases, however, the end-product is qualitatively " inferior ", or at least not the same as that produced by a living, natural inductor. This seems to indicate non-specificity of the inductive stimulus. Such a non-specific action is now conceived of as an " evocator ". A living organizer, besides being an evocator, must also be able to " individuate ", i.e., to have the power to call forth definitive reactions from the resultant tissue, in order to form regional specializations characteristic of the organ or structure in question. For instance, the chorda-mesoderm not only induces formation of neural tissue, but also the various parts of the brain. An inductor or organizer possesses the power of both evocation and individuation. The former usually consists of histological changes produced by the evocating stimulus while the latter is concerned with production of regional organization of embryonic tissues.

Another important concept is that of " competence ". Induction involves the close association of two tissues with each other, and although only one of them (the inductor) plays the active role, the other must be able to respond adequately to the inductive stimulus. The term " competence " refers to this state of reactiveness on the part of the tissue being induced. For instance, a piece of head ectoderm or even belly ectoderm from an early neural stage is considered competent because, when it is grafted over an eye vesicle, it can be induced to form a complete lens. With time, however, this competence gradually diminishes and is eventually lost. Thus, the same ectoderm taken from a much older embryo (e.g., at the tail bud stage) can no longer form a lens under the influence of an eye vesicle. We may conclude, therefore, that successful induction depends upon, on the one hand, the evocating and individuating capacity of the inductor, and on the other, the competence of the tissue being induced. Such mutual reciprocity is a necessary requirement.

The physical basis of induction is not fully understood, but it appears to involve increased cell membrane permeability and subsequent transfer of material from the inductor to competent cells. Previously it was believed that direct physical contact was essential for induction to occur (e.g., between cells of prospective lens and those of the optical vesicle); recent experiments, however, have shown that such contact is not a prerequisite to successful induction (this has been demonstrated both in lens induction in the chick, and in induction of metanephric tubules in the mouse). Nevertheless, it would appear logical that such contact does facilitate chemical transfer across the membrane barrier.

It is virtually certain that induction involves the diffusion of chemical substances emanating from the inductor cells to the reactive tissue. Such a transfer of material was recently demonstrated by radioactive-labeling techniques. What is the nature of the substance being transferred from one cell to another? Some believe it is steroid or sterol-like chemicals, which are effective in very low concentrations. Others consider it to be nucleoprotein, such as is actually released from mesoderm and taken up by ectoderm cells during neural induction. More recently it has been identified as a cytoplasmic ribonucleoprotein, closely related to ribosomal particles. Regardless of the final chemical expression, induction involves altered reactivity of cells and subsequent specification of their fate. It must, therefore, also involve the genetic equipment (DNA) of the cells, either directly or more likely indirectly.

TERATOLOGY

It is a common observation that certain defects run in families, i.e., they are transmitted through the genes; these form 10% of the total number of congenital abnormalities. A further 10% of deformities of one kind or another are caused by intrinsic factors present in the environment. For example, cyclopia (one median eye resulting from the fusion of the eye primordia) can be induced by lithium ions whereas potassium ions can cause cardiac defects in some invertebrates. Similarly, exogastrulation is induced with lithium salts in the sea urchin, or with hypotonic salt solutions in *Triton* eggs. From such experiments it can be concluded that genes and environmental factors are both discrete causes for abnormal development. To these we may add a third category, namely factors representing the results of interaction between genes and the environment in which development is taking place. Actually, 80% of congenital anomalies can be attributed to this latter category.

Role of environmental factors

Agents known to be capable of affecting developmental processes in one way or another include:

1. Physical factors:
   (a) Gravity.
   (b) Electro-magnetic force.
   (c) Temperature (heat* or cold).
   (d) Light.
   (e) Short-wave or ionizing radiation (ultra-violet, X-ray, betta and gamma rays atomic fall-out).*
   (f) Humidity.
   (g) Centrifugal force.

* also capable of inducing mutations, i.e. mutagenic.

2. Chemical factors:
   (a) Oxygen and water.
   (b) K^+, Mg^{++} ions — essential for fertilization.
   (c) K^+, Ca^{++} ions — essential for muscle contraction.
   (d) Cl^-, Na^+ ions — essential for segmentation.
   (e) Ca^{++}, OH^- ions — essential for securing internal osmotic pressure necessary for growth.
   (f) S^{--}, Mg^{++} ions — essential for alimentary tract and skeletal functions.
   (g) $CaCO_3$ — essential for bone formation.
   (h) Food (carbohydrates, proteins and fat).
   (i) Vitamins.
   (j) Hormones.

The effect of most of these agents, physical or chemical, is limited to somatic tissues, and therefore lasts for only one generation. Certain of them, however, such as extreme temperatures and high-energy radiation are so powerful that they can produce effects on the genes and/or chromosomes, thereby causing mutations. These agents, known as mutagenic substances, have attracted much attention largely because of the concern that radio-active fall-out is a potential danger by increasing the rate of congenital malformations in future generations. Mutations also take place spontaneously in nature (cosmic rays are suspected as being one of the possible causative agents). The rate of spontaneous mutation is estimated at one in 10^{-5} per gene per generation. In man, spontaneous mutation may be caused by (a) failure of gene duplication during cell division (b) irradiation from natural sources and (c) action of chemical mutagenic agents on the parents. Regardless of origin, mutations are inheritable from the start, and, most unfortunately, they are almost always harmful.

The term " phenocopy " refers to those cases in which a certain defect is produced through application of single or combined environmental factors at a certain critical time during development. The result closely simulates the effect of a known gene. For example, wing defects in *Drosophila* can be produced by high temperatures applied at critical periods. Such an experimental approach is obviously of great value in determining the specific action of genes.

The concept of the " critical period "

There are periods in the course of normal development during which a certain tissue or organ primordium is most sensitive to the action of some physical or chemical agent, thereby resulting in specific injuries. The concept may be related to the principle that a tissue undergoing rapid growth is especially susceptible to the deleterious action of various teratogenic agents. Thus, a limb-bud prior to differentiation is particularly vulnerable. The recent investigations relating to the effect of the drug thalidomide in arresting the development of limbs of human foetuses demonstrates the validity of this concept (see Fig. 15–9A, B). Evidence has been fast accumulating that the action of many such teratogenic agents is of a specific nature. To use the example just cited, thalidomide primarily affects the limb primordia although it may also cause minor deformities in long bones, intestinal atresia, and various cardiac abnormalities.

Role of genes in development

Many developmental abnormalities are due to changes in genes or chromosomes. Such changes, whether occurring spontaneously or caused by the action of mutagenic agents, may be located in either the somatic or germ cells of an individual. In the former case of changes involving somatic tissues, although the alteration occurs in the nucleus (gene or chromosome) of the cells, the changes are not inheritable, but will last for only one generation and vanish upon death of the afflicted individual. If the changes are localized in the chromosomes or genes of a sperm or egg cell, however, then the anomalies will be inheritable from the start. These two categories of developmental abnormalities are the result of so-called somatic or germinal mutations, respectively.   Naturally, only the latter kind has survival value.

We know relatively little about gene action.   Genes are responsible for the production of chemical substances (enzymes or coenzymes) which direct specific chemical reactions by altering or controlling the rate of chemical reactions.   In other words, genes regulate the rate and intensity of specific developmental processes (morphogenesis; histo-differentiation, etc.).   This means that correct timing of the action of many genes is very important.   Often, abnormal development results if this timing is altered or thrown out of synchronization with the actions of other genes.

The action of a gene may be modified by conditions which are not well understood at the present.   For example, a dominant gene, which normally should express itself in the heterozygous state, sometimes fails to do so; again, a recessive gene could likewise fail to manifest its effect in individuals homozygous for that gene.   This phenomenon of an apparent sporadic inability of a gene to exert its usual effect is known as " reduced penetration ".

It is known that a gene may produce a multiplicity of effects, involving several morphological or functional defects.   Such action is called " pleiotropism ".   For example, a pleiotropic mutant gene recently discovered in mice produces simultaneously: (a) anaemia (b) albinism and (c) sterility, due to deficient numbers of primordial germ cells in both sexes.   Conversely, in certain instances several genes may cooperate to bring about the realization of a single effect. An example of this is found in the inheritance of eye pigment in *Drosophila*.

As pointed out in the introduction to this section about 80% of all known developmental abnormalities, ranging from extremely severe cases (monstrosities) to mild anomalies, result from the interaction of genes with environmental factors in one way or another.   It will be some time before the exact mode of such interactions can be revealed.   In humans it is possible that intelligence or mental capacity, skin pigmentation and height are examples of this mode of inheritance.   As is well known, these all are subject to the influence of nutrition.   In such cases the role of genes involved is probably to set the upper and lower limits of inherent capability.

Abnormalities due to genes

These may be cases where a single gene, or more than one gene, is involved; mutations in a parental germ cell (arising either spontaneously or from high-energy ionizing radiation) or irregularities occurring during maturation (meiosis) of ova and/or sperm belong to this category.

Many congenital malformations in man are known to be inherited according to Mendelian principles.   In many such cases the abnormality in question is found to have resulted from the mutation of a single gene.   Such single gene mutations are responsible for about 10% of all human malformation known today.   A mutated single gene may act in any of the following patterns:

A. Autosomal dominant inheritance.   The malformation is apparent in either heterozygous (the gene transmitted from either parent) or homozygous individuals (genes transmitted from both parents).   Any child has thus a 50% chance of being afflicted.   Examples: achondroplasia, cleidocranial dysostosis, lobster claw (of hands and/or feet) and imperfect oesteogenesis.

B. Autosomal recessive inheritance.   The gene for the malformation must be in the homozygous condition (i.e., transmitted from both parents) in order to express itself.   Since the gene must come from unaffected heterozygous parents, incidences of malformations involving recessive genes are low.   Each sibling of an affected child has a 25% chance of being affected.   Examples: chondro-ectodermal dystrophy, some forms of microcephaly, and chondro-dystrophia calcificans congenita.

C. Sex-linked inheritance (see p. 19).   The mutated gene in question is located on the X sex chromosome, and it is almost always recessive.   Therefore, the defect shows in all males who have got the " bad " X chromosome from their mother, but only appears in homozygous females. Heterozygous females are called " carriers " for the reason that they will give the " bad " X chromosome to half of their sons. Examples: colour blindness, haemophilia, one form of hydrocephalus, one form of gargoylism, and testicular feminization syndrome.

Abnormalities due to chromosomal aberrations (Fig. 8–11)

The many types of changes that can occur to chromosomes are summarized in Fig. 8–11. The seriousness of chromosome aberrations is emphasized by the fact that recent cytogenetic studies have disclosed that up to half of all spontaneous abortions are the result of one form or another of chromosome aberration in the developing embryo. These studies reveal in addition that there is a growing number of abnormalities which are due to too little (rather than too much) chromosome material (see example below).

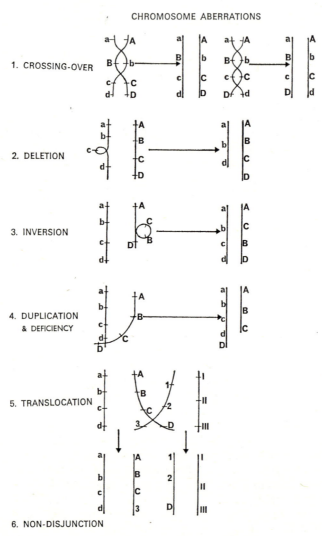

FIG. 8–11. Diagrams illustrating different types of chromosomal aberrations.

A. Involving autosomes:
  1. Mongolism
     45 + XY (man)
     45 + XX (woman)
     The extra autosome is usually chromosome No. 21, hence the name " trisomy 21 ". The condition results from non-disjunction in the first meiotic division.
  2. Monosomy
     43 + XY (man)
     43 + XX (woman)
  3. Translocation: the " cri du chat " (cat cry) syndrome. It involves a missing piece of chromosome No. 5, the missing segment being attached to chromosome No. 13. The translocation produces two modified chromosomes, namely the No. 5⁻ and the No. 13⁺, resulting in three genotypes from different combinations. These are:

     normal 13 and 5⁻ (manifesting the " cri du chat " syndrome)
     13⁺ and normal 5 (mirror image of " cri du chat ", exhibiting a " raucous cry ")
     13⁺ and 5⁻ (" carrier " of the " cri du chat " syndrome)
     The victims of the " cri du chat " disorder are severely retarded and have small heads with widely spaced eyes. The infants have a high-pitched cry, resembling the mewing of a cat, as a result of an underdeveloped larynx. The example cited demonstrates the severe effect of a missing segment of chromosome.
B. Involving sex chromosomes (see p. 18):
  1. Turner's and Kleinefelter's syndromes. These are discussed in Chapter 2.
  2. Mosaicism, which is associated with these syndromes, as the result of errors occurring in mitotic divisions subsequent to conception (e.g., during cleavage).

CONGENITAL MALFORMATIONS AND DISEASES

By definition, a congenital deformity is one present at birth. Though most cases are of a germinal origin (inherited), such a notion is only implied, as environmental factors acting on the foetus during gestation may well be responsible for certain congenital malformations. In general, it can be said that congenital abnormalities are the result of genetic inadequacies or genetic inequalities, or of random alterations in the environment during development, or both. They range in degree of severity from " teratomata " (tumours of developmental origin, usually of the ovary) through monstrosities of various types, to mild forms of anomalies. According to a survey made in 1959, deaths resulting from all kinds of congenital malformations were as high as 12·3% of all births so the seriousness of the problem cannot be denied.

Other factors are known to be implicated in certain human congenital abnormalities. For example, the virus of German measles, *Rubella*, when contracted in early pregnancy is responsible for 5–7% of foetal abnormalities and for 6–10% of still-births. Similarly, diabetes and toxemia (presence of toxic substances in the blood) in pregnant mothers may lead to certain congenital deformities, although the mechanism is not known.

Included in this group are the inborn diseases, or the so-called " errors of metabolism " which involve some malfunction in metabolism which is definitely of a hereditary nature. They include diseases involving almost any phase of protein, fat and carbohydrate metabolism, as well as diseases of the blood. The concept was introduced by Garrod (1858–1936) and today extensive experiments by chemical geneticists have made significant progress towards understanding the causative mechanisms. The responsible genetic action may involve a single enzymatic defect, such as in the case of phenylketonuria (always associated with mental retardation), or in other cases, the production of a single abnormal molecule is the cause, as in sickle-cell anaemia.

From a developmental point of view, congenital abnormalities are classified as follows. Since the name of each category is self-explanatory, no definition is necessary. At least one example is given for each case.

TABLE 8-2.　DEVELOPMENTAL ABNORMALITIES

Category of deformity	Examples
Developmental failure (Agenesis)	Absence of limb, kidney, etc.
	Albinism
Developmental arrest	Dwarfism
	Infantile uterus
Developmental excess	Gigantism
	Extra digits; double penis
	True twins (see below)
Fusion or Splitting	Cleft ureter; horseshoe kidney
Failure to subdivide	Cyclopia
	Syndactyly
Failure to atrophy	Retention of anal membrane
	Cervical fistula
Failure to consolidate	Lobed spleen, pancreas or kidney
Incorrect migration	Undescended testes
	Fused ears
Misplacement	Transposed viscera
	Palatine teeth
Atypical differentiation	Achondroplasia
	Mongolism
	Imperfect osteogenesis
Atavism (ancestral recurrence)	Azygos lobe of lung
	Elevator of clavicle

Teratogenic agents

Numerous teratogenic substances are known. The action of some of them may be unspecific, but it is becoming increasingly evident that most of them act specifically on certain tissues and at critical times during development. As examples one may list cortisone, extracts of sweet peas, insulin, boric acid, pilocarpine, eserine, sulphonamides, selenium and the dye trypan blue; this latter is a good example of a powerful teratogen which induces changes in the configuration of protein molecules, or may act to block sites on the surface of these molecules.

Twinning

The basis for the phenomenon of twinning has already been discussed in the section devoted to experimental embryology (p. 80). It can be either the result of independent development from separated early blastomeres, each of which is totipotent (in species with regulative types of cleavage only), or the result of division or splitting of the "organization centre" at much later stages. In the latter case, complete division of the centre gives rise to complete twins while incomplete division results in all kinds of conjoined twins (Fig. 8–13). Whatever the developmental mechanism involved, twinning has high hereditary tendencies. The characteristics of twinning are summarized below, and in table 8–3.

1. Twinning in mono-ovulatory species (man included):
   (a) Monozygotic: this results in identical twins of the same sex; they arise from separated blastomeres
   (b) Dizygotic:* fraternal twins, which may be of same or different sexes.

* strictly speaking, they are not twins since each develops from a separate zygote from the beginning.

2. Twinning in Di-ovulatory species:
   Examples: marmosets and enphractine armadillos (four complete embryos result).
3. Polyembryony (Multiple births). One fertilized egg may give rise to as many as five complete twin embryos, all of which are " identical ", i.e., from one egg. In such cases, all embryos possess separate amniotic sacs but are enclosed within a common chorion.

This feature distinguishes them from litter mates of normal poly-ovulatory species in which each embryo normally possesses a separate chorion (only in exceptional cases may they fuse into one).

TABLE 8–3. CLASSIFICATION OF IDENTICAL TWINS (Fig. 8–12)

Origin	Description	Frequency (%)
(a) Separated first two blastomeres	With separate placentae and chorionic sacs	25–30
(b) Reduplication of inner cell mass	Single placenta and chorionic sac; but separate amniotic cavities	70–75
(c) Reduplication of embryonic axis	Single placenta and chorionic sac, and a common amniotic cavity	1·0
(d) Incomplete separation of embryonic axis*		1·0
(e) Unequal division of embryonic axis†		Very rare

* Gives rise to all kinds of " Siamese " or conjoined twins (Fig. 8–13).
† Usually gives rise to 1 normal embryo and an acardiac monster (Fig. 8–12D).

Frequencies of human multiple births

Triplets	1 in 7600 pregnancies
Quadruplets	1 in 670,000 pregnancies
Quintuplets	Result of " incomplete triple one-egg twinning " — extremely rare.

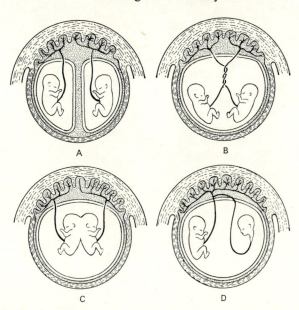

FIG. 8–12. Schematic representations of relationships of foetal membranes in different types of monozygotic twinning.

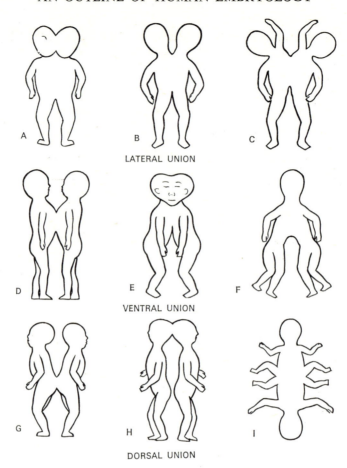

FIG. 8–13. Outline drawings showing different types of conjoined (Siamese) twins.

PART II

SPECIAL EMBRYOLOGY (ORGANOGENY)

CHAPTER 9

THE DIGESTIVE SYSTEM

Introduction

The vertebrate body is built on the fundamental plan of " a tube within a tube ". The two tubes are separated by the body cavity, and merge at both ends (Fig. 9–1). The digestive system and respiratory system are derived from the inner tube, being formed from both the endodermal epithelium and splanchnic mesoderm surrounding the latter; this double-layered wall is compositely known as the splanchnopleure. Only true digestive tissues, mucosa and glands are derived from the endoderm; the rest of the gastrointestinal tract, comprising such structures as smooth muscle cells connective tissues and an outer covering, the serosa, is all derived from the splanchnic mesoderm. This is also true of the respiratory system: only the epithelial lining and its derivatives are of endodermal origin.

The prospective inner tube is not a tube at all in the beginning; instead, it resembles an elongated saucer inverted over the yolk sac (Fig. 9–1). It has a complete roof lined with endoderm, and an open floor and will form the entire gastrointestinal tract with accessory organs and the entire respiratory tract.

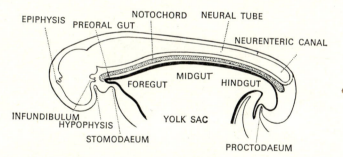

FIG. 9–1. A generalized vertebrate embryo to show the basic body plan with special reference to the endodermal derivatives (in heavy black); median sagittal view.

The first step towards establishing the alimentary tract, which coincides with the formation of the cephalic and caudal amniotic folds (Fig. 6–1), is a closing-off of a fore-gut in front and a hind-gut behind, the latter taking place considerably later than the former. This is accomplished by a similar process of under-cutting by body folds extending from the two ends towards the middle of the embryo. The two ends of the are closed by a layer of both ectoderm and endoderm which form respectively, the bucco-pharyngeal membrane and cloacal membrane (Fig. 4–13 and Fig. 4–15B). The former breaks through during the fourth week (2·4 mm), the latter about four weeks later when the embryo has a length of 30 mm.

The open area of the gut (mid-gut) becomes increasingly smaller whilst the closed fore- and hind-gut undergo rapid growth and increase in length. The under-cutting, first anterio-posteriorly by means of the cephalic and caudal folds, gradually extends circumferentially from the sides with the result that the mid-gut is narrowed down almost to a point connected with the yolk sac stalk (Fig. 9–2).

(Note: Incidentally, the formation of the gut is one of three consequences resulting simultaneously from the upward arching and lateral folding of the early embryo. The other two are the establishment of the definitive coelom from the intra-embryonic coelom and the formation of the primary mesenteries).

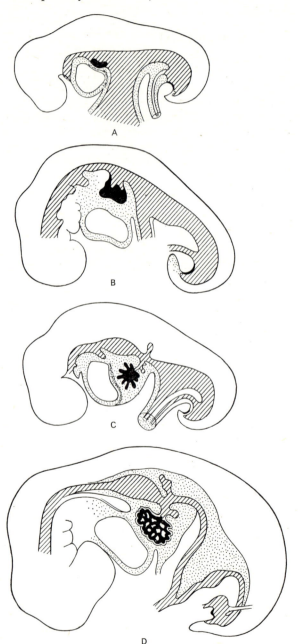

FIG. 9–2. Sagittal sections of human embryos showing four stages in the development of the alimentary canal and its derivatives. The extent of the tract is shown diagonally striped; the liver is in black and the mesoderm stippled
    A. 3 mm.; B. 4 mm.; C. 5–6 mm. D. 9–10 mm. approximately.

Further development of the gut is accomplished through extensive coiling, especially of the small intestine, followed by a period of umbilical herniation, which lasts some 7 weeks.

Another basic developmental process involved is budding or outpocketing of the tube (Fig. 9–3). The lungs, liver, gall bladder, pancreas all represent diverticula formed in this manner.

The anterior end of the tube, the region of the pharynx, presents special features due to the development of a series of pharyngeal arches (Fig. 9–3). These arches are functional structures in the Anamniotes (the gill arches), but in man they appear briefly and are functionless, but do give rise to important structures (see Chapters 15 and 16). The pharyngeal pouches and pharyngeal clefts, which are closely associated with the arches, also give rise to important structures (see Chapter 21), including some of the important endocrine glands (see Chapter 17).

The rotation of the stomach is an interesting phenomenon. It, coupled with the rotation of the intestinal loop upon its return to the peritoneal cavity at the end of the hernia, produces a lasting effect on the formation of the mesenteries.

Finally, the division of the cloaca into the dorsal rectum and the ventral urogenital sinus, together with the developmental relationships of the latter to some of the terminal urogenital structures, are features worthy of attention (Fig. 9–3).

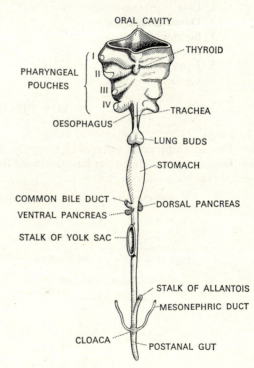

Fig. 9–3. Endodermal derivatives in a 5 mm. human embryo, ventral view.

Regional divisions of the gut and their constituents

Fore-gut:
    (a) Cranial part (from buccopharyngeal membrane to tracheobronchial diverticulum)
        1. Oral cavity
            (a) Hypophysis
            (b) Teeth
            (c) Salivary glands
        2. Nasal cavity

   3. Pharynx
    (*a*) Tongue
    (*b*) Pharyngeal clefts and pouches and their derivatives.
  (*b*) Caudal part (extending to liver bud)
    1. Thyroid gland
    2. Oesophagus
    3. Stomach
    4. Liver
    5. Cranial portion of duodenum.
Mid-gut (from anterior intestinal portal to posterior intestinal portal):
    1. Remaining (caudal) portion of the duodenum
    2. Jejunum and ileum
    3. Ascending colon
    4. First $\frac{2}{3}$ of transverse colon
    5. Pancreas.
Hind-gut (from posterior intestinal portal to cloacal membrane):
    1. Last $\frac{1}{3}$ of transverse colon
    2. Descending colon
    3. Sigmoid colon
    4. Rectum
    5. Upper part of anal canal
    6. Certain urogenital structures

THE PHARNYX (Fig. 9–4)

1. Tongue

This develops as an outgrowth from the floor of the pharynx. Its covering is endodermal epithelium, but the remainder has developed from the mesenchymal core of the first four pharyngeal (branchial) arches as follows:

Arches (No.)	Primordia	Definitive part of tongue
1	{ two lateral lingual swellings: Medial single tuberculum impar }	anterior $\frac{2}{3}$
2, 3 and part of 4	one median swelling: the copula	posterior $\frac{1}{3}$

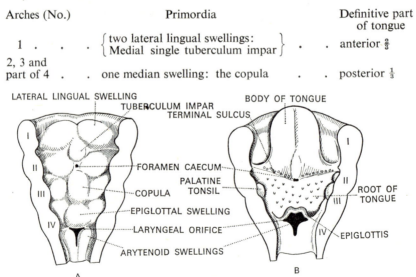

FIG. 9–4. The floor of the pharyngeal region seen from above, to show development of the tongue; A, at 5 weeks; B, at 5 months.

Anomalies

True " macroglossia ", an abnormally large tongue due to an oversized muscle mass, is often associated with mongolism and cretinism. A small tongue, (microglossia) or absence of the tongue (aglossia) may result from increasing degrees of failure of growth and development of the tongue.

Bifid or trifid tongues are caused by failure of the second lateral lingual swellings to fuse; the condition is often associated with a cleft of the lower lip.

2. Derivatives of the pharyngeal clefts (invaginations from the body surface lined with ectodermal epithelium)

Four pairs of pharyngeal clefts have developed in 5-week embryos. The first pair becomes the external auditory meatus (p. 253). Clefts Nos. 2, 3 and 4 become covered and buried by an overgrowth of the second branchial (pharyngeal) arch, resulting in the formation of a cervical sinus, which disappears later.

3. Derivatives of the pharyngeal pouches (lined with endoderm) (see Chapter 17)

Five pairs of pharyngeal pouches are formed along the lateral walls of the pharynx as a series of evaginations. Each pouch develops a dorsal and ventral wing (recess), comes into contact with the ectoderm of the corresponding invaginated pharyngeal cleft; this contact forms a closing epithelial plate. This plate, lined externally with ectoderm and internally with endoderm, perforates in fish to form a gill slit, but not in the human. The fate of these pouches in man is summarized below:

Pouch (No.)	Derivatives
1	Tubotympanic recess (definitive Eustachian tube of middle ear) Tympanic membrane
2	Palatine tonsillar fossa
3	dorsal: inferior parathyroid / ventral: primordium of thymus
4	dorsal: superior parathyroid / ventral: primordium of thymus (soon disappears)
5	Ultimobranchial bodies (incorporated into the thyroid for a while, but eventually completely lost).

In between the pharyngeal clefts and pharyngeal pouches, five pairs of branchial or pharyngeal arches are formed (see Chapters 15 and 16).

The thyroid gland (see Chapter 17)

This originates from the floor of the pharynx as a median diverticulum. Its point of origin migrates to the level of the first tracheal ring during a period from the 17th day to about the 7th week of development. The thyroid is unquestionably endodermal epithelium, and is generally regarded as an outgrowth from the floor of the pharynx at the level of the second branchial arch (Fig. 17–1) marked in the adult by the position of the foramen caecum on the surface of the tongue.

The oesophagus

The posterior limit of the pharynx is marked by the point at which the trachea becomes confluent with the intestinal tract. The portion of the gut from this point until the dilatation marking the beginning of the stomach is the oesophagus. During its elongation its lumen be-

D

comes obliterated, only to be re-canalized later, the event coinciding with the differentiation of a definitive epithelial lining composed of stratified squamous cells.

Anomalies

Sometimes the oesophagus is divided into a proximal and a distal part with a fibrous cord connecting the latter to the trachea. The condition is known as atresia of the oesophagus (Fig. 9–5). This defect is serious because it prevents passage of amniotic fluid into the intestinal tract, resulting in the accumulation of excess amniotic fluid, leading to an enlarged uterus. The baby may be born with the anomaly undetected until milk, overflowing from the proximal part of the oesophagus, fills the lungs. Early surgical correction may be helpful. Communication of oesophagus with trachea (rare) involves a direct connection of the proximal and distal parts (not separated) to the trachea by a narrow passage.

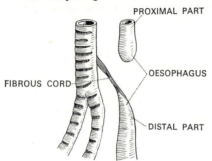

FIG. 9–5. Atresia of the oesophagus. (After Langman.)

Development of the stomach

The stomach is just discernible in 4 mm. embryos. During subsequent weeks it becomes markedly dilated and develops both cardiac and pyloric ends and its faster-growing dorsal surface becomes the greater curvature (Fig. 9–6). During development the stomach descends from the neck region downwards through 16 segments to its final permanent position. During that time it has undergone the following significant changes:

1. It leaves the medial sagittal plane so that its longer axis lies diagonally across it. As a result, its cardiac end lies to the left of the middle line.
2. Concomitantly, it rotates about its own long axis 90° counter-clockwise (viewed from the dorsal or posterior aspect) so that its greater curvature changes from the dorsal to the left side of the embryo. Also, the greater curvature comes to be directed somewhat caudally as well as to the left. (The definitive ventral surface of the stomach is supplied by the left gastric (vagus) nerve). The rotation of the stomach is generally attributed to two causes: (*a*) a differential growth of both the stomach and liver; (*b*) cavitation in the surrounding mesoderm.

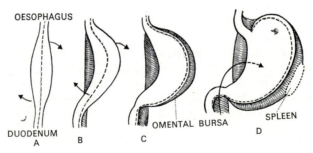

FIG. 9–6. Stages in the growth and differentiation of the stomach in ventral view, showing its rotation and consequent formation of the omental bursa. The broken line indicates approximately the stomach's mid-dorsal line (primary axis) along which the dorsal mesogastrium is attached between the stomach and the dorsal body (abdominal) wall. The arrow in D passes dorsal to the stomach into the omental bursa.

3. During these axial and rotational changes the stomach is carried further caudad.

The rotation of the stomach has two immediate consequences: first, the dorsal mesogastrium is pulled after the stomach and forms a pouch, the omental bursa (Fig. 11–8); second, the duodenum is carried to the right, fuses with the dorsal parietal peritoneum (thereby losing its mesentery) and becomes retroperitoneal.

It has been suggested that the first of the three changes listed above may be due to two factors; these are thought to be a change in position of the enlarging left umbilical vein and a fundamental symmetry determination originating during early development (neural stage).

> Pyloric stenosis is a common lesion in the infant, involving hypertrophy of the muscles (circular, longitudinal, or both) in the region of the pylorus. The pyloric lumen is narrowed down to the point of obstructing the food passage with the consequence that severe vomiting results.

DEVELOPMENT OF THE INTESTINE

Umbilical herniation

The primitive mid-gut is a straight tube with its mid-point communicating ventrally with the yolk sac. During the third to tenth weeks this primitive mid-gut loop elongates into the form of a hair-pin and enters the umbilical cord (containing the original extra-embryonic coelom) (Fig. 9–7). At the tip of this loop the original attachment with the yolk sac is present, demarcating the cranial limb which will form the entire jejunum and the first 18–20 feet of the ileum. The caudal limb will give rise to the terminal few feet of the ileum together with the ascending and transverse colon (approximately two-thirds). The duodenum and the prospective descending colon are not involved in the mid-gut herniation. Thus, the yolk sac marks an approximate point of transition between the future small and large intestines, which coincides with the ileocaecal valve. Much of the coiling of the small intestine occurs during the period of herniation. The large intestine acquires its characteristic diameter in the fifth month; prior to that, it actually is smaller than the small intestine.

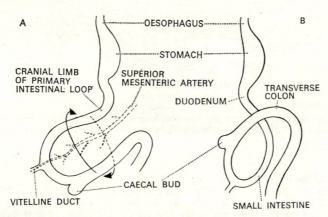

FIG. 9–7. Position of the primitive intestinal loop before (A), and after (B) rotation; lateral view from left side.
   A. This shows the superior mesenteric artery forming the axis of the intestinal loop; the arrow indicates the counterclockwise direction of rotation as seen from the ventral aspect.
   B. This represents the condition after the primitive intestinal loop has rotated through 180°; as a result of the rotation, the transverse colon passes in front of the duodenum.

The proximal limb of the mid-gut elongates greatly, coils and comes to occupy the right side of the umbilical sac. The distal limb of the loop occupies the left side of the sac and develops into the caecum with the appendix marking its apex.

Three factors account for the termination of the mid-gut herniation and return of the intestine back to the peritoneal cavity. They are (a) regression of the mesonephros; (b) regression of the fast-growing liver and (c) sufficient growth and expansion of the peritoneal cavity to accommodate the greatly lengthened intestine (especially the cephalic limb of the loop) by the end of the 10th week.

The final positions occupied by the small intestine and colon, relative to each other in the peritoneal cavity, are determined primarily by two factors. One is a twist in the U-shaped bend of the gut in the body-stalk (counter-clockwise when viewed from the ventral aspect). As a result, the proximal limb of the primary loop, which re-enters first, emerges below the transverse colon and passes to the right of the future descending colon and its mesentery. The other is that during retraction of the hernia, the coils of the small intestine tend to slip into the abdominal cavity ahead of the protruding part of the colon. This is also responsible for the establishment of the characteristic positions of the colon (Fig. 9–8). The descending colon (belonging to the hind-gut) is displaced to the left of the posterior abdominal wall, loses its mesentery and becomes retroperitoneal (p. 119). The caecum and appendix enter the peritoneal cavity last of all and, as they return, pass to the right upper quadrant below the liver, and carry the transverse colon across the abdomen ventral to the retroperitoneal duodenum.

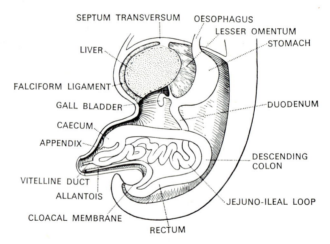

FIG. 9–8. Umbilical herniation of the intestinal loop in a 8-week embryo (this figure also shows the relationships of the growing liver and the septum transversum to developing mesenteries in this area).

Malformations of the intestinal tract

1. Remnants of the vitello-intestinal duct: Meckel's diverticulum. Normally, the vitello-intestinal duct disappears about the 6th week. Sometimes, however, a portion of it persists forming an outpocketing of the ileum known as the Meckel's diverticulum (Fig. 9–9A). If it is located 2–3 feet away from the ileocaecal valve, it is usually symptomless, but if it should contain heterotopic pancreatic tissue or gastric mucosa, it may ulcerate, bleed and even perforate. In more severe cases the entire duct remains patent, forming a communication between the umbilicus and the intestinal tract known as an umbilical or vitelline fistula (Fig. 9–9C). This has the severe consequence of faecal discharge occurring at the umbilicus. If both ends of the duct are transformed into fibrous cords, the middle portion then forms a large vitelline cyst (Fig. 9–9B). Possible intestinal strangulation may follow.

2. Omphalocoele (Fig. 9–9D). This is caused by failure of the intestinal loop to return to the abdominal cavity. The herniated loops are contained in a membranous sac formed by the amniotic membrane.

3. Abnormal rotation of the primary intestinal loop (90° instead of 270° counterclockwise).

4. Congenital hernia into the umbilical cord.

5. Duplication of the gastro-intestinal tract. This may be anywhere along the elementary canal but is most frequently located in the ileum. It is caused by the failure of localized vacuoles to fuse.

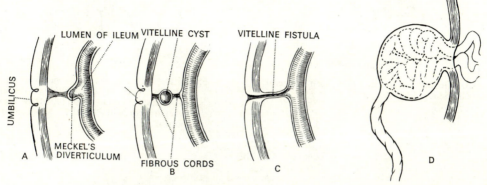

FIG. 9–9. Anomalies of the intestine.
A. Meckel's diverticulum combined with a fibrous cord (vitelline ligament).
B. Vitelline cyst attached to the umbilicus and the wall of ileum by a vitelline ligament.
C. Vitelline fistula connecting the lumen of the ileum with the umbilicus.
D. Umbilical hernia.

THE LIVER

The primordium of the liver is a ventral outgrowth from the cranial tip of the duodenum at an angle between the fore-gut and yolk sac (beginning of the fourth week; 17 somites). This diverticulum divides into two portions: a cranial bud, which gives rise to the hepatic parenchyma and bile ducts, and a caudal portion from which the gall bladder and cystic duct are derived; these are the endodermal components of the gland.

Relationship with the developing septum transversum

The hepatic diverticulum grows into the septum transversum (Fig. 9–10) at a time when the mesenchymal cells of the latter are engaged in vascularizing activity. This vascular mesenchyme is thus invaded by cords of endodermal hepatic cells with the result that the latter are intimately supplied with a system of blood vessels characteristic of the liver. These vessels comprise the hepatic artery, hepatic vein and portal vein, the latter two of which constitute a unique dual venous supply found in no other organ (Fig. 9–11). There is also a system of dilated capillaries (hepatic sinusoids) lined with reticulo-endothelial (Kupffer's) cells (Fig. 9–12). The hepatic cords (Fig. 9–12) are arranged in a spongework with the sinusoids closely applied to the individual hepatic cells. This makes possible a continuous flow of venous blood from the proximal portion of the portal system into the distal hepatic portion of the sinusoids, circulating around the hepatic parenchyma before the blood (loaded with food) enters the heart via the hepatic vein. (The lymphatics are also derived from the vascular mesenchyme of the septum transversum).

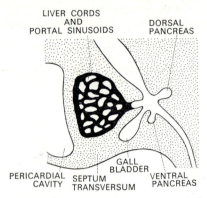

FIG. 9–10. The human liver at 5 mm., seen in lateral sectional view. (After Arey.)

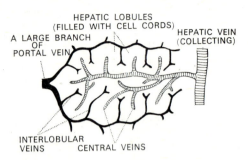

FIG. 9–11. Diagram to show the arrangement of the branches of the portal vein (black) and hepatic vein (blank) and how they encircle the hepatic cords in a lobule. (Modified from Bloom.)

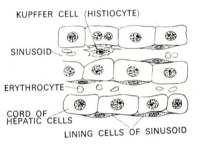

FIG. 9–12. Drawing of a section to show the arrangement of the hepatic cords and the sinusoids. The cells of these cords constitute the parenchyma of liver, which occupies the blank spaces between the incoming portal vein and outgoing hepatic vein in Fig. 9–11.

Growth of hepatic lobules

The liver is divided into structural units, the hepatic lobules. The lobules increase in number as a function of the sinusoids. When the hepatic cords elongate beyond the functional limit of the sinusoids between (supporting) the cords, the central vein divides and the resulting two branch sinusoids assume the place of a new central vein, supporting the two daughter hepatic lobules, and so on. The formation of four such lobules from one original lobule is illustrated in Fig. 9–13.

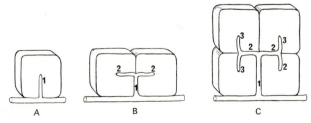

FIG. 9–13. Diagram illustrating the mechanism by which the number of hepatic lobules is increased.

Bile duct and canaliculi

The hepatic lobules are separated by portal canals each of which contains derivatives of the hepatic artery, portal vein and bile duct. The hepatic cells begin to secrete typical bile in the fifth month. The bile leaves the hepatic cells via a system of tiny channels or canaliculi, which permeate between the individual cells and reach the lumen of interlobular bile ducts (Fig. 9–14). The latter eventually empty into a bile duct from which the bile flows into the gall bladder where it is stored. Thus, the hepatic cells have an extensive exposure to both the hepatic sinusoids and the bile canaliculi (cf. Fig. 9–12 and Fig. 9–14).

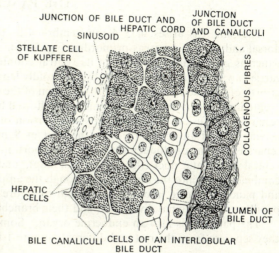

FIG. 9–14. Drawing of a section through the margin of a human liver, showing the juncture of a terminal bile duct with the hepatic cords (heavily granular cells) and direct connections at two places between the bile canaliculi and the lumen of the bile duct.

While these developments are taking place, the mesenchymal cells of the septum not involved in the vascularization process, give rise to a capsule and form a fibrous stroma. The connective tissue elements of the liver are, therefore, of splanchnopleuric mesodermal origin.

The liver is an haemopoietic organ for the foetal period (Fig. 14–2). Blood cells are actively differentiated between the hepatic cords and the sinusoidal lining. Later, some of the latter cells become transformed into the cells of Kupffer, which form a part of the reticulo-endothelial system and are noted for their phagocytotic properties.

Anomalies of gall bladder and bile duct: obliteration of the common bile duct (Fig. 9–15). This condition leads to distention of the gall bladder and hepatic ducts distal to the obliteration, and to atresia of gall bladder, all attributable to failure of the epitheloid cords to canalize. Increasingly severe jaundice will follow after birth.

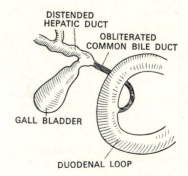

FIG. 9–15. Anomalies of the gall bladder and bile duct; obliteration of the common bile duct resulting in distention of the gall bladder and hepatic ducts distal to the obliteration.

The primary attachment of the liver to the septum transversum causes it to descend with the latter and finally it bulges caudad into the abdominal cavity. At the same time the gut is also drawing away from the septum. The consequence of the close association of the liver with the septum on the one hand, and with the ventral mesenteries of the stomach on the other, are related in Chapter 11.

THE PANCREAS

The pancreas arises in 3–4 mm. embryos as two outpocketings from the duodenum, the dorsal and ventral pancreas primordia (Fig. 9–16). During the fifth to seventh weeks the dorsal pancreas grows much faster than its ventral counterpart whilst the latter, being the smaller, is carried away from the duodenum by the rapidly lengthening common bile duct. Due to unequal growth of the duodenal wall, and the rotation of the stomach and duodenum, the ventral pancreas eventually unites with the dorsal pancreas followed by anastomoses of their respective ducts. The result of this fusion is that the proximal portion of the dorsal pancreatic duct mostly vanishes, leaving behind an accessory duct (the duct of Santorini), as a functional tributary. It has its separate opening on duodenum. The distal portion of the dorsal pancreatic duct is joined by the ventral pancreatic duct (the duct of Wirsung), and meets the common bile duct; the two thus combined open into the duodenum through the ampulla of Vater. The discharge of both the bile and pancreatic juice into the duodenum therefore takes place through the common duodenal papillae. The original diverticula and their branches form the duct system within the pancreas.

The pancreas is also an endocrine organ. Some of its parenchymatous cords remain solid; they separate from the rest and differentiate into Islets of Langerhans which secrete insulin.

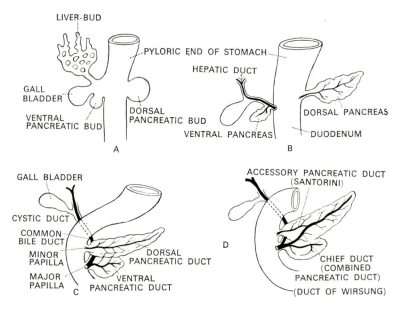

FIG. 9–16. Four stages in the development of the human pancreas and its ducts; lateral view from the left side. A. at 6 mm.; B. at 8 mm.; C. at 12 mm.; D. at 16 mm.

Anomalies of the Pancreas

1. Annular pancrease. Part of the ventral pancreas, instead of shifting dorsally, migrates along the normal path whilst the remainder moves in an opposite direction. The result is that the duodenum becomes surrounded by pancreatic tissue; in severe cases, this may form a duodenal stenosis.
2. Heterotopic pancreatic tissue. This may be found anywhere from the end of oesophagus to Meckel's diverticulum, but most frequently it occurs in the mucosa of the stomach and in Meckel's diverticulum.

Such heterotopic pancreatic tissue usually shows pathological characteristics.

THE HIND-GUT

The hind-gut begins with the last one-third of the transverse colon and terminates with the cloaca. The division of the latter into the anorectal canal and urogenital sinus will be described in Chapter 13.

Before the rupture of the cloacal membrane, the cloaca is surrounded by mesenchyme derived from the caudal end of the primitive streak. The manner in which this source of mesoderm contributes to certain parts of the external genitalia will be described in connection with the genital system (Chapter 13). In the ninth week an ectodermal depression, the proctodaeum (p. 39), deepens and becomes the prospective anal canal and provides the latter with anal folds originating as mesenchymal swellings. Upon rupture of the anal membrane a connection between the rectum and the outside is finally established. The upper third of this canal is endodermal, hence supplied by the inferior mesenteric artery; the lower end, being ectodermal in origin, is supplied by the internal iliac artery.

Malformations of the hind-gut

1. Imperforate anus (Fig. 9–17A). The anal membrane persists as a diaphragm between the upper and lower portions of the anal canal.
2. Rectovaginal fistula combined with rectal atresia. The condition is caused by a defect of the urorectal septum (Fig. 9–17B).

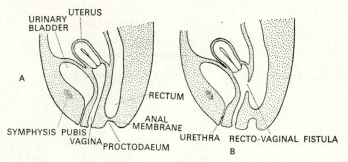

FIG. 9–17. Two anomalies of the hindgut; A. Imperforate anus; B. Rectovaginal fistula.

CHAPTER 10

THE RESPIRATORY SYSTEM

The earliest rudiment of the respiratory organs appears in 2·5 to 3·0 mm. (4 week) embryos as a thickening, the laryngo-tracheal ridge, which bulges ventrally from the cranial end of the prospective oesophagus (Fig. 10–1). The lower part of the ridge soon expands into a bi-lobed primordium of the primary bronchi or lung bud. At that time two longitudinal grooves form in the side walls of the oesophageal part and gradually deepen until they meet, thereby dividing the region into a dorsal digestive tract and a ventral respiratory tract. This process of splitting-off starts at the level of the lung bud and spreads cranially to the future tracheal portion. After separation the proximal portion of the laryngo-tracheal ridge proceeds to differentiate into the larynx, while its distal end forms the trachea and lungs. A primitive glottis communicates with the posterior end of the pharynx.

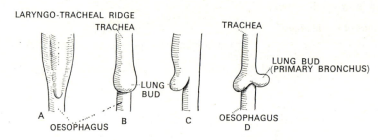

FIG. 10–1. Stages in the development of the human respiratory primordium.
A. at 2·5 mm., ventral view; B. at 3·0 mm., ventral view;
C. at 3·0 mm., lateral view; D. at 4·0 mm., ventral view.

The larynx (Fig. 10–2)

This is a cartilaginous " box " housing the vocal cords and also sustaining the epiglottis as a cover for the primitive glottis. The lower portion of the larynx is organized around the cranial end of the trachea, whilst its upper portion (above the level of the vocal cords) develops from the pharyngeal floor. While the epiglottis is contributed from the ventral portion of branchial (pharyngeal) arches 3 and 4, the larynx as a whole is derived from the mesenchymal cores of branchial arches 4 and 5. Mesenchyme from this source first forms pronounced swellings surrounding the glottis. By the end of the seventh week, these swellings have given rise to primordia of the thyroid, arytenoid and cricoid cartilages. The origin of the latter two cartilages is open to question. One view is that they are derived from arch 5 whilst others maintain that they may not be of branchial origin at all. Both the vocal cords (elastic tissue) and the laryngeal muscles originate from these same branchial arches. The larynx is innervated by the vagus nerve X. Dense mesenchyme from branchial arches 4 and 5 also provides the epithelial lining of the larynx.

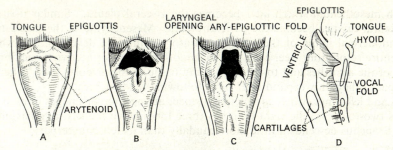

FIG. 10–2. Stages in the development of the human larynx.
A. at 30 mm.; B. at 55 mm.; C. at 30 mm.; D. sagittal hemisection, at birth

The trachea and lungs (Fig. 10–3)

The lung bud undergoes a period of repeated branching. The bronchi and bronchioles are established from the fifth week to the fourth month; the respiratory bronchioles are laid down between the fourth and sixth month. The extension from the smallest bronchioles into a system of alveolar ducts and the differentiation of early alveoli and their vascularization is accomplished in many generations of pulmonary branching (18 generations are completed by the end of sixth month; 24 generations by mid-childhood) (Fig. 10–3E).

The greater part of the unpaired portion of the respiratory rudiment gives rise to the epithelium of the trachea. The surrounding mesenchyme (originally ventral mesentery of the oesophagus, later incorporated into the mediastinum) (p. 114) develops into the supporting (cartilaginous) and muscular parts of the trachea.

The right and left bronchial buds grow laterally out into their respective pleural cavities (Fig. 10–4), carrying before them dome-shaped investments of mesenchyme of the mediastinum,

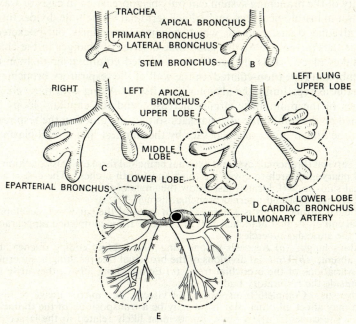

FIG. 10–3. Stages in the development of the human bronchi (A to D) and lung (E), seen from the ventral aspect. (After Arey).
A. at 5 mm.; B, at 7 mm.; C. at 8·5 mm.; D, at 10 mm.; E, at birth.

surfaced with mesothelium which later becomes the visceral pleura. Similar tissues lining the completed pleural cavities become the parietal pleura. Mesenchyme of the mediastinum within which the endodermal lining of the whole respiratory primordia develops, and which actually encases the entire respiratory tree, gives rise to smooth muscle, connective tissue fibres, cartilage plates, walls of the air tubes and to the supporting tissue of the alveolar sacs. The air sacs are, at first, compact; they only expand after birth following the first breath.

The right and left lungs, when completely formed, are not mirror images of each other. The asymmetry is two-fold: (a) the right lung has three lobes while the left lung has only two, and (b) the right bronchus descends a little more caudally than its left counterpart.

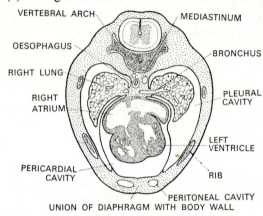

FIG. 10–4. Transverse section showing growth of the human lungs and pleural cavities, with consequent extension of the pericardium at 7 weeks.

Finer structural changes

Each respiratory bronchiole develops a series of sacculations extending out in all directions. The full complexity of the branching system can only be appreciated in casts or wax-plate demonstration models (not in histological sections). Each terminal bronchiole divides into 3–6 irregular passages, called alveolar ducts, each of which becomes irregularly out-pocketed to form the numerous alveolar sacs (alveoli). At the same time a series of changes in the character of their epithelial lining takes place. This changes from a ciliated columnar epithelium (in the wall of bronchioli) to a cuboidal type (non-ciliated) in the wall of the respiratory bronchioles, and finally to the simple squamous type lining the alveolar duct itself. Along with these changes the meshwork of capillaries of the pulmonary circuit increases, and the capillary loops begin to bulge through the thinned epithelium of the alveolar sacs so that the blood in the respiratory capillaries is separated from the lumen of the alveolar sacs by the thinnest film of cytoplasm possible.

Anomalies

1. Lateral cervical (branchial) cyst and external branchial fistula. This condition is due to failure of the second pharyngeal arch to cover the third and fourth arches. The cyst is a remnant of the normal cervical sinus (p. 97), located just below the angle of the jaw.

2. Lateral cervical cyst and internal branchial fistula.

3. Pre-auricular fistula. This is a narrow pit in front of the ear which develops possibly either from the dorsal end of the first branchial cleft or is due to the incomplete disappearance of one of the sulci between the auricular tubercles.

4. Anomalous lungs: (a) Agenesis of one lung with a blind ending trachea; both lungs may sometimes be absent. (b) Unusual divisions of the bronchial tree resulting in supernumerary lobules (rare); other variations of the bronchial tree. (c) Ectopic lung lobes; they arise from trachea or oesophagus outside the respiratory bud.

5. Situs inversus. Complete transposition of viscera, i.e., mirror image of normal condition. The condition may affect all other organs, or may be a transposition of the thoracic or abdominal viscera alone. The cause is little known, but is most likely related to the larger problem of how bilateral symmetry and asymmetry are established (see Chapter 8).

6. Congenital cysts of lung (" honeycomb "). The defect causes poor drainage and may possibly lead to chronic infection. Some measure of correction may be achieved by surgery.

CHAPTER 11

BODY CAVITIES AND MESENTERIES

The systems discussed so far have been derived from the endoderm, but the majority of the organ systems are of mesodermal origin. Table 11–1 presents in summarized form the mesodermal components and their respective derivatives. It may be helpful at this time to review Fig. 5–2 preparatory to a more systematic study of the developmental processes involved in the organ systems derived from mesoderm.

Differentiation of a somite (see Fig. 5–2)

A succession of transverse splits cuts the paraxial mesoderm into segmentally arranged somites. The first occipital and the last few coccygeal pairs of somites are evanescent, after being transient for some time.

TABLE 11–1. COMPONENTS OF MESODERMAL ORIGIN AND THEIR DERIVATIVES

A. HEAD MESODERM ——————→ Extrinsic muscles of eyeball; ciliary muscles; tunics of eyeball including ciliary
   (mesenchymal)   body and iris; possibly participating in forming the meningeal coverings of brain;
                          membrane bones of skull (cranium and jaws).

B. MESODERM (mesenchymal)→ Cartilages, bones (cartilage bones), and certain muscles of the neck, face and head.
   of BRANCHIAL ARCHES   (Some of these structures can possibly be contributed by endodermal epithelium of
                          the branchial pouches)

C. MESODERM PROPER

Paraxial:
   Epimere (somite)
   - Dermatomes→Dermis and hypodermis of skin; Contributions to skeletal muscles of limbs;
   - Myotomes →bulk of skeletal muscles;
   - Sclerotomes →Vertebrae (axial skeleton of vertebral column).

Intermediate mesoderm:
   Mesomere
   - Nephrotomes→Secretory tubules and collecting duct system of kidneys
   - Gonads and their ducts←——————— The entire urogenital system

Lateral mesoderm:
   Hypomere

   Somatic mesoderm (parietal)
   - Portion of hypodermis: subcutaneous tissues and derivatives;
   - Limb muscles;
   - Limb skeleton;

   Splanchnic mesoderm (visceral)
   - Mesenteries;
   - Entire cardio-vascular system, lymphatic system and vessels;
   - Mesothelia, lining all body cavities; serosa, covering all viscera;
   - All connective tissues, cells and fibres;
   - All smooth (involuntary) muscles of viscera and intestinal tract;
   - Stroma of all viscera;
   - Germinal epithelium of gonads

The epithelial cells of the somite are initially radially oriented around a central cavity which is subsequently reduced to a thin vertical split, separating outer and inner walls, corresponding to the parietal and visceral layers of the lateral plate mesoderm. The ventral part of the inner wall breaks up into a mass of mesenchymal cells, the sclerotomes, which besides forming the vertebrae, also contribute to the axial skeleton and the meninges. Cells proliferating from the dorsal part of the inner wall of the somite form the myotomes from which most striated (skeletal) muscles are derived. A segmental nerve grows out from the neural tube to each myotome. The remaining outer wall of the somite becomes dermatomes (see Chapter 18 and Table 11–1).

Introduction to coelom and mesenteries

The earliest body cavity (primitive coelom) results from a splitting of the lateral mesoderm extending no further cephalically than the level of the pharynx; the paired cavity thus formed is bounded medially by the splanchnic mesoderm and laterally by the somatic mesoderm (Fig. 11–1A). In the Amniotes with highly developed extra-embryonic membranes this coelom extends beyond the confines of the developing embryo. The extra-embryonic coelom thus comes into existence earlier than the intra-embryonic coelom.

The early embryo, in an attempt as if to free itself from attachment, tends to arch itself upward from the underlying yolk sac. It is assisted in this process by a constriction at the region

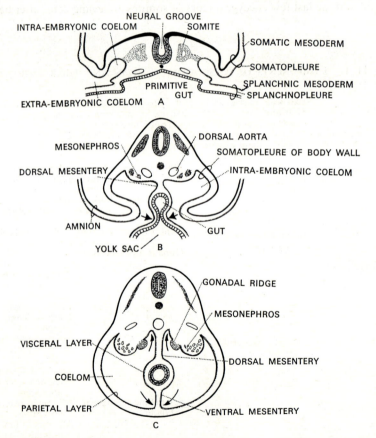

Fig. 11–1. A diagrammatic transverse section to show the closing-off of the embryonic gut from the primitive gut, separation of intra-embryonic from extra-embryonic coelom, and the development of the primary mesenteries by means of the closing-in of the body folds: A. at 2·0 mm.; B. at 4·0 mm.; C. at 8·0 mm.

of the lateral body folds (Fig. 11–1B), which involves both the body wall and the primary gut. When complete, the process will have established three structures simultaneously (Fig. 11–1C):

(a) The intra-embryonic coelom, now completely separated from the extra-embryonic coelom, becomes the definitive coelom of the embryo.

(b) The gut, by acquiring a floor in this process, is completely closed off.

(c) The primary mesenteries are established. These consist of the dorsal mesentery above, and the ventral mesentery below the closed gut. Each of them represents the splanchnic mesoderm of the two sides, which having swung medially, meets and fuses with the other along the mid-line.

The trunk

In this process of under-cutting and under-folding, the combined somatopleures form the sides and ventral surface of the cylindrical trunk. In the young embryos this trunk is flattened somewhat by the compression of the lateral body folds (resulting in a rather irregular contour caused by the fast-growing liver and heart) but when muscles and skeleton of the trunk appear, this visceral-organ dominance soon loses importance. The trunk then acquires a somewhat ovoid form in the foetal period, which more or less persists until in the middle foetal period the abdominal region between the pubis and the umbilicus acquires its characteristic expanse. Upon assuming the erect posture, the lumbar region gains dominance and relative length at the expense of the thorax-abdomen dominance.

Malformations of the trunk (Fig. 11–2)

A. Gastroschisis, with protrusion of the abdominal viscera, resulting from faulty closure of the body wall along its midventral line.

B. Retention of tail in an infant. This may be up to 3 inches long in a new born baby (in one case, it reached 9 inches in a 12-year child).

C. Rachischisis (cleft spine), with gaping skin and exposed spinal cord, due to failure of the vertebral column to close properly.

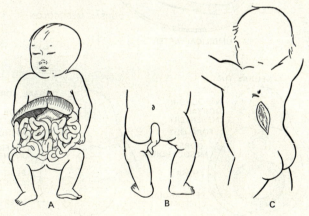

Fig. 11–2. Malformations of the human trunk. (After Arey.)
A. Gastroschisis with protrusion of abdominal viscera;
B. Persisting embryonic tail (shown in the contracted state);
C. Rachischisis (cleft spine) exposing a flat spinal cord with an adventitious tuft of hair and a separate opening.

The coelom, when first formed, is divided into left and right halves (Fig. 11–1C) by the mesenteries, but soon the ventral mesenteries, posterior to the liver, break through and disappear, thereby establishing the single confluent coelomic cavity characteristic of the body cavity of the adult. The dorsal mesenteries, on the other hand, persist to support the gut and serve as a pathway for blood vessels and nerves to the viscera (Fig. 11–3B, C).

THE COELOMIC CAVITIES

Partitioning of the coelom

Three definitive cavities result from changes in the early embryonic coelom. They are (1) the pericardial cavity (2) the pleural cavity and (3) the peritoneal or abdominal cavity (Fig. 11–3A). The formation of these three cavities involves three partitioning membranes or folds as follows:

(a) the single septum transversum (Fig. 11–3A)

(b) a pair of pleuro-pericardial membranes ⎫

(c) a pair of pleuro-peritoneal membranes ⎭ (Figs. 11–3A and 11–4)

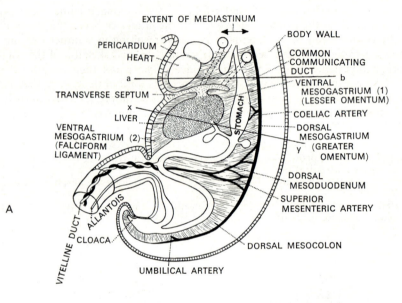

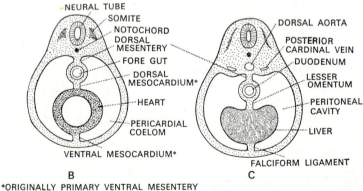

Fig. 11–3. A. Scheme to show the primitive dorsal and ventral mesenteries, lateral view of left side.
The dotted outlines in this diagram indicate future positions of pleuro-pericardial and pleuro-peritoneal membranes;

     B. Relations of the human mesenteries showing in diagrammatic transverse section through the level a and b indicated in Fig. 11–3A;

     C. Relations of the human mesenteries, through the level x and y indicated in Fig. 11–3A.

The septum transversum

This arises very early in embryos of 9 to 12 mm., and extends from the ventral body wall dorsally, forming a semi-circular shelf with the growing liver below it and the developing heart above it. It is considered the forerunner of the diaphragm, although it forms only one of its definitive components. As the septum does not grow all the way to the dorsal body wall, the region occupied by the heart and the lungs is, at first, confluent with the space occupied by the more caudally developing gastrointestinal tract and the liver. The two regions communicate with each other via a duct, the pericardio-peritoneal canal, or common communicating duct (Fig. 11–3A).

The pleuro-peritoneal membranes (Fig. 11–4A)

These arise as folds from the dorso-lateral body wall, and rapidly acquire a triangular shape with their apices extending toward the septum transversum; eventually they meet and fuse with the latter, remaining separated from it only by the mediastinum at the centre. (In a sense, therefore, the mediastinum participates in the formation of the definitive diaphragm, although it is not generally regarded as one of its components). The pleuro-peritoneal membranes serve as partitioning wall to separate the confluent anterior and posterior portions of the coelom into the pleural cavities in front and the peritoneal cavity behind.

The pleuro-pericardial membranes (Fig. 11–4A)

In similar manner the separation of the pericardial cavity from the pleural cavities is completed by the growth of a partition formed by the pleuro-pericardial membranes across the cephalic end of each of the communicating ducts. Unlike the pleuro-peritoneal membranes, which grow toward the septum transversum, these membranes grow out from the latter and unite with the dorso-lateral body walls during the 6th week (11 mm.). After that, the ducts form two blind extensions (pleural recesses) into which the developing lungs push and fill.

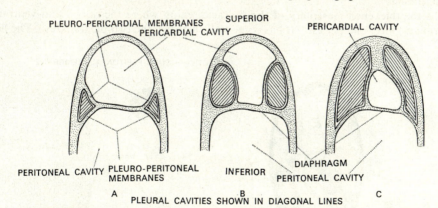

FIG. 11–4. Diagrams to show the result of formation of the pleuro-peritoneal membranes (A) and how differential growth of the parts concerned brings about the adult relations of the definitive pleural, pericardial and peritoneal cavities (B and C). (After Dodds.)

The definitive diaphragm

The last component added to the diaphragm is the paired narrow secondary ingrowth from the dorso-lateral body wall. To summarize, the definitive diaphragm consists of the following parts (Fig. 11–5):

1. The Septum transversum, ventrally, making up its greater part.
2. The two pleuro-peritoneal membranes, each somewhat triangular in shape.
3. The narrow lateral areas which originate from ingrowths of the dorsal body wall.

The musculature of the diaphragm is contributed by two pre-muscle masses probably arising from the fourth cervical myotomes. This is suggested by the fact that the phrenic nerves have their origin from the third and fourth cervical nerves. The diaphragm undergoes extensive migration caudally along with other organs, particularly the heart and its pericardium. The migration covers a distance from the third cervical to the twelfth thoracic segments during a period in which the embryo increases in length from 2 to 24 mm.

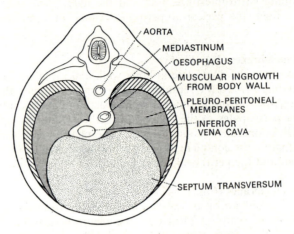

Fig. 11–5. Schematic transverse section to show the definitive diaphragm, with the origin of its various components.

The mediastinum

This is the thickened mesentery of the thoracic region where the dorsal and ventral mesenteries (primary) meet and persist. It has come to lie between the two pleural sacs. The heart and

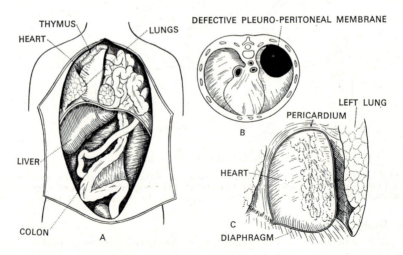

Fig.–6. Anomalies of the human coelom. (After Arey.)
   A. Herniation of the intestine into the left pleural cavity;
   B. Cranial surface of the diaphragm showing a defect in the pleuro-peritoneal membrane, which could lead to a hernia as in Fig. 11–6A;
   C. Incomplete pericardium showing the heart and left lung occupying a common cavity (possibly the result of a defective pleuro-pericardial membrane).

pericardium with the bases of the large blood vessels, the trachea, oesophagus, lymphatics and nerves all lie in it, embedded in a piece of massive mesenchyme of splanchnic mesoderm origin.

Anomalies of the coelom

1. Diaphragmatic hernia (Fig. 11–6A).
2. Defective pleuroperitoneal membrane (Fig. 11–6B).
3. Incomplete pericardium (Fig. 11–6C). This condition possibly results from a lack of complete separation between the pleural and pericardial cavities due to defective pleuro-pericardial membranes.

THE VENTRAL MESENTERIES

The urinary bladder is suspended by a short ventral mesentery. Another organ that retains a ventral mesentery is the liver. Before completion of the diaphragm, the liver bud grows into, and greatly thickens, the septum transversum. Whilst the proximal (dorsal) part of the septum becomes a portion of the diaphragm, its distal (ventral) margin containing the liver becomes greatly reduced and some of its remnants, besides forming the peritoneal covering or capsule of the liver, participate in the formation of some of the hepatic mesenteries, as summarized below (see Fig. 11–7):

1. Falciform ligament. This is the original mesentery between the liver and the ventral body wall. (But later, as the liver turns upward above the stomach, the ligament takes up a dorsal position secondarily).
2. Ligamentum teres. The caudal margin of the falciform ligament contains the umbilical vein, which after birth, degenerates into a solid fibrous cord known as ligamentum teres, or the round ligament of the liver.
3. Coronary and triangular ligaments. These are derived from a segment of the ventral mesentery between the liver and the septum transversum, which later becomes the central tendon of the diaphragm.
4. Gastro hepatic or lesser omentum. This is the mesentery between the liver and stomach. Due to the rotation of the stomach and consequent shift in position of the liver, it takes up a final dorsal position. This mesentery is also known as the ventral mesogastrium or the hepato-gastric ligament. Because of its involvement with the duodenum, the mesentery may also be considered as having two components; hepatogastric and hepatoduodenal.

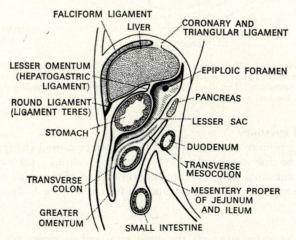

FIG. 11–7. Sagittal section through an adult to show especially the mesenteries of the liver, the greater omentum and associated structures.

THE DORSAL MESENTERIES

Mesenteries of the stomach (Figs. 11–7 and 9)

The stomach has both dorsal and ventral mesenteries. The dorsal mesogastrium is greatly complicated by the formation of the greater omentum, and the fact that it also has two other minor components. They are the gastrosplenic (gastrolienal) ligament and the lienorenal ligament (between the spleen and kidney) (Fig. 11–8). The spleen, which develops as a circumscribed thickening of the dorsal mesogastrium, is involved in the complex of the dorsal mesentery of the stomach. The important causal factor in the formation of the greater omentum is the rotation of the stomach. The greater omentum descends from the caudal portion of the greater curvature of the stomach, and due to its rapid growth, doubles back upon itself and attaches to the dorsal mid-line of the body wall like an apron (or the hood of an academic gown!). For this reason it is sometimes called the omental apron (Fig. 11–7). The cavity within it is the lesser sac, or omental bursa, which communicates with the peritoneal cavity through a narrow passage, the epiploic foramen. The ventral mesogastrium or lesser omentum has been described above in connection with the liver. As the greater omentum drops and hangs over the small intestine and colon, it fuses with the mesentery of the transverse colon (Fig. 11–10B); the extended mesentery, so formed, is known as the gastro-colic ligament (Fig. 11–10B).

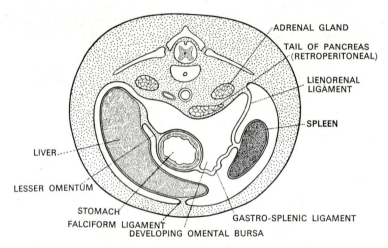

FIG. 11–8. Transverse section through the rotating stomach, liver, pancreas and spleen and their associated mesenteries at a time when the pancreas has already been fixed in its definitive retroperitoneal position. This diagram also shows the formation of the lesser peritoneal sac resulting from the rotation of the stomach.

Mesenteries of the small intestine

The mesentery of the primitive intestinal loop undergoes profound changes from its original disposition. This may be due to several reasons, among which are: (*a*) a rotation during the return of the herniated intestinal loop, (*b*) concomitant coiling of the small intestine, (*c*) surface apposition between two adjoined membranes, and (*d*) fusion with the body wall.

The mesoduodenum

As a result of rotation of the stomach, the duodenum and its mesentery come to lie closely applied to the dorsal body wall. In this position, and with increasing pressure against the latter

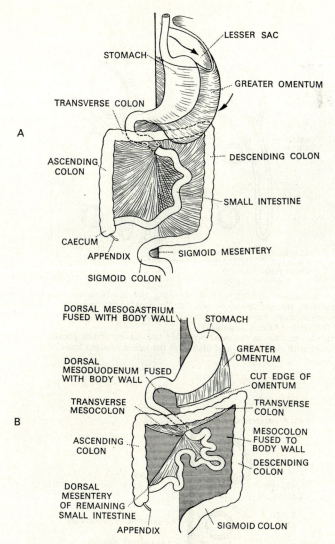

FIG. 11–9. A. Schematic representation of the embryonic alimentary canal (at about end of third month) as seen from the ventral aspect, following the descent of the caecum to its adult position. The upper arrow points into the omental bursa; the lower arrow indicates the direction of rotation of the stomach. (Modified from Harrison.)
B. Condition in the newborn (or adult) with the greater omentum cut away (crosshatched areas denote parts of the primitive dorsal mesentery which have fused with the abdominal wall).

encountered after the return of the herniated gut, the mesoduodenum becomes finally fused with the body wall (Figs. 11–9B and 11–10), thereby making the duodenum retroperitoneal.

Mesentery of jejunum and ileum

The mesentery of the remainder of the small intestine, however, does not become fused to the posterior body wall, but acquires a new line of attachment after the ascending colon becomes retroperitoneal (see below). This line extends from the area of the retroperitoneal duodenum to the iliocaecal junction. The mesentery so formed assumes the shape of a broad fan (Fig. 11–9B).

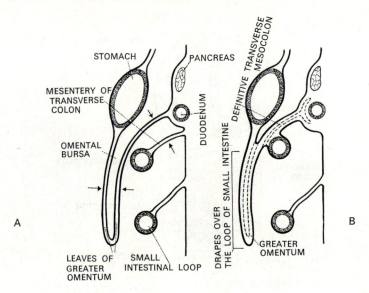

FIG. 11–10. A. A schematic representation showing the relationship between the greater omentum, stomach, transverse colon, and the loop of small intestine at 4-months; the pancreas and duodenum have already become retroperitoneal (the arrows indicate the directions of fusion).   (After Langman.)
B. Similar section in the newborn after the leaves of the greater omentum have fused with each other and also with the colon (dotted lines).

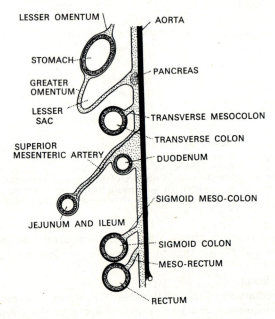

FIG. 11–11. Sagittal section of the embryonic alimentary canal at about end of third month. (After Harrison.)

Mesenteries of the large intestine

1. Mesocolon of caecum and ascending colon. These become apposed and then they fuse to the dorsal body wall on the right side so becoming obliterated (Fig. 11–9B).

2. Mesocolon of the descending colon. This, likewise, becomes obliterated by being apposed to and fused with the dorsal body wall (Fig. 11–9B). In both these cases the colon is permanently fixed in a retroperitoneal position after the fusion.

3. The appendix and lower end of the caecum retain their mesentery intact (Fig. 11–9B).

4. Transverse mesocolon. As the greater omentum pouches downward and forwards over the transverse colon and its mesentery (Fig. 11–10A), the apposed surfaces of the two mesenteries meet and fuse (Fig. 11–10B). This fusion actually is a contributing factor to both the fusion of the duodenum with the dorsal body wall described above, and the fusion of the leaves of the greater omentum (dotted line, Fig. 11–10B). Only the cut edge of the latter mesentery (omental apron) is shown in Fig. 11–10B.

5. Sigmoid mesocolon. This is a small mesentery passing from the dorsal body wall of the lower abdominal and pelvic cavities to the sigmoid (terminal) colon (Figs. 11–9B; 11–11).

6. Meso-rectum. This is transitory (Fig. 11–11).

Anomalies

Mobile caecum and colon. This defect is caused by persistence of a portion of the mesocolon of the descending colon; in extreme cases, there is failure of the mesentery of the ascending colon to fuse with the posterior body wall. The situation permits movements of the gut, and even volvulus of the caecum and colon.

CHAPTER 12

THE URINARY SYSTEM

Introduction

The urinary and reproductive (urinogenital) systems develop from the mesomeres or intermediate mesoderm, with the exception of some caudal portions which are endodermal. In the
vertebrates three distinct and progressively more elaborate renal systems are found, which are of
considerable evolutionary significance; the pronephros, which is the most primitive, is the functional kidney in the cyclostomes and Dipnoi, whilst the mesonephros is functional in fish and
amphibians. The metanephros is characteristic of only the reptiles, birds and mammals. It is
preceded in development by both the pro- and mesonephros. In man the pronephros is never
functional, and the definitive kidney (a metanephros) replaces the functional mesonephros by
the end of the third month of gestation. The relative position of these three kidneys is shown in
Fig. 12–1. A common excretory duct has a continuous course throughout the entire nephric
system in the early embryo, but the definitive ureter consists of only the very terminal portion of
the common duct.

The intermediate mesoderm, from which all kidney tissue is derived, is that portion of the
mesoderm located between the somites and the lateral plate (Fig. 12–2A). This segmented
retroperitoneal mesoderm lies in the dorso-lateral body wall and in the cervical and upper
thoracic regions it gives rise to the pronephros. More caudally, it continues as a pair of unsegmented longitudinal bands, the nephrogenic cords, which contribute to the formation of both the
mesonephros and metanephros. The intermediate mesoderm develops into excretory tubules, and
a duct system of collecting tubules. These two distinct sets of structures may be likened,

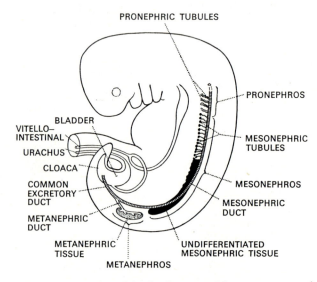

FIG. 12–1. A schematic representation of the development of the pro-, meso-, and meta-nephros
and their ducts at about the 5 mm. stage.

in the Pronephros, to the bristles (which represent the tubules) joining the handle of a toothbrush (which represents the duct). The succession of the pro-, meso-, and metanephros is characterized by a progressive shift caudad, as well as an increase in the number and complexity of the secretory elements involved. The most important features of their development are summarized in Table 12–1.

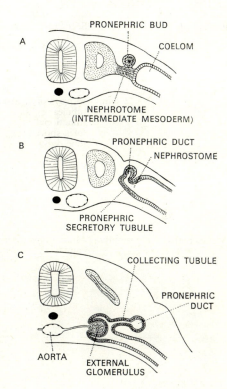

FIG. 12–2. Semi-diagrammatic representation of the stages in the development of a functional pronephric tubule in a lower vertebrate.

The pronephros

Seven segmentally-arranged pairs of pronephric tubules (Fig. 12–1) develop in the region of the neck and thorax. The pronephric tubules initiate the formation of the pronephric duct, which develops by caudal growth of the distal portion of each tubule (Fig. 12–2B), and continues to grow caudally between the ectoderm and nephrogenic tissue. The pronephric duct extends as far as the cloaca with which it communicates. The pronephric kidney is characterized by secretory tubules which open into the coelomic cavity at one end and join the pronephric duct at the other. This coelomic opening constitutes a nephrostome, and is often provided with cilia (Figs. 12–2B; 12–13A). Adjacent to, but entirely separate from each tubule, a branch of the aorta gives rise to an external glomerulus which protrudes into the coelom. The pronephros appears around the third week, and by the fifth week it has completely degenerated with the exception of its duct, which persists to become the mesonephric duct.

The mesonephros

The mesonephric tubules, each longer and more tortuous than a pronephric tubule, develop from the nephrogenic cord of the entire thorax together with the first three lumbar segments; the tubules total 83 pairs by the end of the 7th week (Figs. 12–3B; 12–4). The primordia of mesonephric tubules are situated close to the mesonephric duct (the former pronephric duct) and extend laterally to establish connections with it. The proximal portion of each tubule grows

TABLE 12–1. DEVELOPMENTAL FEATURES OF THE KIDNEYS

Kidney type	Appearance	Position and fate	Segmentation	Morphology		
				Duct	Tubules and fate	Characteristics
Pronephros	3–4½ weeks; 1·7–4·3 mm.	Segments 7–14 (vestigial)	Tubules paired and segmentally arranged	Pronephric duct (retained)	None functional; degenerate completely	1. External glomerulus 2. Tubules open to coelom and possess a nephrostome
Mesonephros	3½–7½ weeks; 2·5–21 mm.	Segments 10–26 83 pairs of tubules (functional for a short time only)	Not segmentally arranged	Mesonephric duct	$\frac{5}{6}$ cranial tubules lost by 2nd week; remnants become ligament of gonad. Remaining $\frac{1}{6}$ gives rise to new tubules by 10th week which later connect to male genital ducts	1. Internal glomerulus 2. No nephrostomes 3. Urogenital ridge subdivides into genital and nephric ridges 4. Separate primordia give rise to the secretory tubules and collecting duct
Metanephros	1–5 months	Much more caudal	All traces of metamerism lost	Completely new duct system	New secretory tubules from metanephrogenic mass; each with Bowman's capsule and joining an arched collecting tubule	1. Two separate primordia involved 2. Ureteric bud gives rise to entire collecting duct system 3. Metanephrogenic mass gives rise to: nephrons, stroma, and kidney capsule

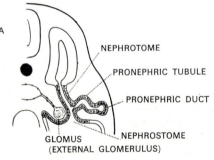

A

NEPHROTOME

PRONEPHRIC TUBULE

PRONEPHRIC DUCT

NEPHROSTOME

GLOMUS (EXTERNAL GLOMERULUS)

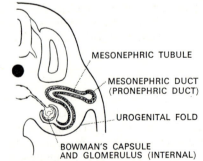

B

MESONEPHRIC TUBULE

MESONEPHRIC DUCT (PRONEPHRIC DUCT)

UROGENITAL FOLD

BOWMAN'S CAPSULE AND GLOMERULUS (INTERNAL)

FIG. 12–3. A. Schematic drawing of functional pronephric tubule
B. Semi-diagrammatic drawing of a transverse section of a 5 mm. human embryo to show the form and relation of a mesonephric tubule.

extensively, ultimately differentiating into a double-walled cup-shaped Bowman's capsule (Fig. 12–4). The latter receives a tuft of arterial capillaries (branches of the renal artery), thereby forming a glomerulus (internal type). The Bowman's capsule and its associated glomerulus together constitute a mesonephric renal corpuscle, which functions as a filtering plant for the first step in the removal of nitrogenous wastes from the blood.

The mesonephric kidney develops in a urogenital ridge which protrudes into the coelom. Shortly after the mesonephros is established the ridge subdivides into a lateral mesonephric ridge and a medial genital ridge. By this time degeneration has begun in the cranial portion of the mesonephros; this progresses caudally, and by the end of the second month, about five-sixth's of the tubules have already degenerated and serve as the suspensory ligaments of the gonad. The remaining sixth of the tubules undergo budding and continuous splitting. Some of the resulting tubules become incorporated as part of the genital duct system in the male (Fig. 13–18; Table 13–1).

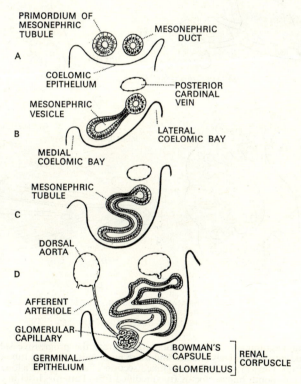

FIG. 12–4. Semi-diagrammatic representation of stages in the differentiation of a human mesonephric tubule.

The metanephros

The metanephros (Figs. 12–5; 12–6), the definitive kidney, originates from two primordia (a) the secretory primordium, which arises from the most caudal portion of the nephrogenic cord (known as the metanephrogenic mass) (b) the collecting system, which arises as an outgrowth (the ureteric bud) from the basal part of the mesonephric duct. The ureteric bud makes its appearance at four weeks as an evagination of the lower mesonephric duct just proximal to the point where the latter enters the cloaca. Due primarily to growth of the ureteric bud, the primordia of the bud and metanephrogenic mass meet at a level slightly higher than the site of their origin. The stalk of the bud forms the future ureter, whilst its distal end is distended to become the primitive renal pelvis.

Derivatives of the ureteric bud

The renal tubules of the collecting system are formed as a result of continuous branching of the renal pelvis. The major subdivisions of this branching are as follows: pelvis; calyces; papillary ducts; straight collecting tubules; arched collecting tubules. By the end of the fifth month, a total of 12 generations of such branching are completed, the first three of which are indicated in Fig. 12–5A, B, C. The distal convoluted tubule of each excretory unit or nephron is precisely united with one arched collecting tubule (Fig. 12–5D; Fig. 12–6).

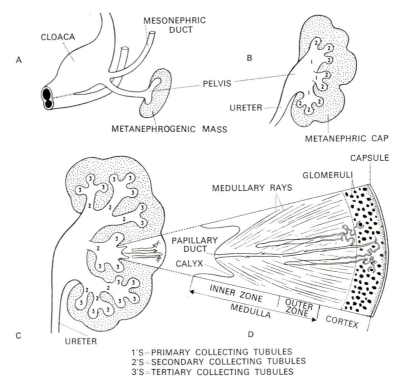

Fig. 12–5. Semi-diagrammatic representation to illustrate the progressive subdivision of the ureteric bud into successively smaller and more numerous collecting tubules (A, B, and C—modified from Davies); a further magnified section of a portion of a lobe of metanephric kidney of a 6-month human foetus (D—modified from Patten). Inset in C shows the part of the kidney in D.

Derivatives of the metanephrogenic mass

An external looser layer of metanephric tissue develops into the interstitial tissue of the kidney and the enveloping connective tissue capsule (Fig. 12–5), whilst the inner tissue (a solid mass of tissue known as the metanephric blastema) covers the distal end of each newly formed collecting tubule. Parts of this blastema separate from the main tissue mass, and form small cell clusters known as renal vesicles, on each side of the tubule. The step-by-step differentiation of one such vesicle into a complete nephron is portrayed in Fig. 12–6. The differentiated components of a nephron, from proximal to distal, are:

(*a*) The Bowman's capsule with a glomerulus, the two forming a renal corpuscle.

(*b*) The proximal convoluted tubule.

(*c*) Henle's loop with its ascending and descending limb.

(*d*) The distal convoluted tubule, which is connected to an arched collecting tubule.

The substance of the completely formed kidney is divided into three zones, termed the inner zone of the medulla, the outer zone of the medulla, and the cortex (Fig. 12–5D) which contains most of the renal corpuscles and convoluted tubules. The medulla mostly houses the loops of Henle and the straight collecting tubules.

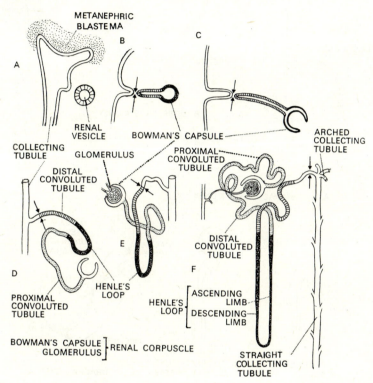

Fig. 12–6. Schematic representation of the development of a metanephric excretory unit, nephron. Arrows indicate the place where the excretory tubule comes into open communication with an arched collecting tubule.

Anomalies

Many forms of abnormal or subnormal development of the renal structures are known to occur. The severest case of all is renal agenesis, which may be either unilateral or bilateral. The failure of development of a kidney may be caused either by early degeneration of the ureteric bud, or by failure of the mesonephric duct to descend. If this happens in a female foetus the Müllerian ducts may also be involved, resulting in the absence of a uterus and major portion of the vagina. Babies born without kidneys die soon after birth.

During normal development the definitive kidneys ascend from the pelvic to the lumbar region. Sometimes, however, one of them fails to do so and remains in its initial position as a pelvic kidney (Fig. 12–7A). In even rarer cases, both kidneys are pushed close together during their upward passage and their lower lobes touch and fuse so that a horseshoe kidney results (Fig. 12–7B). A cystic kidney (Fig. 12–7C) is the result of failure of proper union between collecting and excretory tubules (cf. Fig. 12–6). The resulting accumulation of urine in the nephrons causes the convoluted tubules to dilate and become cysts lined with a degenerated cuboid epithelium.

Cases of incomplete and complete splitting of the ureteric bud are illustrated in Fig. 12–8A and B, respectively.

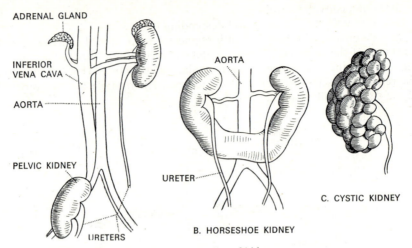

ADRENAL GLAND

INFERIOR
VENA CAVA

AORTA

PELVIC KIDNEY

URETERS

AORTA

URETER

B. HORSESHOE KIDNEY

C. CYSTIC KIDNEY

FIG. 12–7. Anomalies of kidney.

A. UNILATERAL PELVIC KIDNEY

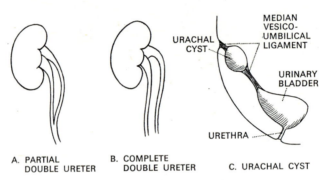

URACHAL
CYST

MEDIAN
VESICO-
UMBILICAL
LIGAMENT

URINARY
BLADDER

URETHRA

A. PARTIAL
DOUBLE URETER

B. COMPLETE
DOUBLE URETER

C. URACHAL CYST

FIG. 12–8. Anomalies of ureter.

CHAPTER 13

THE REPRODUCTIVE SYSTEM

Introduction

Sex is genetically determined, but the realization of this chromosomal determination with respect to the gonads and their ducts depends on the specific action of sex hormones. Sex differentiation therefore is not the same as sex determination; the former process can be altered, modified or even reversed regardless of the chromosomal sex of the individual (p. 140–42). Normal development of the entire sex apparatus occurs only when the required hormones are present in the right concentration at the right time.

Early development is characterized by an indifferent stage in which the sex of the gonads and the male or female nature of the duct system cannot be readily distinguished. At this time each gonad, which is neither a testis nor an ovary, is provided with both a Wölffian (mesonephric) and a Müllerian duct. These are, respectively, the potential male and female genital duct systems. Under the preponderant influence of male sex hormones the Wölffian duct differentiates into the definitive male duct system, whilst the Müllerian duct regresses and vanishes almost completely. Conversely, under the influence of the female sex hormone, the Müllerian duct differentiates into the definitive female duct system, whilst the Wölffian duct in its turn degenerates. At the same time the gonad develops into either a testis or an ovary as the case may be. Certain vestiges of the atrophied ducts do, however, remain. By the end of the second month, the sex of the foetus is recognizable by the differentiation of the external genitalia. The homologous structures of the two sexes at an early stage are illustrated in Fig. 13–1.

This concept of a bi-potential hormonal control mechanism in sex differentiation has stood the test of numerous experiments performed both by nature and by man, beginning with the study of the classical case of the freemartin. A freemartin is the name given to the female member of fraternal twins in cattle. It is sterile, because its initial female sex apparatus has been modified in the male direction; the gonad (genetically an ovary) has been transformed into an ovotestis. This may be of various degrees of severity, short of being capable of producing spermatozoa. The results of extensive studies by Lillie and others show that the freemartin is a case of dominance of the male twin. The latter is far ahead of its female partner in sex differentiation, with the result that its testis produces the male sex hormone long before the ovary of the female twin begins to secrete the female sex hormone. The male hormone is able to reach the female twin across the placenta and thereby masculinizes it. This experiment of nature produces similar results to that of ovariectomy in birds (p. 4). The exact reverse is the production of an ovo-testis from the left gonad of a genetic male chick by treatment with female sex hormone. The role of sex hormones in the differentiation of gonads is thus clearly demonstrated.

The gonads

The testis begins to differentiate earlier than the ovary. Functionally, however, the male reaches sexual maturity a little later than the female.

A well accepted concept with regard to the gonadogenesis of mammals (and even of vertebrates in general) is that an embryonic indifferent gonad develops two components, a centrally located medulla and a peripheral cortex. The two components are endowed, respectively, with male and female developmental potencies. In the course of subsequent differentiation, the

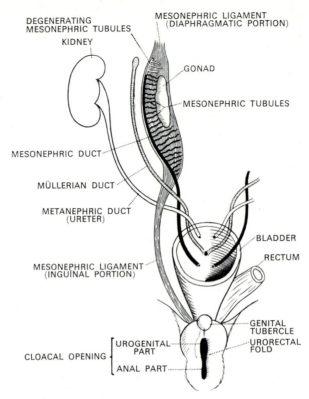

DEGENERATING
MESONEPHRIC TUBULES
KIDNEY
MESONEPHRIC LIGAMENT
(DIAPHRAGMATIC PORTION)
GONAD
MESONEPHRIC TUBULES
MESONEPHRIC DUCT
MÜLLERIAN DUCT
METANEPHRIC DUCT
(URETER)
BLADDER
RECTUM
MESONEPHRIC LIGAMENT
(INGUINAL PORTION)
GENITAL
TUBERCLE
UROGENITAL
PART
URORECTAL
FOLD
CLOACAL OPENING
ANAL PART

FIG. 13–1. Schematic diagram to show the basic structural pattern of the urogenital system at the sexually indifferent stage. (Modified from Patten.)

medulla in a prospective testis assumes dominance over its cortex with the result that the latter vanishes and the germinal epithelium is replaced by a connective tissue membrane known as the tunica vaginalis (p. 142). These changes take place under preponderant action of the male sex hormone. Thus, the definitive testis is actually all medullary in origin. The definitive ovary, on the other hand, is the result of dominance of the cortex over the medulla under the preponderant influence of the female sex hormone. The two gonads differ however in that whereas a cortical component is completely lacking in a testis, the medullary component of the ovary, though greatly reduced in size and importance almost to the point of vanishing, often persists and is represented by some dormant medullary cords (p. 3–4). This explains the basic working mechanism of the bi-potential theory of sex differentiation.

Germ cells vs. structural elements in gonads

The most important function of the gonads is to produce gametes. The spermatozoa and ova therefore, are the primary constituents of the testis and ovary, respectively. The primordial sex cells (p. 2) accordingly represent the foremost component of the gonad whilst the remaining gonadal tissues originate from another component, the structural component. This latter may be further divided into (1) the germinal epithelium (representing a specialized coelomic epithelium lining the peritoneal cavity), which completely covers the developing gonad and (2) the mesenchymal cells of the splanchnic mesoderm which contribute to the bulk of the non-germinal gonadal tissues (Table 13–2) (Fig. 13–12c). The definitive gonad (testis or ovary) is the product of differentiation of the structural component.

When the primordial sex cells first arrive at the genital ridge, the sex of the gonad and of the gametes to be produced is not, as yet, determined. We refer to this early stage in sex differentiation as " indifferent ", meaning that the gonad may become either a testis or an ovary. The available data from experimental studies on gonadogenesis overwhelmingly support the view that the primordial sex cells at this stage, regardless of whether they come from either a genetic male or genetic female embryo, are sexually bi-potential, i.e., they could give rise to either spermatozoa or ova, depending on the eventual sex of the gonad which the primordial sex cells have entered. In other words, the fate of the primordial sex cells as prospective gametes depends on the differentiation of the structural elements of the early gonad; which direction such differentiation may lead, depends in turn, on the sex hormones as just discussed (Fig. 13–2c).

Origin of germ cells (p. 2)

It is now established beyond any doubt that in the human, as well as in the chick, mouse and rat, the sex cells are of an external gonadal origin; they arise very early from the yolk sac endoderm as large spherical cells rich in alkaline phosphatase. After they detach from the yolk sac (Fig. 13–2) they migrate by way of the gut mesentery, and possibly also via blood vessels, to their final destination where they enter the gonadal blastema (Fig. 13–2A, B). It is not known what factors, if any, might guide these cells to their destination. It is known, however, that these cells are sensitive and susceptible to various adverse agents, e.g., X-ray irradiation. Sterility of an individual may result from (a) the destruction of the primary sex cells on their way to the gonad

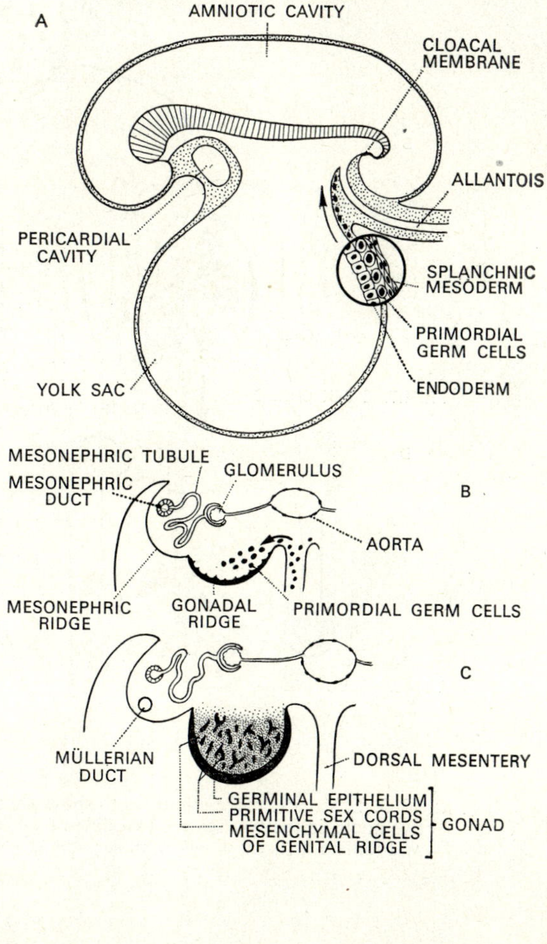

FIG. 13–2. A. Diagram of an early somite embryo showing the primordial germ (sex) cells in the wall of the yolk sac, close to the attachment of the allantois (after Langman). The arrow indicates the direction of migration of the primordial germ cells from the site of origin to the gonadal ridge. The cellular composition of the wall of the yolk sac (inset) is shown enlarged at the lower right.

B. A transverse section through the lumbar region of a 5-week embryo showing the arrival of the primordial germ cells at the gonadal ridge via the mesentery (arrow).

C. A similar section of an older embryo (approx. 8-weeks), showing the establishment of the three definitive components of the developing gonad.

E

or after their arrival (*b*) insufficient number of cells penetrating the gonad and (*c*) failure of the sex cells to increase their initial number during the early differentiation of the gonad (see Chapter 1).

The indifferent stage

The sexually indifferent stage as represented by 5–12 mm. embryos (about 5–6 week) consists of a pair of gonads with two sets of duct systems, with the same macroscopic appearance in both sexes. Soon significant changes begin to take place; firstly, the peritoneal epithelium covering the gonad greatly thickens, giving rise to several layers of actively proliferating cells which cause the blastema to bulge into the coelom. Secondly, as the gonadal blastema becomes thus transformed into a gonad primordium, the primordial sex cells (1400 have been counted at the 4 mm. stage) arrive at the site and penetrate the gonad (Fig. 13–3A).

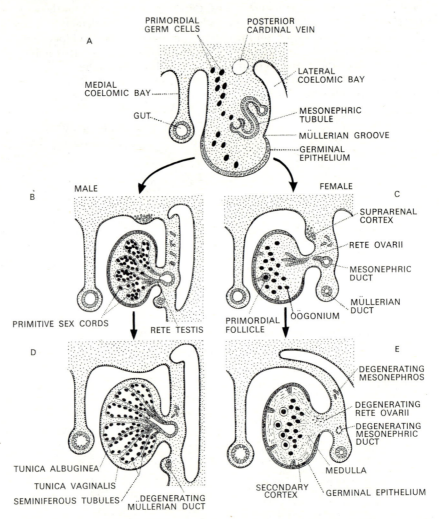

FIG. 13–3. Schematic representations to show the development of the gonads, with their respective ducts, in the two sexes. (Modified from Hamilton, Boyd and Mossman.)
A. Indifferent stage; B and D, male; C and E, female.

Primitive genital ducts

A pair of Müllerian or paramesonephric ducts appears in both sexes. Each arises as a circumscribed thickening of the coelomic epithelium (the Müllerian plate (Fig. 13–4A)) at the cranial end of the urogenital ridge. The plate then sinks in to form a funnel (Fig. 13–4B). The caudal extremity of the diverticulum thus formed then extends caudally along the ventral surface of the ridge in close relationship with the Wölffian or mesonephric duct (Fig. 13–4C). The two Müllerian ducts later enter the unsplit mesoderm of the pelvis and come together in the mid-line and fuse with each other (see Fig. 13–9C). Thus, a double set of genital ducts is present in all embryos throughout the second month (Fig. 13–1). After sex is definitely established, the provisional ducts of the opposite sex regress and mostly disappear. In the male, utilization of the mesonephric duct system as part of the sperm duct is completed by the end of the fifth month (Fig. 13–6), and the urethra is established as a terminal sexual passage.

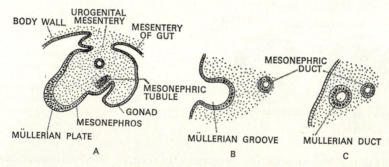

Fig. 13–4. Origin of the human Müllerian duct as seen in transverse sections of the urogenital ridge.
   A. 9 mm. embryo showing thickened peritoneal epithelium, the Müllerian plate (modified from Arey); B and C, 12 mm. embryo at successively lower levels showing, respectively, the closing of the Müllerian groove and the completely formed tube. (Modified from Davies.)

Differentiation of the testis (Figs. 13–3 and 5)

As the testis gradually takes shape, it becomes covered with a germinal epithelium, develops a fibrous tunica albuginea underneath the latter and, most characteristically, its interior becomes filled with anastomosing cords, the testis cords (Fig. 13–5A, B). A new structure, the so-called rete testis, arises from a separate primordium; the rete testis consists of a network of fine tubules (Figs. 13–5B and 13–6), which will soon link the testis cords with the persisting mesonephric tubules. Mesenchymal cells from the splanchnic mesoderm migrate in to fill the spaces between the testis cords and become the indifferent cells, which eventually give rise to the structural elements listed in Table 13–3.

The testis cords are the forerunners of seminiferous tubules. At first they are solid (Fig. 13–5C) and contain cells from two different origins. The majority of these cells are descendants of the primordial sex cells. They actively proliferate and finally become the spermatogonia. Scattered among the latter are the Sertoli cells (p. 9), which are derived from the germinal epithelium.

The testis cords undergo a repeated process of longitudinal splitting to increase their number. At the same time the tubules also increases their length and so become convoluted. In the definitive testis the highly convoluted tubules are contained in hundreds of lobules which are separated from one another by connective tissue septa. Each lobule houses a number of seminiferous tubules. Canalization of the seminiferous tubules does not occur until puberty (Fig.

13–5D). Soon after establishment of the tunica albuginea, the germinal epithelium reverts to an ordinary type of flattened peritoneal mesothelium so that the adult testis is devoid of a germinal epithelium (Fig. 13–5D).

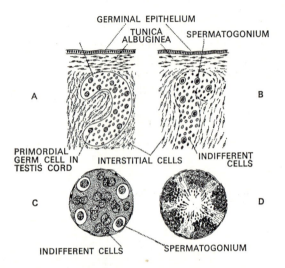

FIG. 13–5. Differentiation of the testis. (After Arey.)
A. Structural details at 8-weeks;
B. Structural details at 14-weeks;
C. Section of a seminiferous tubule of a newborn;
D. Section of a seminiferous tubule of an adolescent.

Within the testis, the formation of connections between the seminiferous tubules and the duct system for passage of spermatozoa continues until the process reaches completion by the end of the 5th or 6th month of gestation. Table 13–1 gives a summary of the origin and anatomy of this continuous sperm pathway (see also Fig. 13–6).

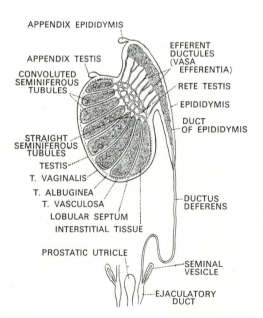

FIG. 13–6. Diagram of the fully developed male genital system, showing the complete pathway for the sperm and the definitive connective tissues of the testis. (Modified from Harrison.)

TABLE 13–1. ORIGIN AND ANATOMY OF THE SPERM PATHWAY

Ducts	Origin
Seminiferous tubules	gonadal
Rete testis	Separate gonadal primordium
Straight portion of efferent ductules (vasa efferentia) }	
	persisting mesonephric tubules
Head . . . Convoluted portion of efferent ductules }	
Epididymis . . . { Body . . . Ductus epididymis (convoluted) }	
Tail . . . Ductus deferens (straight) }	mesonephric duct
Ejaculatory duct (straight) (extends into urethra) }	

Differentiation of the ovary (Figs. 13–3 and 7)

The ovary, suspended by a mesentery (the mesovarium), settles to a more caudal position than the testis. At the blastema stage it contains both clusters of indifferent cells and primordial sex cells. Soon a primary cortex becomes recognizable beneath the germinal epithelium, and a primary medulla, filled with an internal cell mass, is also discernible (Fig. 13–7A). At this time there are neither epithelial cords nor a tunica albuginea in the cortex. A separate primordium gives rise to a non-functional rete ovarii (Fig. 13–3C), which is homologous to the rete testis in the male.

Beginning about the third month, rapid growth of the ovary results in the transformation of its primary cortex into a definitive cortex (Fig. 13–3E). With this change, many cells of the internal cell mass in the medulla move up to the cortex where most of them are converted into egg follicles (Fig. 13–7B; see also Fig. 1–6), which contain closely associated cells of large size, the oögonial A tunica albuginea soon appears by ingrowth of connective tissue, migrating together with blood vessels from the peripheral region of the rete ovarii. The primary (primitive) medulla then declines and degenerates; its place is taken by a definitive medulla (Figs. 13–3E; 13–7C) which is highly vascularized and rich in connective tissue.

Further follicular activity is confined to the cortex and commences under the action of the hormones discussed in Chapters 1 and 7. The question of whether or not cells proliferated from the germinal epithelium ever actually form new ova (i.e., ova developed in addition to those derived from the primordial sex cells) has not been unequivocally settled. Some believe that this is the case. From the histological study of fixed material they would interpret an ovigerous tube (Fig. 13–7D) as being entirely contributed by the germinal epithelium. From this localized accumulation of cells, one actually differentiates into a germ cell (oögonium) while the rest become follicular cells and surround the former in the formation of a typical primary follicle. It is only fair to state, however, that this view has not been satisfactorily substantiated by experimental evidence. In fact, the most recent research on this subject using improved techniques and better experimental controls tends rather to strengthen the opposite view, namely that the cells derived from the germinal epithelium, while definitely giving rise to the follicular cells and some other non-germinal elements of the ovary (Table 13–3), do not form oögonia. Supporters of this view maintain that the germinal epithelium is not a secondary source of ova and that the primordial sex cells constitute the only source of definitive sex cells in both sexes. One may recall that in the case of " pleiotropism " in mice (p. 87), discussed in Chapter 8, one of the effects of the mutated gene is to reduce the initial number of primordial sex cells so that even though these cells do arrive at the gonad, their number is not sufficient to yield a fertile gonad. These circumstances provide an excellent opportunity to test the potency of the germinal epithelium to form germ cells. The fact is, however, that the germinal epithelium, despite the great need imposed on it, does not show itself capable of forming any ova.

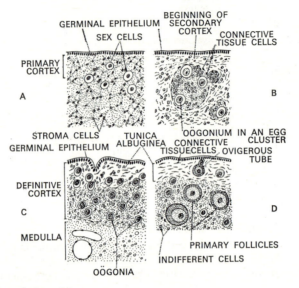

FIG. 13–7. Differentiation of the ovary.
A. The primary cortex and primary medulla with sex cells scattered among them (11–14 week stage);
B. The beginnings of a secondary cortex and formation of egg clusters (4-months);
C. The development of a definitive cortex and formation of tunica albuginea (6-months);
D. The follicular development beginning (newborn).

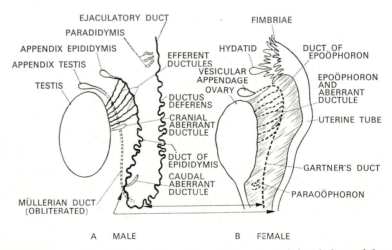

FIG. 13–18. Diagrams illustrating the diverse fates of the mesonephric tubules, and the mesonephric and Müllerian (paramesonephric) ducts in the two sexes. (Modified from Arey.)
A. Definitive condition in male;
B. Definitive condition in female.

TABLE 13–2. HOMOLOGOUS STRUCTURES OF THE TWO SEXES (Fig. 13–18)
(Non-functional structures are underlined)

A. COMPONENTS OF DUCT SYSTEM

MALE	INDIFFERENT	FEMALE
Cranial aberrant ductules Efferent ductules (vasa efferentia) Caudal aberrant ductules and paradidymis	Mesonephric tubules	Epoöphoron and aberrant ductules
		Paroöphoron
Appendix epididymis		Vesicular appendages
Duct of epididymis		Duct of epoöphoron
Ductus deferens	Mesonephric duct	Gartner's duct
Ejaculatory duct		
Appendix testis	Paramesonephric (Müllerian) ducts	Fimbriae and hydatid Uterine tube Uterus Vagina (upper ⅘)
Prostatic urethra Membranous urethra Penile urethra	Urogenital sinus	Vagina (lower ⅕) hymen vestibule

B. EXTERNAL GENITALIA (Fig. 13–14)

MALE	INDIFFERENT	FEMALE
Glans penis	Genital tubercle	Glans clitoris
Urethral surface of penis	Urethral folds (inner genital swelling)	Labia minora
Scrotum	Outer genital swelling	Labia majora

C. ACCESSORY REPRODUCTIVE GLANDS

MALE		FEMALE
Prostate		Para urethral
Bulbo-urethral (Cowper's)		Vestibular (Bartholin)
Urethral (Littre's)		Lesser vestibular

D. GENITAL LIGAMENTS

MALE		FEMALE
Mesorchium		Mesovarium
Ligamentum testes		Ligament of the ovary proper
Scrotal ligament		Broad ligament of the uterus

(The gubernaculum is formed jointly by the ligamentum testes and the scrotal ligament.)

Formation and derivatives of the urogenital sinus (Fig. 13–8)

The embryonic digestive tract terminates in a blind sac-like space, the cloaca. In 15 mm. embryos (7th week) the cloaca is divided into a dorsal anorectal canal (prospective rectum) and a ventral urogenital sinus by the downgrowth of a connective tissue known as the uro-rectal septum. The rectum is, of course, continuous with the hind-gut whereas the urogenital sinus is continuous with the allantois. Both divisions of the cloaca are covered with ectodermal cells where they come into apposition with the body wall of the embryo, thereby forming double-layered (ectoderm and endoderm) membranes, known as the anal membrane and the urethral membrane, respectively. These membranes rupture shortly afterwards.

The urogenital sinus differentiates into three regions, the vesico-urethral, the pelvic and phallic portions. In both sexes the vesico-urethral portion, which represents the proximal part of the allantois, becomes dilated to form the urinary bladder. The remaining two portions of the sinus give rise, respectively, to the urethra and part of the external genitalia of the respective sex. In the male, the urethra consists of a proximal pelvic part and a distal penile portion, this latter

TABLE 13–3. HOMOLOGOUS COMPONENTS OF THE GONADS

Component		Testis	Ovary
A. Germinal	Primordial sex cells (bi-potential; sex of gonad realized by structural elements)	Same in both sexes; originate from yolk sac endoderm, migrating via mesentery and/or blood vessels to reach and penetrate the indifferent gonadal blastema	
B. Structural (Sex-determining)	Germinal Epithelium	A cortex never develops	Initial medulla, represented by medullary cords, recedes; a cortex, developed later, dominates
		Early — Testis cords ↓ Seminiferous tubules	Medullary cords (dormant, if any left)
		Early — Rete testes	Rete ovarii
		Late — Complete regression; replaced by tunica vaginalis	Persists as such; gives rise to follicular cells, and possible other non-germinal elements in cortex
	Mesenchyme of Splachnic mesoderm	Tunica albuginea (early) . . . Tunica vasculosa Intersitial tissue Septa	Tunica albuginea (much later) Theca externa Theca interna General stroma

part is lacking in the female.   Various accessory reproductive glands (Table 13–2c) arise as outgrowths from the urogenital sinus into the mesenchyme along the wall of the urogenital sinus.

The junction between the vesico-urethral and pelvic portions of the urogenital sinus is a region of some special interest, particularly in the male. In this region the male duct (the original mesonephric duct) expands and dilates to form an ampulla from which the seminal vesicle originates. The region is known as trigonum vesicae (Fig. 13–8c), and since mesodermal and endodermal epithelia converge at this point, the structures formed from the trigone may have a mosaic mesodermal and endodermal lining, at least in their proximal portions. The definitive position where the ureter opens into the bladder is slightly above the mesonephric duct (Fig. 13–8b, c). Prior to this, however, the mesonephric and metanephric duct (the forerunner of the ureter) empty into the base of the bladder through a single opening, the metanephric duct (which appears later) arising from the base of the mesonephric duct. The two ducts eventually separate and furthermore switch their original positions, resulting in the final definitive position of the opening of the ureter as just described (cf. Figs. 13–1 and 8).

Anomalies will result from the persistence of the lumen of the urachus. If this involves the latter's entire length, it is a case of urachal fistula, in which urine may drain from the umbilicus. A urachal cyst (Fig. 12–8c) will be the result if only part of the urachus retains its lumen.

Formation of the genital cords (Fig. 13–9)

Near the cloaca the two urogenital ridges swing toward the mid-line (Fig. 13–9A, B) and fuse into the so-called genital cord. In this process the progressively elongating paramesonephric (Müllerian) ducts, which were originally lateral in position, come to lie side-by-side in the mid-line, leaving the mesonephric ducts (originally more medial than the paramesonephric ducts) to assume a lateral position (Fig. 13–9c). The paramesonephric ducts eventually fuse within the

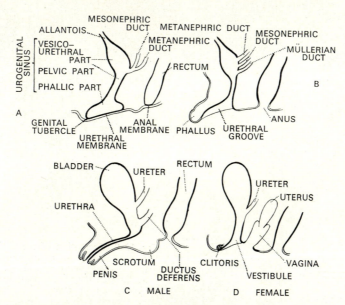

FIG. 13–8. Diagrams illustrating the development of the bladder, urethra and external genitalia, shown in sagittal sections. (After Dodds.)
A. Early stage prior to rupture of the anal and urethral membranes and with a low genital tubercle;
B. Later stage (still sexually indifferent) characterized by ruptured anal and urethral membranes and the appearance of a phallus;
C. The definitive male condition;
D. The definitive female condition.

genital cord (by the ninth week) and end blindly at the Müllerian tubercle, which is a median protuberance projecting from the dorsal wall of the urogenital sinus. The fused common portion of the paramesonephric ducts is the first indication of a uterus and vagina. The more cranial portions of the ducts, however, remain separate and are destined to become the uterine (Fallopian) tubes, together with the fimbriae and hydatid (Fig. 13–18).

Approximately, the upper four-fifths of the vagina are derived from the fused paramesonephric ducts. The terminal one-fifth, plus the hymen and vestibule is derived from the urogenital sinus (Fig. 13–10; Table 13–2).

Anomalies

Many forms of congenital anomalies of the uterus and vagina result from various deviations from the normal developmental course taken by the paramesonephric ducts. Some of the most common and best known cases are illustrated in Fig. 13–11, which is self-explanatory as to the cause of each.

Development of the external genitalia

Parts of the external genitalia in both sexes are derived from the terminal portion of the urogenital sinus (Fig. 13–8). During the third week of development, mesenchymal cells of primitive streak origin (Fig. 13–13A) surround the cloacal membrane to form a pair of elevated folds, the cloacal folds. These subsequently fuse with each other in front of the cloacal membrane, resulting in the formation of a cloacal eminence (Fig. 13–12B). At first, the cloacal membrane faces ventrally (Fig. 13–12A) but, due to localized proliferations of mesoderm which converts the cloacal eminence into a genital tubercle, it undergoes a rotation until it faces caudally (Fig. 13–12B, C). Likewise, the underlying mesodermal cloacal folds split into the anterior

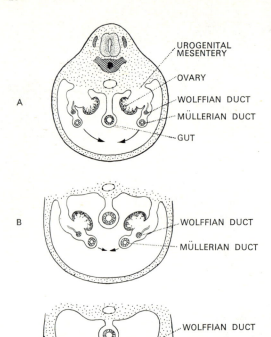

A

UROGENITAL
MESENTERY

OVARY

WOLFFIAN DUCT

MÜLLERIAN DUCT

GUT

B

WOLFFIAN DUCT

MÜLLERIAN DUCT

C

WOLFFIAN DUCT

FUSED MÜLLERIAN
DUCTS

TRANSVERSE
PELVIC FOLD
(GENITAL CORDS)

Fig. 13–9. Formation of the genital cords as seen in transverse sections of the urogenital ridge at three levels. (Modified from Davies.)
A. through the metanephric kidney;
C. through the lower caudal region;
B. midway between levels A and C.
The urogenital ridges are shown to pass ventrally and medially (arrows in A and B) so that the Müllerian and Wolffian (mesonephric) ducts approach each other (B). The Müllerian ducts and their surrounding mesoderm then fuse (C), thereby coming to lie in a transverse pelvic fold. During this process the ovaries are carried onto the posterior face of the pelvic fold, making them lie dorsal to the broad ligament in the adult woman.

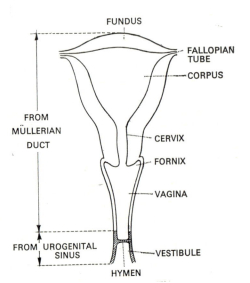

FUNDUS

FALLOPIAN
TUBE

CORPUS

FROM
MÜLLERIAN
DUCT

CERVIX

FORNIX

VAGINA

FROM UROGENITAL
SINUS

VESTIBULE

HYMEN

Fig. 13–10. The derivation of the uterus and vagina from the Müllerian duct and urogenital sinus (definitive condition in a newborn).

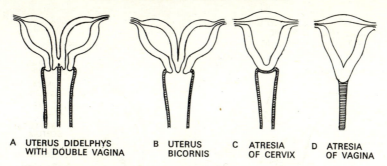

A UTERUS DIDELPHYS
   WITH DOUBLE VAGINA

B UTERUS
   BICORNIS

C ATRESIA
   OF CERVIX

D ATRESIA
   OF VAGINA

FIG. 13–11. Anomalies of the uterus and vagina. (After Langman.)
A. Failure of the entire Müllerian ducts to fuse;
B. Failure of fusion of the upper portion of the Müllerian ducts;
C. Persistence of the urovaginal septum;
D. Obliteration of the lumen of the urovaginal canal.

genital folds (or urethral folds) and posterior anal folds (Fig. 13–13B). In the meantime, the urogenital sinus has differentiated into three portions as described above.

Thus two of the three primordia, from which the external genitalia are derived, are established. These are the median genital tubercle and a pair of genital folds immediately surrounding the

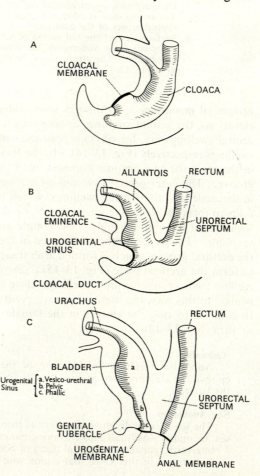

FIG. 13–12. Changes in the cloaca region. (After Davies.)
A. Before division of the cloaca;
B. Formation and growth of the urorectal septum (arrow);
C. Resultant formation of the urogenital sinus and rectum.

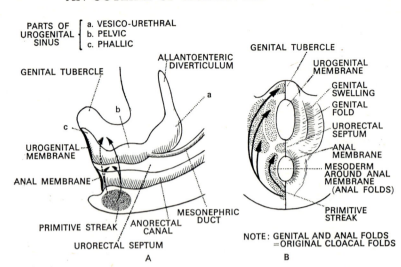

FIG. 13–13. Origin and migration of mesoderm (from the primitive streak) concerned in the formation of the external genitalia. (After Harrison.)

    A. Diagrammatic appearance of the tail region (left side) following division of the cloaca. The arrows show the direction of migration of mesoderm from the primitive streak to the ventral aspect of the embryo;

    B. Surface view of the tail region of an embryo to show the proliferations of mesoderm (stippled) lying underneath the ectoderm and surrounding the anal and urogenital membranes. The arrows show the direction of growth and migration of the mesoderm as in Fig. 13–13A.

urogenital membrane. To these is soon added a third primordium, which consists of a pair of elevations, the genital swellings arising on each side of the genital folds. The genital folds and genital swellings are, for obvious reasons, sometimes referred to as the inner and outer genital swellings respectively (Fig. 13–14). In the female the former give rise to the labia minora, whilst in the male the two become apposed, with their ventral edges fusing along the entire urethral groove. The outer genital swellings which form the labia majora in the female, are transformed in the male into the scrotal swellings, which fuse subsequently after the manner of the urethral folds to form the definitive scrotum, leaving their line of fusion as the raphe which is continuous with that of the urethral folds. The female urethral groove is open to the surface and forms the vestibule. The penile urethral is formed in the following manner. The endoderm at the base of the urethral groove, which is formed after disappearance of the urogenital membrane, proliferates to form the urethral plate (Fig. 13–15A). At the end of the third month, the two urethral folds (genital folds or inner genital swellings) close over the plate to complete the urethral canal of the penis. In this way, the urethral groove eventually comes to open terminally on the glans penis. In contrast to this, the clitoris in the female is turned downwards and is not traversed by the urethra (Fig. 13–14).

Anomalies

    Anomalies resulting from failure of the urethral folds to close properly (hypospadias and epispadias) are illustrated in Fig. 13–15B and C. The former occurs with a higher frequency than the latter.

Sex Anomalies

    The sex of an individual may deviate from total maleness or total femaleness in a wide range of sex anomalies which fall into two principal categories as follows.

1. Intersexes (gonads and genital ducts of both sexes are present in the same individual). A typical " intersex " of this kind, that is one with complete and functional sex apparatus of both sexes

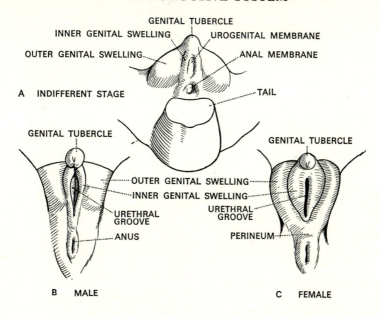

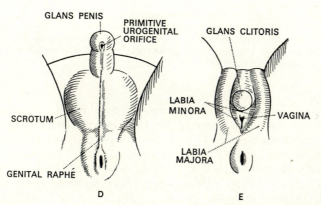

FIG. 13–14. Formation of the external genitalia. (After Davies, originally adapted from Spaulding, 1921.)

    A. External genitals of an embryo before its sex can be determined (cf. Fig. 13–12c);

    B. and C. External genitals, respectively of the male and female embryos of 23 mm.;

    D and E. Final form of external genitals respectively in the male and female embryos of 65 mm.

is exceedingly rare (perhaps non-existent in humans). The condition is known as true hermaphroditism; it is the normal way of reproduction in some invertebrates (worms and mulluscs). However, human cases displaying varying degrees of hermaphroditism (none of them fertile) have been described. Briefly these can be characterized as follows:

Gonads: separate ovary and testis; or a pair of combined ovotestes; or an ovary or testis paired with an ovotestis.

Genital ducts: double ducts on one or both sides.

External genitalia: intermediate between male and female.

Secondary sexual characteristics: mixed and changeable.

    Other cases, sometimes labeled as false (pseudo) hermaphroditism, are of usually one dominant sex accompanied by genital structures of the opposite sex, hence the term male hermaphrodite or female hermaphrodite. On this basis, one individual may have a pair of ovaries, but male

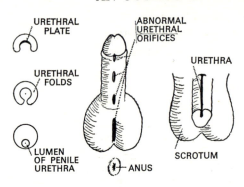

URETHRAL PLATE

ABNORMAL URETHRAL ORIFICES

URETHRA

URETHRAL FOLDS

LUMEN OF PENILE URETHRA

ANUS

SCROTUM

A NORMAL PROCESS OF FORMATION OF PENILE URETHRA

B HYPOSPADIAS

C EPISPADIAS

FIG. 13–15. Formation of the penile urethra.
A. Three stages in the closure of the urogenital folds, resulting in the formation of a normal penile urethra. (After Langman.)
B. and C. Consequences of failure of proper closure of the urethral groove; various locations of unclosed urethra, opening ventrally (B), opening dorsally (C). (After Arey).

external genitalia and secondary sexual characteristics to a varying degree, or vice versa. Another individual may have the internal reproductive tract of either sex, doubled or mixed.

The causes of intersexness are of a complex nature, but are generally attributable to an abnormal genic balance (cf. p. 18).

2. Sex-reversal (a modification in the direction of the opposite sex). All cases of feminized males and masculinized females belong to this category. The causative agent responsible for these abnormalities is a sex hormone (cf. p. 72). For example, excessive production of the androgenic hormone in a woman due to either an enlarged cortex of the suprarenal gland or tumour-growth in the ovarian medulla (cf. hypertrophied medullary cords, p. 4) often can change the woman into a female pseudo-hermaphrodite. Conversely, an inadequate suppressive or inhibitory influence of the testicular hormone during the foetal period may well result in feminization of an otherwise male pseudo-hermaphrodite.

Descent of the testes

The testis, with the epididymis, develops as an abdominal organ. At about the eighth month of foetal life, the testes, each accompanied by its epididymis, begin to descend through the inguinal canal into the scrotum guided by two extensions of the coelom, known as the processus vaginalis (Fig. 13–16A) and a fibrous band or gubernaculum. Both the testes and the latter processes are covered with peritoneum. After the descent, the testicular epithelial covering is the tunica vaginalis, which completely replaces the former germinal epithelium. The tunica is divided into a parietal layer, lining the scrotal sac, and a visceral layer which covers the testes and epididymis. After birth the inguinal canal closes, thereby separating the vaginal process from the peritoneal cavity. Figure 13–16B shows the development of the diverticulum of the peritoneum (the processus vaginalis) in relation to the anterior surface of the gubernaculum. This diverticulum penetrates the abdominal wall of the testis (arrow, Figs. 13–16A and B). The testis and epididymis are caudally displaced for approximately ten segments, so enclosing them in the scrotal sac, the testis finally coming to rest dorsal to the lower end of the processus vaginalis (Fig. 13–16C). The whole process of events normally terminates by obliteration of the communication of the processus vaginalis with the peritoneal cavity. The sperm duct, nerves and blood vessels of the testes are also drawn with the testes during the descent, and when they are invested with connective tissue, they collectively form the so-called spermatic cord.

Three factors play a role in this testicular descent. They are (a) degeneration of the mesonephros (b) restraint by the gubernaculum, and (c) rapid growth of the body wall. In addition, possibly gonadotrophic and androgenic hormones may act as supplementary controlling factors in this process.

The descent of the testes, aside from developmental and anatomical considerations, also has a physiological significance. It has been demonstrated that testes which fail to descend (a

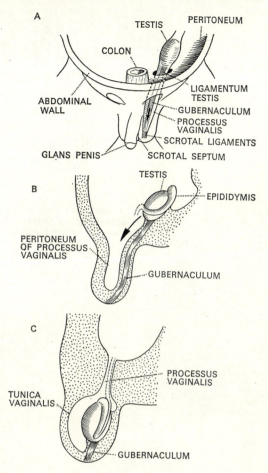

FIG. 13–16. Descent of the testis.
A. View of caudal end of coelomic cavity showing the topographical relationships of the structures involved in descent of the testis. (After Williams and Wendell-Smith.)
B. Early stage in development of the processus vaginalis. The arrow indicates the direction of caudal displacement of the testis and epididymis to the scrotal sac. (After Davies.)
C. Final position of testis in the scrotal sac and beginning of the obliteration of the processus vaginalis. (After Davies.)

condition known as cryptorchidism) are not capable of carrying on spermatogenesis. This is due to the fact that the temperature inside the scrotum is two to three degrees (Fahrenheit) lower than that of the body, and the temperature of the latter is evidently too high for spermatogenesis. It is also known that a cryptorchid, even though he is sterile, nevertheless exhibits normal secondary sexual characteristics as well as a normal libido. Histologically, the testis of such an individual shows degenerate seminiferous tubules, but normal amounts of interstitial tissue between the degenerate tubules. This observation forms the basis for concluding that the interstitial tissue (cells of Leydig) constitutes an endocrine gland for the elaboration of the male sex hormone, testosterone. As stated before (Chapter 7) the function of the male sex hormone is to maintain the accessory sex glands, male behaviour and sex drive, and all the secondary sexual characteristics.

Anomalies

A cryptorchid testis may lie in any position along the normal descent pathway, or occupy various other ectopic locations, e.g., superficial abdominal, femoral, superficial inguinal, pubic, peritoneal, etc.

Aside from these cases of failure of testicular descent, complications involving congenital inguinal hernia may result and, as shown in Fig. 13–17A, the intestinal loop descends into the scrotum. In yet other cases, the closure of the passage from the coelomic cavity to the scrotal sac takes place irregularly, leaving small cysts along its course (Fig. 13–17B). These cysts may later secrete excessive fluid, resulting in the formation of a hydrocoele.

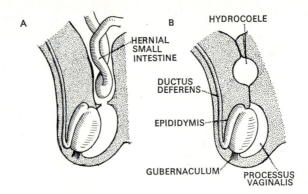

Fig. 13–17. Congenital anomalies accompanying the failure of testicular descent.
A. Congenital inguinal hernia.   (After Arey.)
B. Hydrocoele.   (After Langman.)

CHAPTER 14

THE CARDIOVASCULAR SYSTEM

Blood vessel formation

The earliest blood vessels to be formed are extra-embryonic. The process begins in the third week at three well circumscribed sites, the wall of the yolk sac, the connecting stalk and the chorion (Fig. 14–1A). The process consists of three steps (*a*) an aggregation of mesenchymal cells to form blood islands (Fig. 14–1B) (*b*) a confluence of intercellular clefts filled with a fluid (Fig. 14–1C)

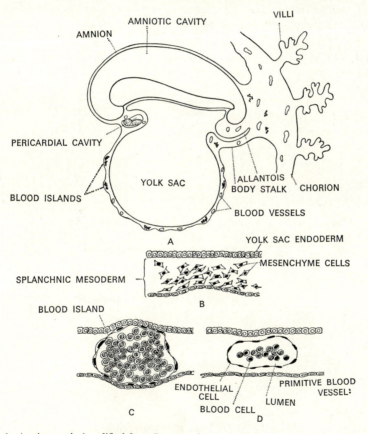

Fig. 14–1. Angiogenesis (modified from Langman);
  A. Diagrammatic median sagittal section of a 19 day (presomite) embryo, showing the extra-embryonic blood vessel formation in the yolk sac wall, the connecting stalk and the chorion. Histological details of the wall of the yolk sac (inset) are magnified in B, C, and D to show three successive stages in blood vessel formation;
  B. Undifferentiated mesenchymal cells of the extra-embryonic mesoderm;
  C. Blood island formation;
  D. Differentiation of a blood island into primitive blood vessel containing blood cells and lined with endothelial cells.

and (c) a separation of the endothelial cells (endothelioblasts) lining the primitive blood vessel from those enclosed within it; these latter cells give rise to blood cells (haemocytoblasts) (Fig. 14–1D). The process just described is exactly the same in the later differentiation of all the intra-embryonic blood vessels.

In this manner a network of vascular primordia is established *in situ* wherever called for. Further progress depends on a process of " selective differentiation ", whereby new vessels may arise through continual sprouting of pre-existing vessels. Existing vessels may also either coalesce with one another or become obliterated. In this way the embryo is provided with a system of vitelline vessels serving the yolk sac and umbilical vessels for the supply of the chorion. These extra-embryonic blood vessels keep on sprouting and gradually establish connections with the intra-embryonic blood vessels formed *in situ*.

Haemopoiesis

It is now generally accepted that all kinds of blood cells are derived from a common stem cell, the haemocytoblast (Table 14–1). This cell, which is present in all haemopoietic centres, originates from the primitive (embryonal) undifferentiated mesenchyme, which also gives rise to fixed mesenchyme cells, the precursors of all kinds of connective tissue cells, including the macrophages.

TABLE 14–1. LINES OF BLOOD-CELL FORMATION ACCORDING TO THE MONOPHYLETIC
THEORY

Undifferentiated mesenchyme cell
(reticulo-endothelial)

Stem Cell
(Haemocytoblast)

1	2	3	4	5
Early primitive erythroblast	Monoblast	Megakaryocytoblast	Myeloblast	Lymphoblast
Definitive erythroblast	Monocyte	Megakaryocyte	Promyelocyte	Small Medium } Lymphocytes Large
		platelets	Myelocytes	
Intermediate polychromic			Metamyelocytes	
Late polychromic			Granulocytes { Eosinophilic Neutrophilic Basophilic	
Reticulocyte (no nucleus)				
Erythrocyte (no nucleus)				

Haemopoietic centres

The definitive haemopoietic organs are bone marrow (cell lines 1–4, Table 14–1) and lymphatic tissues (cell line 5, Table 14–1). These organs start to manufacture the various types of blood cells beginning from the fourth month (Fig. 14–2) but they are preceded in the early embryo by three other organs (yolk sac, liver and spleen), which assume haemopoietic functions one after another with considerable overlapping in time; this is especially true for the liver (Fig. 14–2). In addition to these, the endothelium of embryonic blood vessels serves as the earliest haemopoietic tissue up to about the sixth week (this is not shown in Fig. 14–2).

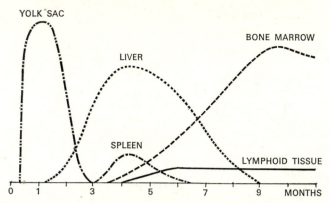

FIG. 14–2. Graph showing the extent and functional period of the haemopoietic tissues in succession from the embryonic to the foetal and postnatal stage. (After Williams and Wendell-Smith.)

DEVELOPMENT OF THE HEART

A. Origin

In the chick the heart is formed between 25 to 29 hours of incubation from cells detached from the splanchnic mesoderm on both sides of and immediately caudal to the anterior intestinal portal. On each side, mesenchymal cells are given off to form a tube; the two endothelial tubes thus formed meet and fuse beneath the closed elongating pharynx. Simultaneously, surrounding splanchnic mesoderm closes in on the single endocardium, thereby forming the epimyocardium of the heart. In so doing, the dorsal mesocardium is formed, but only temporarily; it soon fenestrates and disappears. The ventral mesocardium either never forms or has only a very brief existence. Thus the heart is left without any mesenterial support, but freely suspended within the pericardial cavity (Fig. 14–3A–F).

In the human embryo the heart comes from a single primordium, known as the cardiogenic plate. At the pre-somite stage, this primordium lies in front of the head, within the splanchnic mesoderm and beneath a single pericardial chamber (this constitutes the earliest coelom). At seven somites, due to the rapid forward growth of the head, a reversal in position takes place, resulting in the heart primordium coming to lie beneath the enlarging fore-gut, and the pericardium further below the heart. The single cardiogenic plate then splits into two longitudinal strands, each with a cavity. The two tubes, thus formed from the mesenchymal cells, are comparable to the paired endothelial tubes found at an early stage in the chick. Subsequently, as in the chick, the two endothelial tubes fuse into a single tube, and the surrounding mesenchyme encloses the endothelial tube with a double wall, the epimyocardium. In mammals the embryonic heart is suspended by a dorsal mesentery for some time, but a ventral mesentery is never formed (Fig. 14–4A–C).

B. Establishment of the external form

The heart, when first formed, is a tubular structure (Fig. 14–5A) with four differentiated regions; listed in the order of direction of blood flow these are, from behind, the sinus venosus, atrium, ventricle and truncus arteriosus or bulbus cordis (Fig. 14–7A). A number of steps are involved in the transformation of such an embryonic heart into a definitive adult heart. Many factors are responsible for this transformation of which the three most important are (a) the faster growth of the heart than the pericardium (b) the differential growth of the heart itself,

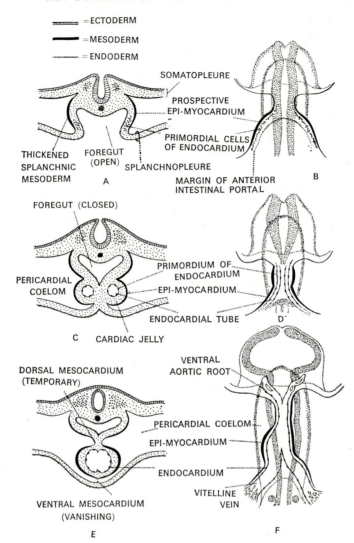

FIG. 14–3. Diagrammatic cross sections (A, C, E) and their respective ventral views (B, D, F) through the pericardial region of chicks, to show the formation of the heart (after Patten): A and B, at 25 hours; C and D, at 27 hours; E and F, at 29 hours of incubation.

and (c) the division of the heart into right and left halves.   The following stages are recognized.
1. Disappearance of the dorsal mesocardium (this takes place at the 7–16 somite stage).
2. A single bending, tilting the heart with its future cephalic end towards the right (Fig. 14–5B).
3. A second bending, turning it into an " S " shape with a sharp flexure between the atrium and ventricle, with the latter lying ventral and caudad (Fig. 14–5c, D).
4. A double-folding (at about the 22 somite stage) resulting in the formation of a U-shaped loop (Fig. 14–6A) during the 4th week, and so shifting the atrium to a position cephalic to the ventricle.   At the same time the sinus venosus is carried dorsally (Fig. 14–6B) and the truncus arteriosus and ventral aorta ventrally, so shortening the heart considerably.   This process fixes the definitive position of the future atria and ventricles in proper relation to

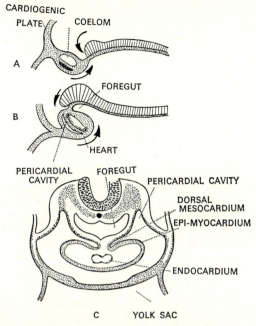

FIG. 14–4. Formation of the human heart (modified from Arey); A and B represent diagrammatic sagittal sections at a presomite stage and at 17 somites, respectively, showing the reversal of the heart and pericardial cavity. The arrows indicate the directions of growth of the embryonic head relative to that of the heart primordium as a factor responsible for the reversal.
C is a transverse section.

each other. By this time, the sinus venosus has withdrawn from the septum transversum, its right and left horns partially merge, and the right horn shows a tendency to enlarge more rapidly than the left horn. The ventricle rapidly increases its size and the thickness of its wall (myocardium) and as a result of internal changes, a ventral groove soon appears (Fig. 14–6c, D).

C. Other changes

The embryonic heart at this time receives blood via the sinus venosus from six veins, 2 common cardinals, 2 vitelline and 2 umbilical veins (Fig. 14–7A). This primitive condition evolves into one

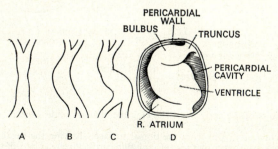

FIG. 14–5. A, B, and C. Diagrams to show the early stages in the development of the vertebrate heart (adapted from several sources): A. Fused cardiac tube; B, primary flexure; C, the " S " stage; D, in situ human heart in early flexion, ventral view at 11 somites.

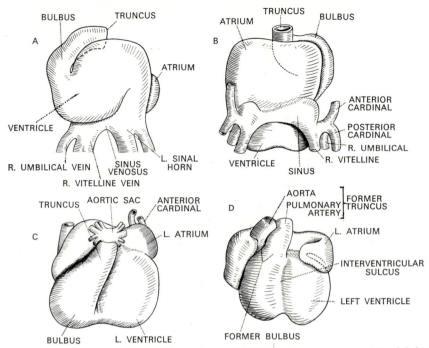

FIG. 14–6. Human hearts in further advanced stages of flexion, progressing toward the definitive external form (after Arey);
A. Ventral view at 16 somites;
B. Dorsal view at 22 somites;
C. Ventral view at 5 mm.;
D. Ventral view at 12 mm.

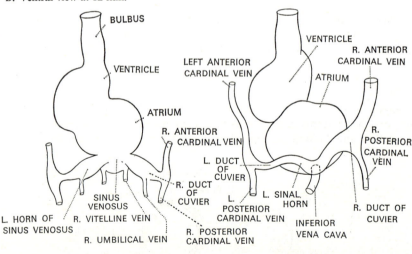

FIG. 14–7. Two views of the early heart showing the changes undergone by the sinus venosus and the veins entering it (after Davies);
A. Primitive condition, seen from the dorsal surface, showing the cardinal veins entering the sinus venosus at the sides via the common cardinal veins (ducts of Cuvier) and a pair each of vitelline and umbilical veins entering it posteriorly after traversing the septum transversum;
B. Later stage (see text for explanation).

in which the venous blood empties directly into the right atrium via two new large veins, the superior vena cava and the inferior vena cava following almost complete absorption of the sinus venosus into the atrium (Fig. 14–7B). Meanwhile, the atrium and the ventricle both become partitioned and separated into right and left halves by internal septa, with valves guarding the passage from atrium to ventricle on both sides. The anterior end of the heart (the ventral aorta and aortic sac) also undergoes appropriate changes so as to complete the final structural adaptations for separating the venous blood (on the right side) from the oxygenated blood (on the left). The final result is that instead of having blood entering the heart and leaving it at opposite ends, the big veins and arteries now make their connections all at the cranial end of the heart (Fig. 14–27).

D. Internal changes

The single ventricle will become the right and left ventricles, separated by an interventricular septum. Concurrently, the bulbus cordis is partitioned by means of a spiral bulbar ridge into a pulmonary trunk connected with the right ventricle, and an aortic trunk connected with the left ventricle.

The first indication of the closing of the interventricular foramen linking the two ventricles is the development of two flaps of endocardial tissues, the dorsal and ventral atrioventricular cushions. The two face each other like lips (Fig. 14–8B), thus narrowing down the original circular interventricular foramen into a shape of the letter " I " lying on its side. As a result of this dorso-ventral compression, the dorsal and ventral portions of the cushion undergo considerable thickening with their free edges moving toward each other (Fig. 14–10). They finally fuse in the middle, thereby leaving two orifices, one on each side, as the right and left atrioventricular canals (Figs. 14–8C and 14–10). Each orifice is surrounded by localized proliferations of mesenchymal tissue which together with the chordae tendinae contributed from the papillary muscle of the ventricle wall, forms the atrioventricular valves, the tricuspid valve (on the right) and the mitral valve (on the left) (Fig. 14–11).

In the meantime the interventricular septum deepens (Fig. 14–8B), and important changes are taking place also in the bulbus cordis. Either through slower growth and/or atrophy of the bulbo-ventricular fold (Fig. 14–9A, hatched portion), the lower (basal) portion of the bulbus cordis becomes absorbed and incorporated into the right ventricle (Fig. 14–9B), following which the bulbus itself becomes aligned with the free margin of the interventricular septum, lying only slightly to the right of the septum.

The completed (adult) interventricular septum is thick and muscular except a small portion below the fused atrioventricular cushions (Fig. 14–9), which is the membranous part of the septum (Pars membranaca septi) (Fig. 14–9). This is thin and develops from the under surface of the endocardial cushion and the two bulbar ridges. It is composed only of fibrous tissue and, because of its delicate nature, this area is often involved in interventricular defects (p. 169).

Inside the bulbus cordis, two bulbar ridges develop, so marking the beginning of its separation into the pulmonary and aortic channels. The ridges are recognized at their beginning as right and left bulbar ridges (Fig. 14–8B), passing on to the dorsal and ventral walls of the bulbus cordis, respectively. Later, the bulbar ridges fuse along their length (Fig. 14–8C), so forming a spiral bulbar septum. The latter separates the bulbus cordis into an anterior (dorsal) pulmonary channel and a posterior (ventral) aortic channel. The septum is spiral because it lies in the frontal plane in the upper part of the bulbus, but gradually becomes sagittal at its lower end as the septum approaches the interventricular septum. In other words, the bulbar septum rotates through 90°, in a counterclockwise direction when viewed from above (Fig. 14–15); the pulmonary and aortic channels consequently have a similar spiral. These developmental processes finally result in the pulmonary channel becoming linked with the right atrioventricular orifice and the aortic channel with the left atrioventricular orifice. That part of the aortic channel from the region of the bulbar cushion to the interventricular foramen becomes the aortic vestibule (Fig.

14–8c). Similarly, the pulmonary channel also has a vestibular portion; it forms the infundibulum of the right ventricle, or conus arteriosus, with the bulbar septum forming the common
wall between the aortic wall and the infundibulum (Fig. 14–12).

Completion of the spiral bulbar septum is accomplished by the fusion of the right and left
bulbar ridges, assisted by proliferations derived from the ventral atrioventricular cushion on the
right side and from the free margin of interventricular foramen (Fig. 14–8D). This area of
fusion constitutes a critical zone since it completes the interventricular septum and many septal
defects take their origin from here (p. 169). Most of these defects are caused by a failure in the
completion of the lower part of the spiral bulbar septum, rather than to a failure in the closure
of the interventricular foramen.

E. Septum formation in the atrium (Fig. 14–9)

The process of partitioning the single atrium into right and left atria begins in 5 mm. embryos.
The first step is the formation of a sickle-shaped septum, the septum primum, which grows

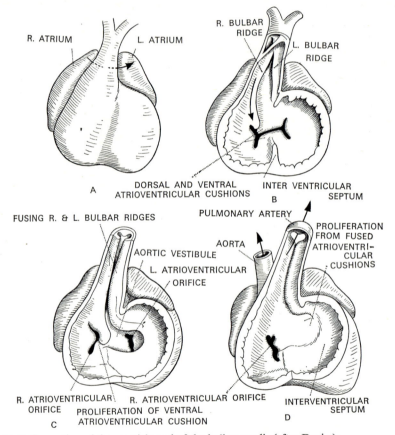

Fig. 14–8. Separation of the ventricle and of the bulbus cordis (after Davies);
    A. External view of the embryonic heart from the front;
    B. After removal of the anterior wall of the ventricle and bulbus, showing an early stage
       in the formation of the spiral bulbar septum and the tubercles of the atrioventricular
       cushions bounding the two atrioventricular orifices;
    C. Later stage in the formation of the spiral bulbar septum and the fusion of the atrio-
       ventricular cushions;
    D. Completion of the spiral bulbar septum, resulting in the formation of the pulmonary
       artery on the right and aorta on the left; note also the contributions by proliferation
       of the medial tubercles of the fused atrioventricular cushions during this process.

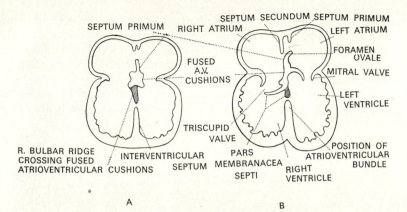

FIG. 14–9. Frontal sectional views of the developing heart to show partitioning of the atrium and ventricle (after Davies);
A. Early stage, showing the formation of the septum primum and the beginning of the septum secundum, fused atrioventricular cushions and the interventricular septum;
B. Later stage showing the final disposition of the two atrial septa (with the foramen ovale extending through both), and the formation of the atrioventricular valves.

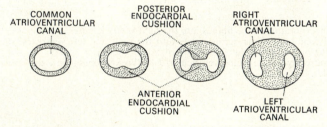

Fig. 14–10. Diagrammatic transverse sections of the developing heart showing formation of the septum in the atrioventricular canal as seen in embryos of 4, 6, 9, and 12 mm., respectively, from left to right. (After Langman.)

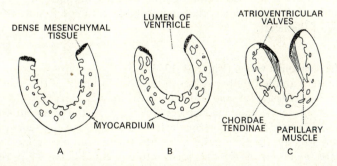

FIG. 14–11. Successive stages (from left to right) in the formation of the atrioventricular valves and chordae tendinae. Each valve is developed from localized proliferation of mesenchymal tissue (A) surrounding the atrioventricular orifice. Subsequently, the valves become hollowed out, but remain attached to the ventricular wall by means of muscular cords, the chordae tendinae (B and C). (After Langman.)

down from the middle of the roof in the sagittal plane. Its opening, the ostium primum, or foramen primum, is soon closed by its further downward extension from its free border. But soon
the upper part of the septum primum ruptures, resulting in the formation of a new opening, the
ostium or foramen secundum. Meanwhile, a second septum, the septum secundum, arises from
the roof of the right atrium and grows down slightly below the upper limit of the lower part of
the septum primum. The two septa, closely applied to each other, leave an oblique pathway (the
foramen ovale) from the right to the left atrium which remains until shortly after birth.

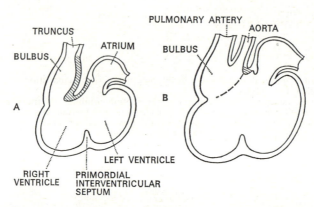

Fig. 14–12. Incorporation of the bulbus into the right ventricle (after Arey);
    A. Initial condition of the bulbus relative to the right and left ventricles, showing slow-
        growing bulbo-ventricular fold (hatched);
    B. After atrophy of the bulbo-ventricular fold (broken lines mark the former extent of
        the fold).

F. Division of the truncus arteriosus (Fig. 14–15)

As noted above, the bulbar ridges run a spiral course, and their fusion, therefore, produces a
spiral aorto-pulmonary septum. Consequently, the aorta and pulmonary trunk are virtually
twisted around each other 180°. The result is that in the distal portion of the truncus the pulmonary artery is located to the left and dorsal to the aorta (14–15D), whilst in the region of the
conus the pulmonary artery is situated to the right and ventral to the aorta (Fig. 15B). The final
outcome of this mode of development is that the aorta enters the left side, and the pulmonary
artery the right side of the heart.

G. Formation of the semilunar valves (Figs. 14–13, 14)

The fusion of the right and left bulbar ridges in the establishment of the pulmonary and aortic
trunks as just described (Figs. 14–8 and 15) involves primarily a pair of bulbar cushions (Fig.
14–13A–D), which constitute the major trunco-conal ridges. At the junction of the bulbus cordis
and truncus arteriosus, however, another smaller pair of ridges are formed; these minor ridges
alternate in position with the major ones. The subsequent fusion (face to face) of the major
ridges divides each of the two trunco-conal ridges into two equal halves (Fig. 14–13E and F). As
a result, the aorta and pulmonary artery are each provided with three thickenings of loose connective tissue covered by endocardium (Fig. 14–13F). In time, their bulbar cushions become
hollowed out on their upper surface, thereby forming the definitive semilunar valves (Fig. 14–14),
which are so named because of their characteristic cusps.

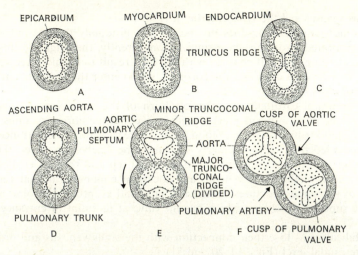

FIG. 14–13. Successive stages in the partitioning of the truncus arteriosus to form the descending aorta and pulmonary trunk (A, B, C and D), and the formation of the semilunar valves at the levels where the two vessels join their respective ventricle. This diagram also indicates the spiral rotation involved in the process (arrows, E) and the final separation of the two great vessels (arrows, F). (Refer also to Figures 14–8 and 15.) (Modified from Patten.)

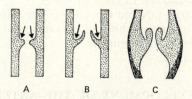

FIG. 14–14. Formation of the semilunar valves at 6, 7 and 9 weeks (from left to right). The arrows indicate the hollowing out of the endocardium-covered trunco-conal ridges to form the valves.

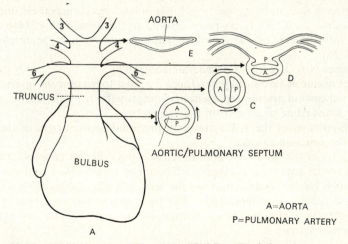

FIG. 14–15. Division of the truncus arteriosus (modified from Davies);
A. Frontal view of the embryonic heart with the 3rd, 4th and 6th aortic arches;
B. C. D. and E. Transverse sections, at four different levels, through the truncus arteriosus (arrows). (See the text for explanation.)

H. Fate of sinus venosus and the veins entering it (Fig. 14–7)

The embryonic sinus venosus does not persist but gradually flattens out and is eventually completely incorporated into the right atrium. Concurrently, the original veins which enter the sinus venosus undergo a series of changes with the final result that only three veins (the superior vena cava, the inferior vena cava and the coronary sinus) enter the right atrium. These changes may be summarized as follows.

1. The left common cardinal vein, the left horn of the sinus venosus and the transverse portion of the sinus venosus are reduced to become the coronary sinus and the oblique vein of the left atrium, returning blood from the heart wall. The entrance of the coronary sinus is guarded by a valve, formerly known as the Thebesian valve. The only remnant of the sinus venosus is a contribution to the atrial septum from its left horn.
2. The right horn of the sinus venosus and the right common cardinal vein enlarge at the expense of the same structures on the left side, and eventually become modified into the definitive superior vena cava which has no valve at its point of entrance into the atrium (Fig. 14–2).
3. The umbilical veins lose their connection with the sinus venosus and drain into the liver at a more caudal level (Figs. 14–20 and 21).
4. The vitelline veins degenerate; their disappearance is associated with the replacement of the vitelline circulation by the portal system (Figs. 14–20 and 21). During this process, the part of the right vitelline vein that remains becomes the most anterior segment of the future inferior vena cava (Fig. 14–4). The entrance of the latter into the atrium is guarded by a valve, sometimes called the Eustachian valve.
5. The valve of the coronary sinus and the valve of the inferior vena cava are both derived from the original valve of the right horn of the sinus venosus; what is left of this becomes a ligament, known as the crista terminalis.

DEVELOPMENT OF THE ARTERIES

A. The aortic arches and their derivatives (Fig. 14–16)

The aortic arches originally developed in connection with an aquatic respiratory mechanism; seven pairs develop in fish, all being functional, but in land vertebrates these undergo a process of reduction and simplification. Only six pairs develop in the human (Fig. 14–6A); their fate and transformation into arteries of the definitive adult condition may be briefly summarized as follows (Fig. 14–16).

1. Aortic arches Nos. 1, 2 and 5 degenerate completely.
2. The dorsal aortae at levels of arches 1 and 2 persist to become the internal carotid arteries.
3. The external carotid arteries represent new outgrowths from the aortic sac. After formation their bases come to arise from the 3rd arches.
4. The common stem of the 3rd aortic arch proximal to the origin of the external carotid becomes the common carotid.
5. The two sides of the 4th aortic arch develop along different courses. On the right — the right half of the aortic sac enlarges and becomes transformed into the brachio-cephalic artery (which has no counterpart on the left), the main stem from which the common carotid and subclavian artery arise. The right subclavian artery has three components: (a) the right 4th aortic arch (b) a portion of the dorsal aorta, and (c) the 7th cervical intersegmental artery.

   On the left — the left half of the aortic sac (corresponding to the brachio-cephalic artery) and the left 4th aortic arch (corresponding to the proximal portion of the right subclavian artery) constitute two of the five components of the definiti ve aortic arch (s below). The left subclavian artery is a branch of the aortic arch, equivalent to the 7th intersegmental artery.

6. The 6th aortic arches become the pulmonary arteries, which open into the right ventricle via the pulmonary trunk. Each pulmonary artery consists of two components: (a) a new vessel growing from the middle of the 6th arch toward the lung primordium; (b) the ventral end of the 6th arch vessel. The components of the definitive aortic arch from proximal to distal, are;

    (1) A truncus portion, the distal part of the arteriosus.
    (2) The left half of the ventral aorta.
    (3) The left-half of the aortic sac.
    (4) The 4th aortic arch on the left side.
    (5) The left dorsal aorta caudal to the 4th arch, or the descending aorta.

Subsequent to these changes (Fig. 14–17A), the vessels undergo further shifts in position relative to one another and finally arrive at a totally different configuration. One important factor involved in this process is the caudal migration of the vessels in order to keep pace with the lengthening neck. Another factor is the asymmetry of the two sides, caused by the fact that the aortic arch is on the left and the brachio-cephalic artery on the right. The outcome is that three large arteries arise directly from the adult aortic arch (Fig. 14–17B) (a) the left subclavian (b) the left common carotid and (c) the brachio-cephalic artery.

The asymmetry of the right and left subclavian arteries is produced by the degeneration of that part of the right dorsal aorta between the right subclavian and the union of the aortae. This same degeneration also accounts for the arch of the aorta being on the left side.

B. Branches of the descending (dorsal) aorta (Fig. 14–18)
    These may be tabulated as follows.
    1. Dorsal (intersegmental) branches (Fig. 14–18A)

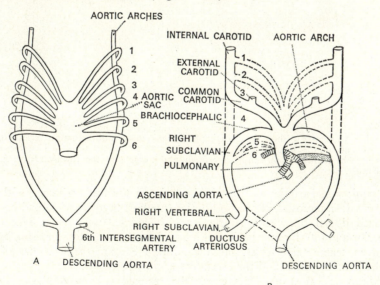

FIG. 14–16. Diagrams (in ventral view) of the transformation of the human aortic arches (modified from Arey);
    A. Full set of 6 pairs of aortic arches prior to the onset of degeneration and transformation;
    B. After transformation, showing how the dorsal vessels spread laterally: persisting vessels are shown by continuous lines; discontinued vessels by broken lines; atrophied vessels are stippled (1–6 = aortic arches).

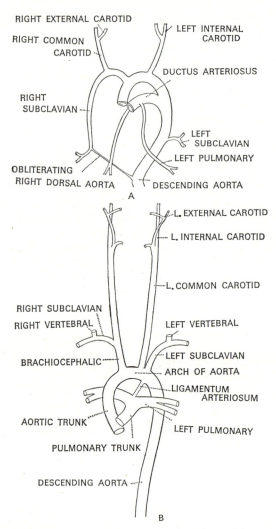

FIG. 14–17. A diagram to show the changing positional relations of the main arteries, especially the subclavian, the diagram is a ventral view (modified from Arey); A, at 17 mm.; B, adult form. The changes from A to B are brought about chiefly by the downwards migration of the heart.

Dorsal rami: spinal arteries and vertebral arteries (in the adult, a branch of the subclavian);
Ventral rami: intercostal (thoracic) arteries (lumbar, thyro-cervical and costo-cervical);
Specialized dorsal branches: subclavian (6th cervical); common iliac (5th lumbar); superior and inferior epigastric and internal mammary arteries arising by anastomoses between segmental arteries. In the adult, there are the branches of the brachio-cephalic on the right and the ascending aorta on the left.

2. Lateral branches (most of them segmentally arranged) (Fig. 14–18B).
Renal, suprarenal, inferior phrenic, internal spermatic (or ovarian) arteries.

3. Ventral branches (median and unpaired) (Fig. 14–18C).
(a) Originating from the vitelline arteries: coeliac, superior mesenteric and inferior mesenteric arteries.
(b) Originating from the umbilical arteries: common iliac and hypogastric.

C. Arteries of the head, neck and brain (Fig. 14–19)

The dorsal rami supply the spinal cord, including the dorsal muscles and the skin. The vertebral artery arises from two series of dorsal rami belonging to the neck which undergo longitudinal linkage just dorsal to the ribs; only the very caudal one of the series persists to function as the vertebral artery (Fig. 14–19A). This artery, along with the subclavian, takes its origin from the 7th cervical intersegmental artery (Fig. 14–16B). The vertebral arteries join with certain branches of the internal carotids, the resulting linkage constituting the basilar artery beneath the brain. Anastomoses between the basilar and the internal carotids produce the circulus arteriosus of Willis (Fig. 14–19B), so providing multiple routes of arterial supply to the brain.

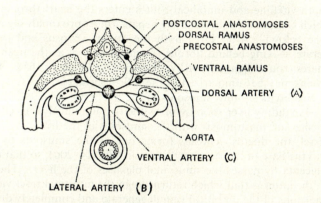

FIG. 14–18. Diagrams (cross sections) through the abdominal region of an embryo showing the three types of arteries arising from the descending aorta (after Davies); A. Dorsal (intersegmental) arteries; B. Lateral (visceral) arteries; C. Ventral (splanchnic) arteries.

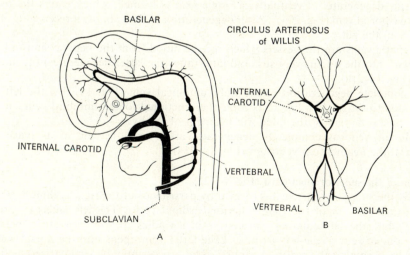

FIG. 14–19. Arteries of the head and neck region in the human embryo (after Arey); A. at 6 weeks, viewed from the left side; B. at 14 weeks, seen in ventral view.

DEVELOPMENT OF THE VEINS

A. The portal circulation (Figs. 14–20, 21).

The development of the portal system, which involves the embryonic liver and the two vitelline veins, provides a means for the blood from the gastrointestinal tract to pass through the liver on way to the heart. When completed it consists of a network of sinusoids inside the liver, which connect at one end (proximal) with the hepatic vein and at the other with one single vessel, the portal vein. At the same time the umbilical veins begin to degenerate in anticipation of a complete abandonment of the placental circulation at birth. The disappearance of the right umbilical vein occurs very early. The left umbilical vein loses its proximal portion and establishes connection with the base of the right vitelline vein through a large oblique vessel, the ductus venosus, so that blood from both vitelline and umbilical routes enters the heart through the base of the right vitelline vein, which is destined to become the hepatic (most proximal) segment of the future inferior vena cava (see below). After birth both the ductus venosus and the functional left umbilical vein degenerate, leaving behind fibrous remnants known as the ligamentum venosum and the ligamentum teres (round ligament of liver), respectively (see p. 165). The formation of the portal system of veins may be summarized in the following steps:

1. Both vitelline veins break up into sinusoids in the liver (Fig. 14–20B).
2. The continually expanding liver soon involves the two umbilical veins (Fig. 14–20c), each of which establishes an anastomosis with the sinusoids of the liver.
3. A diagonal vessel, the ductus venosus, forms out of the sinusoids to connect the left umbilical vein to the base of the right vitelline vein (Fig. 14–20c), so that the blood returning from the placenta by-passes the sinusoidal plexuses of the liver. The only blood that will go through the latter is that which returns from the intestinal tract via the portal vein.
4. The proximal portions of the umbilical vein degenerate and completely disappear, together with the sinus venosus (Fig. 14–20D).
5. That part of the left vitelline vein between the liver and the heart also degenerates so that blood carried by both the vitelline and umbilical veins enters the heart through the base of the right vitelline vein.
6. The two vitelline veins form anastomoses near their entrance to the liver and parts of the two veins degenerate. Eventually, a single vein is formed, which enters the liver as the definitive portal vein (Fig. 20A). After degeneration of the yolk sac it receives the mesenteric veins from the gut.
7. The hepatic veins are the vessels which receive blood from the hepatic sinusoids draining it at first, into the ductus venosus, and later (after the latter degenerates) the inferior vena cava (Fig. 14–21B).
8. After complete degeneration of the right umbilical vein (Fig. 14–21A) the left umbilical vein shifts to the median line to become the functional foetal umbilical vein; it is located in the caudal margin of the falciform ligament of the liver.
10. The ductus venosus completely degenerates after birth, leaving in its place a fibrous remnant, the ligamentum venosum (Fig. 14–21B).

B. Formation of the superior vena cava (Fig. 14–22)

Essentially the superior vena cava is formed by persistence of the right common cardinal vein and the proximal portion of the right anterior cardinal vein. The left anterior cardinal vein degenerates, while the left common cardinal vein dwindles in size, persisting merely as the stem of the oblique vein of the left atrium. (The latter vein opens into the dorsal wall of right atrium, thereby becoming the coronary sinus.) The process may be summarized as follows.

1. An oblique anastomosis develops between the two anterior cardinal veins; this new cross vessel becomes the left brachio-cephalic vein (Fig. 14–22B).

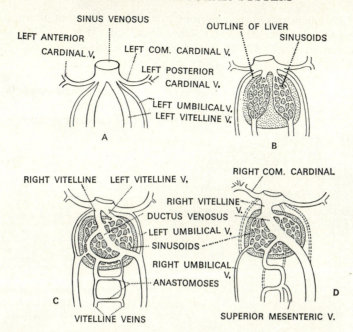

FIG. 14–20. Diagrams to show the early development of the portal system of veins:
A. Initial condition (sinus venosus receives 3 pairs of veins);
B. Formation of the hepatic anastomoses;
C. Involvement of the umbilical veins in the hepatic sinusoids, and formation of anastomoses between the left and right vitelline veins posterior to the liver;
D. Fate of the umbilical and vitelline veins.   Broken lines indicate degenerated vessels.

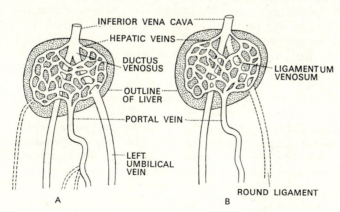

FIG. 14–21. Diagrams to show the foetal (A) and adult (B) stages of the portal system of veins

2. The union between this new vein and the right anterior cardinal vein marks a junction: below this point, the proximal portion of the right anterior cardinal and the right common cardinal form the superior vena cava; above the junction, the distal portion of the right anterior cardinal as far as the base of the internal jugular vein becomes the right brachiocephalic vein.

F

3. Further cephalic extensions of the anterior cardinal from the point of origin of the external jugulars constitute the internal jugular vein on both sides (Fig. 14–22c).
4. The external jugular veins on both sides represent new growths appearing at a later stage of development.
5. The subclavian veins of the two sides are asymmetrical. The left one originates close to the junction of the left internal jugular vein and the left brachio-cephalic vein, whereas the right subclavian opens directly into the right brachio-cephalic vein. These veins attain their final positions as described above only after the caudal migration of the heart has taken place (Fig. 14–22c).

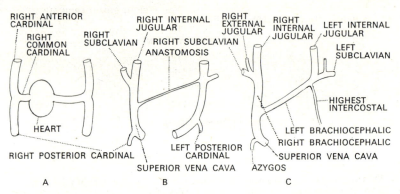

Fig. 14–22. Diagrams in ventral view to show the transformation of the cardinal veins (after Arey):
A. at 6 weeks; B. at 8 weeks; C. adult.

C. Formation of the inferior vena cava (Figs. 14–23, 24)

During the foetal period three pairs of cardinal veins develop in the abdominal region, all of which are associated at one time or another with the mesonephric kidney; these are the posterior, sub- and supra-cardinal veins (Fig. 14–23). Most of the posterior cardinals degenerate, their remnants become part of the azygos system of veins, other parts of the azygos vein system arising from the remains of the supracardinals. Both the subcardinal and supracardinal veins participate in the formation of the inferior vena cava (Fig. 14–24A, B).

The posterior cardinal veins are directly continuous with the anterior cardinal veins and extend along the dorsal surface of the mesonephros. They receive blood from the embryonic kidney, and from segmental veins draining the intercostal and lumbar regions of the body wall. The subcardinal veins, which appear slightly later, run along the ventral sides of the mesonephros, making anastomoses with the posterior cardinal veins. The supracardinal veins which appear even later run along the dorso-medial surface of the mesonephros (Fig. 14–23).

The inferior vena cava, when completely formed, consists of four components with the following origins (Fig. 14–24A):

Component No. 1. This is the hepatic portion consisting of (a) part of the original ductus venosus and (b) a new diagonal vein, connecting the ductus venosus with the proximal end of the right subcardinal vein.

Component No. 2. This is a pre-renal segment, consisting of the right subcardinal vein as far caudally as the anastomoses between the subcardinal veins.

Component No. 3. A short section, consisting of the right inter-subcardinal anastomosis which forms a bridge between the subcardinal and supracardinal veins.

Component No. 4. The post-renal segment originates from the caudal portion of the right supracardinal vein from the renal anastomoses to the iliac anastomoses. Components Nos. 3 and 4 comprise the so-called sacrocardinal segment of the inferior vena cava, receiving tributaries as lumbar veins.

These four component segments of the inferior vena cava finally straighten out to form the definitive inferior vena cava (Fig. 14–24B), a process which is completed by the end of the 8th week. Those portions of the three pairs of cardinal veins which participate neither in the formation of the inferior vena cava nor in the development of the azygos vein system, eventually atrophy and disappear altogether.

The connection between the inferior vena cava and the common iliac veins does not occur in the mid-line, being much closer to the right than to the left. The consequence of this asymmetry is that the left common iliac vein is much longer than its right counterpart (Fig. 14–24A).

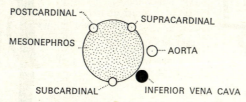

FIG. 14–23. Diagram (transverse view) through the veins at the level of the hepatic segment of the developing inferior vena cava (only the right side is shown) to illustrate the relative positions of the three cardinal veins with respect to the kidney (mesonephros).

D. The azygos system of veins (Fig. 14–24B)
The azygos veins fall into three groups as follows.
1. The azygos — this consists of portions of the right posterior cardinal vein and portions of the right supracardinal vein.
2. The hemiazygos — this originates from part of the left supracardinal vein and from an anastomosis with the azygos.
3. The accessory hemiazygos — this is the adult representative of that part of the left posterior cardinal vein which joins the azygos through the left supracardinal and an anastomosis.

E. The pulmonary veins
The pulmonary veins develop in the mesenchyme surrounding the endodermal lung buds; they grow towards the heart and connect with the left atrium.

STAGES IN THE DEVELOPMENT OF THE CIRCULATION AND ITS CHANGES AFTER BIRTH

Up to the end of the third week of development vessels carry blood between the embryo and chorion. There is also a small nominal circulation in the yolk sac.

Circulation of the embryonic period (Fig. 14–25; cf. also Fig. 14–7) from the 3rd to 8th week.
During this period the heart is tubular and has four chambers which are, caudocephalically, the sinus venosus, auricle, ventricle and bulbus cordis. The sinus venosus receives venous blood from three pairs of veins (Fig. 14–7). These are the systemic common cardinals, the vitelline and the umbilical veins (Fig. 14–25). The latter are the most important because they return blood

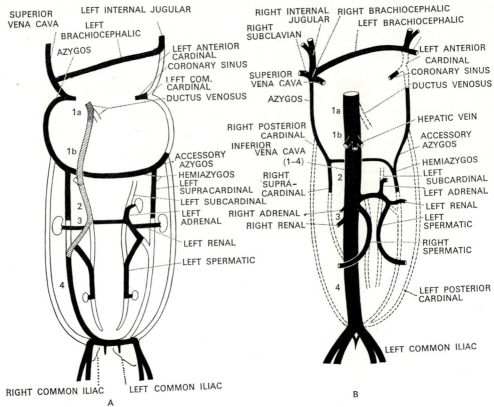

FIG. 14–24. Diagrams to show the development of the superior and inferior venae cavae and
the azygos veins (embryonic veins drawn as if spread out in one plane):
    A. Early stage. Persistent veins are shown in solid black; degenerating vessels, unshaded.
       The five segments of the developing inferior vena cava (1a, 1b, 2, 3, 4) are represented
       differentially in order to indicate their respective origins;
    B. Adult stage. Persistent veins are shown in solid black; degenerating vessels in broken
       lines. The definitive inferior vena cava is formed from corresponding vessels of the two
       sides as indicated by the broken unshaded line in the middle. Its different definitive
       portions bear the same numericals as in Figure 14–24A.

loaded with oxygen and food from the placenta via the umbilical cord; this is immediately
mixed with venous blood brought in by the cardinal veins. Nevertheless, it is this blood of intermediate quality (as far as oxygen content is concerned) that successfully nourishes the growing
embryo. This blood leaves the heart through the ventral aorta and passes via the aortic arches
into the paired dorsal aortae from which various branches (including a pair of vitelline arteries
to the yolk sac) supply the body tissues. The chorionic villi are supplied by the umbilical arteries
which originate from the caudal end of the aorta. The intra-embryonic circulatory pattern at
this stage resembles closely that of the adult fish.

The foetal circulation (from the third month of pregnancy, to about one month postnatal)

Since the foetal lungs are not yet functioning, there is little or no pulmonary circulation in
operation. The oxygenated and food-rich blood carried by the umbilical veins from the placenta
passes via the inferior vena cava to the right atrium where it becomes mixed with the venous
blood that circulates through the systemic system. Part of this blood in the right atrium enters

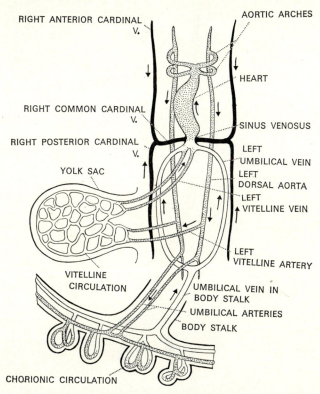

FIG. 14–25. Diagram (ventral view) of human circulation in the embryonic period, showing the main intra- and extra-embryonic blood vessels in an approximately 4 mm. embryo (at the end of the fourth week of development) (modified from Dodds). Arrows show the direction of blood flow. Venous blood, solid black; mixed or intermediate blood, stippled; oxygenated blood, unshaded.

the left atrium through the foramen ovale; part of it goes to the right ventricle. Blood from the left atrium (which has not received any blood from the embryonic lungs) immediately goes into the left ventricle and out into the aortic arch. The foramen ovale thus provides a device for short-circuiting most of the pulmonary circulation. Blood from the right ventricle which should (as in the adult) be sent to the lungs for oxygenation via the pulmonary trunk, is also short circuited into the aortic arch through a short vessel, known as the ductus arteriosus, connecting the aortic and pulmonary trunks. The ductus arteriosus thus serves as a device for preventing blood from entering the yet unprepared lungs and, together with the foramen ovale, is essential for achieving equalization of the systemic circulation in the absence of a functional pulmonary circuit. Thus, the two sides of the heart sustain equal pressure and no damage is done to the lungs (Fig. 14–26).

Changes in the circulation at birth (Fig. 14–27)

It is evident from the above that with the elimination of the placenta at birth the umbilical circulation must be quickly replaced by a pulmonary circulation; as a result of this transformation some vessels become fibrosed and form so-called ligaments. These are (a) the ligamentum teres formed from the left umbilical vein (b) the ligamentum venosum formed from the ductus venosus and later, (c) the lateral umbilical ligaments derived from the two umbilical arteries (Fig. 14–27).

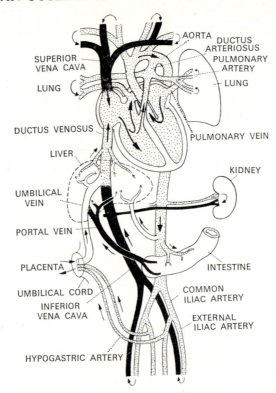

FIG. 14–26. Diagram of the foetal circulation. Arrows indicate directions of blood flow. The degree of oxygenation of the blood is differentiated as follows: completely oxygenated, unshaded; completely venous, solid black; intermediate or mixed, stippled.

With the initiation of the pulmonary function the foramen ovale, ductus arteriosus and ductus venosus are abolished by closure. The closing of the foramen ovale is mechanically facilitated by falling pressures in the pulmonary artery and inferior vena cava, coupled with rising arterial pressure in the left atrium. These factors combine to press the septum primum against the septum secundum, thereby producing an effective closure of the foramen ovale. The closure eventually leaves a scar, known as the fossa ovalis. A ligament, termed the ligamentum arteriosum is what is left of the ductus arteriosus. There is some question as to how quickly this transition from the foetal to adult circulation is accomplished. It was formerly believed that it took place rather quickly, beginning from the initiation of the respiratory movements; the inflation of the lungs brought about a sudden great increase in the capacity of the pulmonary capillaries and from that point, pulmonary and systemic circuits reached an equilibrium. It is now generally held, however, that the transition is a more gradual one, taking possibly a month for the completion of the whole process. A final change is an increase in the thickness of the ventricular wall. The wall of the left ventricle attains greater thickness as a functional adaptation. The typical adult preponderance of the left over the right ventricle is probably not reached until the seventh year.

Fate of the vitelline and umbilical vessels

Unlike the vitelline and umbilical veins which mostly vanish, the vitelline and umbilical arteries persist to become part of the adult arterial system. The transition from the foetal to adult condition takes place gradually without changes in function.

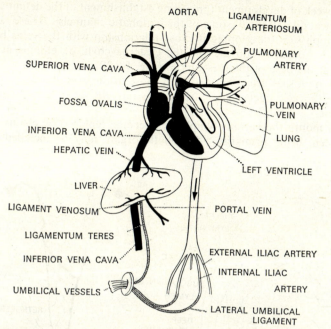

AORTA

LIGAMENTUM ARTERIOSUM

SUPERIOR VENA CAVA

PULMONARY ARTERY

FOSSA OVALIS

PULMONARY VEIN

INFERIOR VENA CAVA

LUNG

HEPATIC VEIN

LEFT VENTRICLE

LIVER

LIGAMENT VENOSUM

PORTAL VEIN

LIGAMENTUM TERES

INFERIOR VENA CAVA

EXTERNAL ILIAC ARTERY

INTERNAL ILIAC ARTERY

UMBILICAL VESSELS

LATERAL UMBILICAL LIGAMENT

FIG. 14–27. Diagram (ventral view) of changes in the human circulation after birth. Oxygenated blood is shown unshaded; venous blood, solid black.

The vitelline arteries of the yolk sac gradually fuse to form the arteries supplying the entire gastrointestinal tract, represented in the adult, by the coelic, superior mesenteric and inferior mesenteric arteries (p. 158).

The umbilical arteries, originally a pair of ventral branches of the dorsal aorta, serve the vital function of bringing the foetal blood to be oxygenated in the placenta. During the fourth week of development each of them acquires a secondary connection with a dorsal branch of the aorta, the common iliac artery (Fig. 14–27), after which their original connection with the aorta completely atrophies. After birth, the proximal portions of the umbilical arteries become the internal iliac and the superior vesical arteries, while their distal portions become fibrosed and remain as the lateral vesicle umbilical ligaments (Fig. 14–27).

THE LYMPHATIC SYSTEM

The lymphatic system consists of a network of channels by which the tissues are constantly bathed in a circulating plasma-like fluid. This fluid, known as lymph, seeps out from the blood into interstitial spaces and returns through the lymphatic channels back into the vascular system via the veins. Because of its close association with the venous system, it may be considered as an " auxiliary " of the latter.

The lymphatic vessels, once thought to be outgrowths of the blood vascular system, arise independently but in similar manner to the blood vessels, i.e., through continuous sprouting from mesenchyme, the cells of which assume an endothelial character. Through subsequent coalescence of adjacent channels a closed system of lymphatics is finally established at the end of the second month.

During the sixth week of development (preceding establishment of the definitive system) lymph sacs are formed as local dilatations of some of the lymphatic channels. These sacs consist of the jugular and iliac lymph sacs (developing in close relationship with the veins bearing the same names) plus a retroperitoneal lymph sac and the Cisterna chyli, developing at the level of the adrenal gland lying at the base of the mesenteries (Fig. 14–28).

The abdominal lymph sacs are connected with those in the neck by means of a longitudinal " trunk " vessel, the thoracic duct. The latter drains into the left internal jugular vein via the left jugular lymph sac.

During the third month the various lymph sacs become replaced by chains of lymph glands or nodes. The spleen, being primarily a lymphatic organ, may be included in this category (Fig. 14–28).

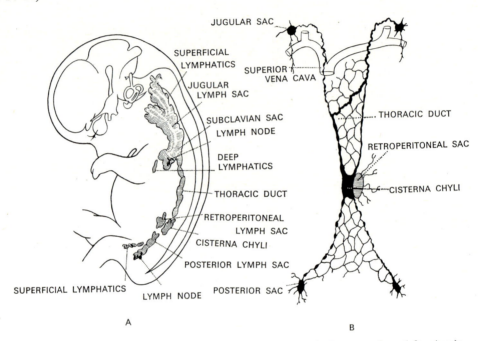

Fig. 14–28. Development of the primary lymphatic vessels in the human embryo (after Arey):
A. Primitive lymphatic system (shown in profile) in an embryo of 9 weeks;
B. Diagram, in ventral view, of the definitive thoracic duct emerging from the definitive lymphatic plexuses.

CARDIOVASCULAR ANOMALIES

In view of the large number of components and rather complicated, yet precise, developmental mechanisms involved in the establishment of the definitive heart and vessels it is understandable that the structural anomalies of the cardiovascular system are high in both frequency and variety. It may be said in general that variations in the pattern of the vessels, arteries or veins, which do not present a functional obstruction are of no consequence; in fact, some of them (e.g., variation in the aortic arches) may go unnoticed. On the other hand, defects and malformations of the heart are usually more serious because it is likely that they will lead to functional disorder or to death. Examples of these will be given below. Modern advances in surgery have, however, proved capable of correcting some of these defects in infancy, thus saving many lives.

As in all other cases of developmental anomalies the causative factors involved here are either genetical, environmental or both. Certain congenital anomalies of the heart are known to run in families, although their exact mode of inheritance is incompletely understood. Further elucidation of this subject depends on the acquisition and study of an increasing number of family pedigree reports.

Recently, there has been increasing experimental evidence that many teratogenic agents (trypan blue, vitamin or oxygen deficiency, x-ray-irradiation, etc.) can produce congenital cardiovascular anomalies in laboratory animals. This does not necessarily mean that the same agents may cause similar defects in human infants. The only positive case well accepted today is that caused by the German measles virus. Many cases of heart malformations (associated with cataract and deafness) in the newborn have been traced to pregnant mothers who contracted German measles during early pregnancy. Some of the most frequent heart abnormalities attributable to this virus are (a) persistent ductus arteriosus; (b) ventricular septal defect; (c) Fallot's tetralogy; (d) atrial septal defect; (e) pulmonary valvular stenosis.

Abnormalities of the heart

A. Severe gross Abnormalities
   1. Acardia. This is complete absence of a heart, a monstrous condition often associated with twins sharing a common placenta (the other twin is usually a normal individual).
   2. Ectopia cordis. A heart with a bifid ventricle. The organ is usually exposed on the surface of the chest with the result that the body wall becomes enclosed only by a non-muscular membranous layer.
   3. Dextro-cardia. This is a transposition involving the left to right reversal of the heart and its great vessels. The condition evidently stems from primary reversal of the primitive cardiac loop. It could be associated with total transposition of the viscera.

B. Multiple defect — tetralogy of Fallot (Fig. 14–29B)
   This is a complex condition which involves four features. (a) Stenosis of the pulmonary artery, with the consequence that only part of the venous blood from the right ventricle goes to the lung. (b) Presence of a permanent interventricular foramen as a result of a ventricular septal defect. (c) Over-riding of the ventricular septum by the mouth of the aorta. In consequence of this the aorta receives blood from both ventricles. (d) Hypertrophy of the right ventricle as a result of its being over-worked in an effort to force blood past the stenosis of the pulmonary artery. The overall result of these combined conditions is poor oxygenation of the blood as a result of little blood reaching the lungs and the blood (of reduced oxygen content) being further degraded in the left ventricle before it is pumped out through the aorta. Fallot's tetralogy results in a typical case of a " blue baby ". The defects can be corrected by open heart surgery performed in time.

C. Septal Defects
   1. Ventricular septal defect (Fig. 14–29A). The persistent ventricular foramen occupies a location which may extend as high as the origin of pulmonary artery. The defect originates from an absent or weakened membranous part of the septum.
   2. Atrial septal defects:
      (a) due to excessive resorption of the septum primum
      (b) as a result of inadequate development of the septum secundum
      (c) a persistent foramen ovale guarded by a defective (multiperforate) valve, or with no valve at all.

D. Anomalies of the great vessels
   (Usually these are cases of failure of vessels to degenerate or fibrose.)
   1. Persistent ductus arteriosus.
   2. Persistent truncus arteriosus. The pulmonary arteries arise from the common trunk whilst the unfused bulbar ridges become a four-cusped valve with a patent interventricular foramen beneath the valve.
   3. Stenosis of pulmonary artery (Fig. 14–29D). This is a narrowing of the lumen with atresia of the valves and usually associated with a patent ductus arteriosus. As a consequence of this anomaly little blood goes to the lung.

E. Anomalies of the atrio-ventricular canal
   1. Persistent atrio-ventricular canal, usually accompanied by a septal defect involving the atrial as well as the ventricular portion of the heart.
   2. Atresia of the tricuspid valve.
   3. Incomplete fusion of the atrio-ventricular endocardial cushions.

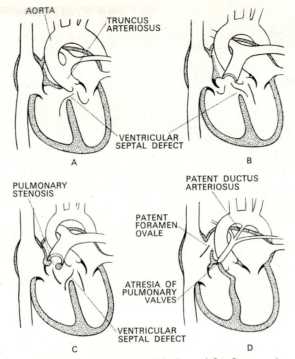

FIG. 14–29. Abnormalities of the heart (after Langman):
A. Ventricular septal defect;
B. Tetralogy of Fallot;
C. Aortic valvular stenosis and atresia;
D. Stenosis of the pulmonary artery.

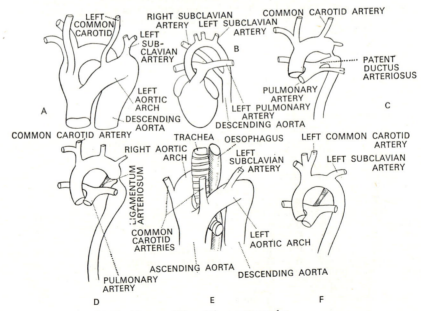

FIG. 14–30. Abnormalities of the great vessels:
A. Double aortic arch;
B. Anomalous right subclavian artery;
C. Preductal coarctation of the aorta;
D. Postductal coarctation of the aorta;
E. Interrupted aortic arch;
F. Abnormal origin of the left common carotid artery.

F. Stenosis of the semilunar valves
    1. Aortic valvular stenosis and atresia (Fig. 14–29c).
    2. See D.3 above.

    Abnormalities of the great arteries and veins. These defects are common occurrences which may be caused by any one of these known factors (a) choice of unusual paths in the primitive vascular plexuses (b) persistence of vessels normally obliterated (c) disappearance of vessels normally retained (d) incomplete development of vascular rudiments (e) fusion and absorption of parts usually distinct.

A. Abnormalities of the great arteries
    1. Persistence of a double aortic arch (Fig. 14–30A).
    2. Anomalous right subclavian artery. This is formed from the distal part of the persistent right dorsal aorta and the 7th intersegmental artery (Fig. 14–30B).
    3. Coarctation of the aorta, usually compensated by the institution of a by-pass system of vessels: (a) preductal (Fig. 14–30c); (b) postductal (Fig. 14–30D).
    4. Interrupted aortic arch. This is caused by obliteration of the fourth aortic arch on the left side. It is frequently combined with an abnormal origin of the subclavian artery. In consequence the aorta supplies the head region only; the remainder of body is supplied by the pulmonary artery by way of the persistent ductus arteriosus. It is a serious defect (Fig. 14–30E).
    5. Aortic arch persists on the right side.
    6. Abnormal origin of left common carotid artery (Fig. 14–30F).

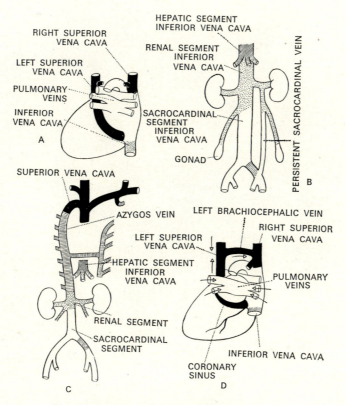

FIG. 14–31. Abnormal venous drainages:
    A. Double superior vena cava;
    B. Double inferior vena cava;
    C. Absent inferior vena cava;
    D. Anomalous pulmonary venous drainage.

B. Abnormal venous drainage
   1. Double superior vena cava (Fig. 14–31A).
   2. Double inferior vena cava (Fig. 14–31B).
   3. Absence of the inferior vena cava (Fig. 14–31C).
   4. Accessory posterior renal vena cava on the left.
   5. Rudimentary pre-renal vena cava, completed with a compensatory development of the azygos veins.
   6. Anomalous pulmonary venous drainage (Fig. 14–31D). The pulmonary veins enter the left superior vena cava, which in turn enters the right superior vena cava by way of the brachio-cephalic vein.

CHAPTER 15

SUPPORTING TISSUES AND THE SKELETAL SYSTEM

Introduction

The cells of all three germ layers are potentially endowed with the property of becoming "mesenchymal". This assumption of mesenchymal characteristics may be of a transient nature, lasting briefly during the course of differentiation (e.g. early neural crest cells, myoblasts, oesteoblasts, etc.) or of a permanent nature (e.g. fibrocytes, phagocytes, melanocytes, etc.). Note that the examples of mesenchymal cells given above are either of ectodermal or mesodermal origin. This is because these two germ layers possess in a high degree the ability to become transformed into mesenchyme in contrast to endoderm, which normally is not transformable in this way. The only exception to this is the case of the migratory primordial sex cells (pp. 2, 129).

Mesenchymal cells have a number of characteristics, four of which are considered here because they are especially relevant to connective tissue. They are: (*a*) stellate cells, i.e., they possess processes (*b*) capable of forming anastomoses with neighbouring similar cells by touching of their processes (*c*) capable of extensive migration (Fig. 15–1) and (*d*) capable of secreting specific chemical substances, which fill the intercellular spaces. Of these, the last characteristic is the most pertinent to the present discussion because this property of secretion is directly concerned with the formation of all kinds of supporting tissues. The different varieties of formed supporting tissues (cartilage, bone, tendon, etc.) are to be recognized by the nature of the substance elaborated by the connective tissue cells in question.

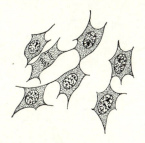

Fig. 15–1. Embryonic mesenchymal cells of mesodermal origin, one of them undergoing mitosis.

Thus, all embryonic connective tissues (the precursors of the definitive supporting tissues) are characterized by a matrix (Fig. 15–4A), which is often spoken of as the "ground substance" of a connective tissue. However, ground substance and matrix when used in this context may not be synonymous terms. A ground substance is generally fluid or semi-fluid; it is only when it becomes impregnated with a hardening substance that a ground substance is transformed or converted into a definitive matrix. The impregnating substances can be cellular products, such as collagenous or elastic fibres, or chemicals such as calcium salts, or both. It is interesting to note that the cells which produce different supporting tissues (e.g., fibroblasts, chondroblasts, oesteoblasts) may not differ much from one another in appearance in their undifferentiated stage, yet their secretions produced structures which are unmistakeably distinct.

Types of connective tissues (Fig. 15–2)
1. Reticular. This is the most primitive and departs least from the embryonic type (excepting the mucous tissue of the umbilical cord). Reticular tissue is argyrophilic, i.e., can be stained with silver; generally it is regarded as the forerunner of collagenous fibres.
2. Fibro-elastic. This contains both collagenous (Fig. 15–2B) and elastic (Fig. 15–2C) fibres, which are believed to be the products of fibrocytes (Fig. 15–2B); the former appear at about the third week, the latter by the sixth month of development.
   Examples of formed connective tissues
       Loose or areolar—mesentery, subcutaneous tissue.
       Elastic—periosteum, fascia.
       Collagenous—tendon, ligament.
3. Adipose. Lipoblasts which are specialized for storing fat (Fig. 15–2A).

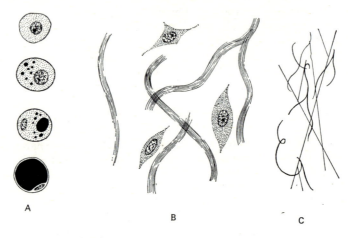

A

B

C

Fig. 15–2. Various connective tissues:
   A. Four successive stages (from top) in the differentiation of an adipose cell (fat shown in black);
   B. Skin of pig embryo showing collagenous fibres amid several fibrocytes;
   C. Elastic fibres such as are present in subcutaneous tissue.

CARTILAGE

Formation of cartilage commences in the fifth week by the activities of the chondroblasts. These cells aggregate and begin to grow by both interstitial growth and appositional growth. In the former, the cells proliferate, each rounds up and starts to secrete a matrix which causes the congested cells to separate from one another; each repeatedly divides to form groups of two or more cells which are confined in capsules (Fig. 15–3). Interstitial growth soon slows down from the centre peripherally. Further growth is made possible by activities of chondroblasts concentrated at the periphery, which form an active layer called the perichondrium. Through their activity of matrix formation, the cartilage increases in size (appositional growth).

Types of cartilage
1. Hyaline cartilage. This has a matrix containing a masked feltwork of collagen fibres. Example: covering the articular surfaces of bones in synovial joints.

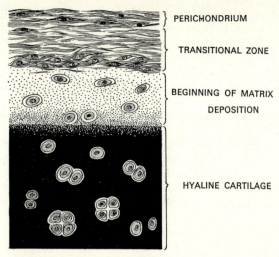

PERICHONDRIUM

TRANSITIONAL ZONE

BEGINNING OF MATRIX
DEPOSITION

HYALINE CARTILAGE

FIG. 15–3. Development of young hyaline cartilage, e.g. trachea.

2. Fibro-cartilage. This has a heavy content of collagenous fibres.
   Examples are the intervertebral disc and the pubic symphysis.
3. Elastic cartilage. This is yellow in colour, due to presence of large numbers of elastic fibres.
   Examples: epiglottis, some laryngeal cartilages, pinna of the ear.

BONE

Bone formation commences from the eighth week and continues until after puberty. The bones in our body are classified into two varieties based on their origin, rather than method of formation. Cartilage bones are those which replace a provisional cartilagenous skeleton; in other words, they have a predecessor in the form of hyaline cartilage. The membrane bones, on the other hand, develop directly from oesteoblasts at sites specifically predetermined by the genes. The method by which membrane bones are formed is the only method of bone formation since even in the case of cartilage bones, the bone is deposited in the same manner as in membrane bones once the cartilage model is eroded and absorbed to make way for the bony structure.

Fundamental processes in osteogenesis

1. Pre-ossein stage. Osteoblasts aggregate at sites of bone formation (e.g., membrane bones of skull) and begin to produce collagenous fibres mixed with a fluid ground substance. This is followed by a maturation process of the fibres in which crystals of hydroxyapatite are formed on and between them. The result is an amorphous young osteoid tissue ready to be mineralized (Fig. 15–4A).
2. Formation of spongy bone. The rounded osteoblasts begin to secrete a calcareous material (calcium salts) which impregnates the osteoid tissue so converting it into a meshwork of bone trabeculae (Fig. 15–4B). Some of the osteoblasts, having been thus slowed down metabolically, become encased or trapped in the spongy bone; others remain to form an osteogenic layer around the trabeculae to carry on further bone-forming activity. In the meantime, the mesenchyme occupying the spaces between the trabeculae forms a primary (primitive) marrow with a high vascularizing activity.

3. Formation of compact (lamellar) bone. Due to the continual activity of the osteogenic layer, the bone trabeculae grow in thickness and extent (Fig. 15–5A, B), and as the ramifying trabeculae coalesce to form a lacework (Fig. 15–5C), more osteoblasts become trapped and imprisoned in them. They are, by now, mature bone cells, the osteocytes, each of which is lodged in a lacuna. The processes of the osteocytes maintain communication with one another through tiny canaliculi. This is the beginning of the process of transforming the spongy (cancellous) bone into compact bone, which is characterized by the formation of series of concentric lamellae, each with a Haversian canal in its centre (Fig. 15–5D).

The definitive bone is reached after a period of growth and maturation during which giant multinucleated cells, the osteoclasts, play an important role. Bone is constantly being destroyed by the activity of these cells followed immediately by reconstruction by the persisting osteoblasts. This process occurs on both the inner and the outer or periosteal surfaces. It is this alternate process of bone resorption and re-deposition that finally moulds the bone into the definitive form, shape and size.

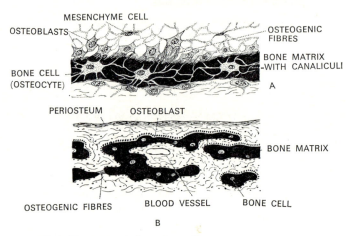

FIG. 15–4. Two stages in bone formation:
    A. Early stage, showing the beginning of matrix formation;
    B. Later stage, with beginning of bone trabeculae.

Cartilage bone

What has just been described is the process of intramembranous bone formation. The end product is known as a membrane bone. The majority of bones, however, are cartilage bones, which are preceded by an embryonic hyaline cartilage model, which more or less corresponds in shape but not in size to the future bone. The process by which a bone is formed from hyaline cartilage is known as endochondral ossification. In endochondral bone formation no cartilage is ever directly turned into bone, but mature cartilage cells and their matrix are first calcified and then give way to bony tissue in fundamentally the same way as in intramembranous bone formation. The osteogenic tissue involved in this process migrates into the calcified cartilage together with blood vessels as the first step in endochondral bone formation. Since there is only one basic mechanism of bone formation (through the activity of osteoblasts) the resulting bone has the same structure whether it is the product of intramembranous or endochondral ossification.

By the seventh week, cartilage models are present for nearly all the bones of the skeleton, and bone has begun to form in a few of them. The process may be described with the aid of

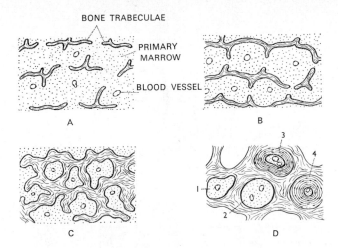

FIG. 15–5. Intramembranous bone formation:
  A. B, and C. Processes in establishing primary cancellous bone;
  D. Transformation of cancellous bone into compact bone (the numbers indicate the sequence of events).

Fig. 15–6. In A, a cylinder of periosteal bone has formed; this represents the first (earliest) bone to be laid down in most long bones and has resulted from the activity of the osteoblasts in the perichondrium (not labeled in Fig. 15–6). After this, the perichondrium becomes the periosteum of the newly-forming bone. This process of periosteal ossification continues and continually adds new bone to the outside of this initial cylinder. At the same time old bone is being eroded from the inner surface by the osteoclasts in the marrow. This process thus constitutes a mechanism for growth in the diameter of long bones. At the same time, this cylinder of periosteal bone also grows in length, extending towards both ends of the cartilage model (Fig. 15–6B, C), but never quite reaches them because the cartilage itself is also steadily lengthening.

In Fig. 15–6B, a periosteal bud (with marrow) has just invaded the cartilage, penetrating the periosteal layer at about the middle of the cartilage. This invasion is the beginning of endochondral ossification, and has two immediate results (a) the dissolution and subsequent calcification of the cartilage matrix, and (b) the destruction of columns of mature cartilage cells by contact with the invading mesenchyme. This is followed by the formation of endochondral bone on the persisting vestiges of the calcified cartilage trabeculae. In this manner, a primary spongy bone with an enlarging marrow cavity, becomes gradually established as the erosion proceeds towards both ends of the cartilage model (Fig. 15–6D), events which are taking place whilst the cartilage is still growing. It is this continual building-up of cartilage, accompanied by the simultaneous breakdown of its oldest part, that eventually produces a definitive cartilage bone of the size and shape genetically pre-determined.

Growth in long bones

In prenatal life and infancy a cartilage bone (Fig. 15–7A) is composed of a bony shaft with cartilagenous ends (Fig. 15–7B). The bony shaft is distinguishable into compact (black), periosteal (or perichondral) and endochondral (stippled) bone. During childhood and youth, secondary or epiphyseal centres of ossification appear in the cartilagenous ends of the long bone (Fig. 15–7C). Further growth of these ossification centres separates each of the cartilage ends into

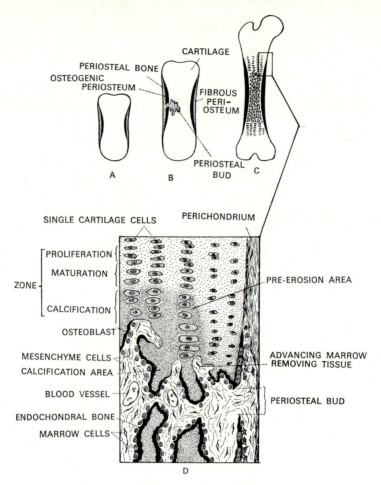

FIG. 15–6. Formation of cartilage bone (adapted from several sources):
  A, B, and C. Early stages of ossification (bone shown in black, cartilage is blank and the periosteum is stippled). The small area in C indicates the location of the area shown further magnified in D;
  D. Histological details of endochondral ossification as seen in the radius of a 125 mm. sheep embryo (bone shown in black, cartilage is lightly stippled and calcified cartilage is heavily stippled).

two cartilagenous parts, one on each side of the epiphyseal ossification centre itself (Fig. 15–7D). They are (a) the terminal articular cartilage, covering the articular surface and (b) the epiphyseal plate. This latter allows the full adult length of the bone to be attained. During the entire period of growth the proliferating epiphyseal plate separates the ossification centres of the epiphysis and diaphysis or shaft of the bone (Fig. 15–7D). Eventually the epiphyseal plate stops growing, starts to get thinner, and finally breaks up, with the result that the spongy bone of the diaphysis and epiphysis merge and become fused (Fig. 15–7E). This marks the end of growth of the bone in length. Subsequently, the epiphysis becomes enclosed in a thin shell of endochondral bone except at the articular surface, where a layer of hyaline cartilage is permanently retained to function as the free surface in a movable joint (see below). The most important factor in control of this timing is the chondrogenic hormone of the anterior pituitary (p. 200).

Growth in diameter of the bone is through resorption at the inner limit of the marrow cavity (Fig. 15–7D) accompanied by renewed activity of the periosteal osteoblasts. A steady increase in the size of the central marrow cavity is thus achieved together with the deposition of additional periosteal lamellae on the surface of the bone shaft. Figure 15–7E shows a human femur at birth superimposed in the marrow cavity of an adult femur to show their relative sizes and the amount of deposition and internal resorption of bone which takes place during growth. The final attainment of the definitive shape and contour of the bone, especially at the ends, depends on resorption and remodelling going on simultaneously with the deposition of new bone. The consequence of the failure of such a corrective measure is illustrated in Fig. 15–7F, which shows what would happen if, during elongation of the femur, the new bony deposits (stippled) were not properly corrected.

Factors regulating oesteogenesis
    (a) Hormones produced by the hypophysis, parathyroid and thyroid (see Chapter 17).
    (b) Alkaline phosphatase produced by the oesteoblasts; this enzyme is essential for the deposition of calcium salts.
    (c) Vitamin D (or sunlight) and mineral salts (calcium, phosphates).
    (d) Certain undetermined local factors.

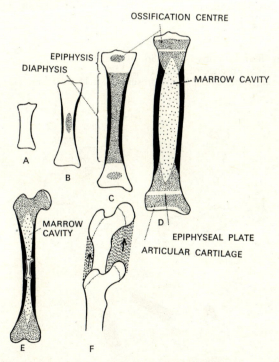

FIG. 15–7. Ossification and growth in a long bone (after Arey):
  A. Cartilagenous stage;
  B. Deposition of spongy endochondral bone (stippled) and compact perichondral bone (black);
  C. Appearance of an epiphysis at each end;
  D. Union of the epiphyses, leaving a plate of articular cartilage at the free ends, and enlargement of the marrow cavity by the resorption of periosteal bone centrally as deposition continues peripherally;
  E. Superposition of a human femur at birth in the marrow cavity of an adult femur to show the relative sizes, and the amount of deposition and internal resorption during growth;
  F. Two periods in the elongation of a femur illustrating the shape (stippled) that would prevail were the steady deposition of bone not corrected by resorption and remodelling.

DEVELOPMENT OF THE SKELETON

A. Appendicular skeleton

The bones of arms and legs, which follow a similar course of development, originate from mesenchyme of somatic mesoderm that migrates into the limb buds. Three developmental stages are recognized. We will take the innominate bone and bones of the leg as examples (Fig. 15–8).

Stage 1. Pre-cartilage (about 9–10 weeks; 11 mm.). The limb bud contains massed chondroblasts in a generalized pattern. The areas of the future pelvic girdle, thigh, lower leg and digits are only vaguely outlined (Fig. 15–8B).

Stage 2. Cartilage (20 mm. embryo). The entire skeleton is laid down in hyaline cartilage, bone by bone (Fig. 15–8C, D).

Stage 3. Ossification stage (35 mm. embryos). Ossification begins with each individual bone showing a centre of ossification from which a wave of endochondral osteogenesis spreads; the process occupies the remainder of gestation and is completed postnatally. The ilium, pubis, and ischium of the innominate bone each has its own centre of ossification, as does the femur, tibia, fibula, tarsals, meta-tarsals and phalanges (Fig. 15–8E).

Anomalies

Malformations of the human limbs (see p. 86 for possible causes)
1. Amelia — complete absence of limbs (Fig. 15–9).
2. Phocomelia — only stumps of limbs present (Fig. 15–9B).

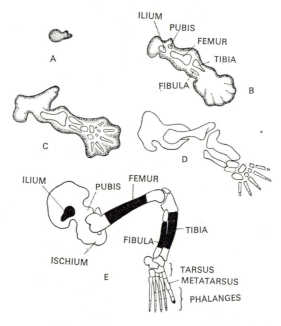

Fig. 15–8. Stages in embryonic development of the human leg:
    A. 9 mm. embryo: primordium;
    B. 11 mm. embryo: pre-cartilage stage;
    C. 14 mm. embryo: beginning of cartilage formation;
    D. 20 mm. embryo: cartilage;
    E. 50 mm. embryo; ossification.

3. Micromelia — very short extremities, which are, however, complete with all segments.
4. Sympodia — fused limbs (Fig. 15–9B).
5. " Lobster claw " (Fig. 15–9C).
6. Syndactyly — fused fingers (Fig. 15–9F).
7. " Double hand " (dichiria) (Fig. 15–9D).
8. Polydactyly — supernumerary fingers (Fig. 15–9E).

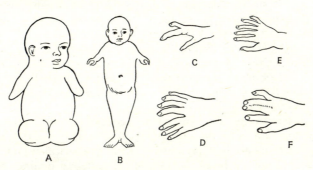

FIG. 15–9. Malformations of the human limb:
    A. Hemimelia in arms; amelia in legs;
    B. Phocomelia in arms; sympodia in legs;
    C. Cleft hand (lobster claw);
    D. Dichiria (double-hand);
    E. Polydactyly;
    F. Syndactyly.

B. Vertebrae and ribs

The vertebral column is not a derivative of the notochord. Rather, it is a new structure formed around the notochord, finally replacing it almost completely. The only remnants of the notochord to be found in the adult are the pulpy nuclei in the intervertebral discs (see below).

Each vertebra is formed by the sclerotomes of one vertebral segment. The latter, however, does not correspond to the extent of one somite of the original metameric arrangement. What happens is that the mesenchymal cells of the sclerotomes depart from the somites and migrate medially towards the notochord (Fig. 15–10). On their way, they split transversely into a cranial and a caudal half (Fig. 15–10A); the caudal half from one segment unites with the cranial half

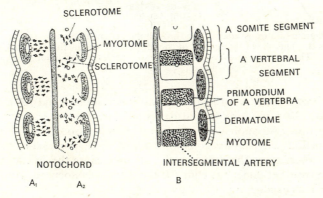

FIG. 15–10. Diagrams to show stages in the differentiation of human vertebrae:
    A₁. Frontal section through the left somites (approx. 4 mm. embryos);
    A₂. The same, but slightly later than A₁.
    B. New combination of the halves of successive sclerotomes into definitive vertebral primordia (about 5 mm. embryos).

from the segment immediately behind to form one vertebral segment (Fig. 15–10B). Consequently, the intersegmental arteries, which were originally located between the segments, now become translocated into the centre of each vertebral segment. Each vertebra is therefore an intersegmental structure.

The sclerotomes on each side of a vertebral segment arch around the spinal cord (Fig. 15–11). Three centres of cartilage formation develop in this primordium of a half-vertebra; one encases the notochord and is destined to form the future body of the vertebra, one is for the costal process or rib and one is for the future neural arch. The sclerotomes from both sides merge and unite in the mid-line both above and below the spinal cord. Some cells from the lower (caudal) half of a vertebral segment move their centre of proliferation cranially to the sides of the intervertebral fissures and contribute to the growth of successive vertebrae by forming the fibrous annuli of the intervertebral discs. The remnants of the degenerating notochordal and annular cells remain as the pulpy nuclei.

Ossification follows later in development. The ribs begin to ossify about the middle of the ninth week (starting from 6th and 7th ribs; others follow in the next few days). Next, the vertebral arches begin to ossify about 4 days later, first in the cervical region, and then spreading rapidly caudally. This is followed by ossification of the vertebral bodies. Slight modifications to this scheme exist in the case of the first (atlas) and second (axis) vertebrae and the coccyx. At birth, the three centres of ossification for these are still distinct (Fig. 15–11), and their ossification is not completed until the individual reaches the age of about twenty-five.

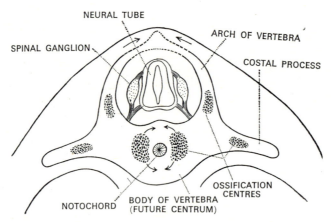

FIG. 15–11. Diagram of a transverse section through the mesenchyme stage of a vertebra at the thoracic level. This shows the pattern of chondrification within the principal sclerotomic extensions. These same centres will become the sites for later ossification.

C. The sternum

The sternum, or breast bone, is formed from two longitudinal bands of mesenchyme which become cartilagenous; these resulting sternal bars unite later with the ventral ends of the first eight or nine pairs of ribs. An anomalous sternum is usually associated with malformations of the chest, whilst anomalous clavicles are commonly caused by hypoplasia of the clavicle (cleidodysostosis). In very severe cases the defective clavicle may cause the shoulders to be so drawn forward that they almost meet under the chin. If the defect is associated with a defective skull, the condition is known as cleidocranial dysostosis.

D. The skull

The neurocranium. Initially, the developing brain is supported by a plate of mesenchyme which encases the cranial end of the notochord and extends further cephalically and laterally

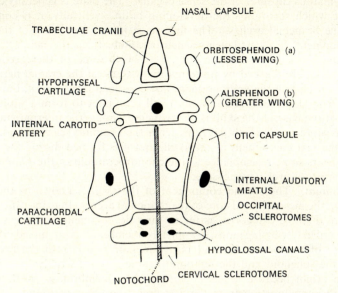

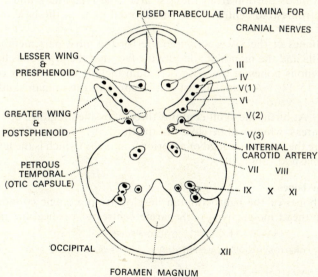

Fig. 15–12. A. Diagram of a cartilagenous neurocranium as seen from the dorsal aspect showing the primordia of cartilagenous bones (after Harrison);
Middle primordia: parachordal plate,
hypophyseal plate,
trabeculae cranii;
Lateral primordia: orbitosphenoid plate (lesser wing),
alisphenoid plate (greater wing),
otic capsule,
nasal capsule;
B. Human cartilagenous neurocranium seen from the ventral surface to show the cartilagenous bones derived from early primordia, and the locations of foramina for the cranial nerves (after Williams and Wendell-Smith).

into the mesenchymatous capsules of the sense organs. The plate is generally confluent with the head mesenchyme which surrounds the developing brain; ventrally, it is continuous with the mesenchyme of the branchial arches. The first stage in the formation of the future complex skull is the development of a cartilagenous neurocranium from the mesenchyme plate by the appearance of centres of chondrification (Fig. 15–12A). Some of these centres subsequently fuse, the sites of which are marked by foramina for the exit of the cranial nerves (Fig. 15–12B).

The cartilagenous base of the neurocranium just described lacks a roof, but three large membrane bones (the frontal, parietal and occipital) will arise later to form a vault. One bone (the occipital) formed at the base of the skull is partly membranous (the interparietal part) and partly cartilagenous (the supra part, which develops from the occipital sclerotomes). The completed neurocranium is the first component of the skull, and it is formed during the second month of development. It bears some resemblance to the chondrocranium of the *Elasmobranchs* (dogfish and sharks), which is however never ossified.

The viscerocranium. The second component of the skull is known as the viscerocranium, and is derived from the mesenchymal core of the branchial arches (Fig. 15–13). The bones of this viscerocranium are of three categories as far as their developmental origin is concerned; they may be either completely cartilagenous, completely membranous or mixed, i.e., partly cartilagenous (from base of neurocranium) and partly membranous (from the arches). Two such mixed bones are the sphenoid and the temporal (Table 15–1). Strictly speaking, the temporal bone has a triple origin because it has an independent membranous portion (the squamous temporal), a membranous portion from the first arch (the tympanic), and a cartilagenous part derived from the petromastoid centre of the parachordal plate in the base of the neurocranium (Fig. 15–14B).

The remaining bones of the viscerocranium are for the most part membranous (the largest ones being the maxilla and the mandible) despite the fact that the jaw bones have a cartilagenous basis. The cartilagenous bones of the viscerocranium include the auditory ossicles, the styloid, and the hyoid (Fig. 15–14). A complete list of the bones of the human skull, with their origin, is given in Table 15–1.

The fontanelles. At birth, the skull contains three unossified regions, covered only by a thin membrane. These areas, which will be closed in the third or fourth postnatal year, are shown in Fig. 15–14B; they are the frontal-parietal or anterior fontanelle (which is the largest), the sphenoid fontanelle and the mastoid fontanelle.

Growth of membrane bones

The membrane bones of the neurocranium develop from a single continuous sheet of condensed mesenchyme (head mesenchyme). Separate centres of ossification appear in this mem-

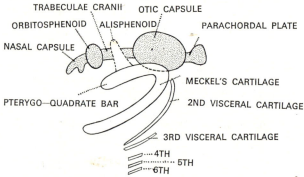

FIG. 15–13. Schematic representation of the relations of the parts of the primordial chondrocranium seen from the lateral aspect (neurocranium, stippled; viscerocranium, blank). (After Hamilton, Boyd and Mossman.)

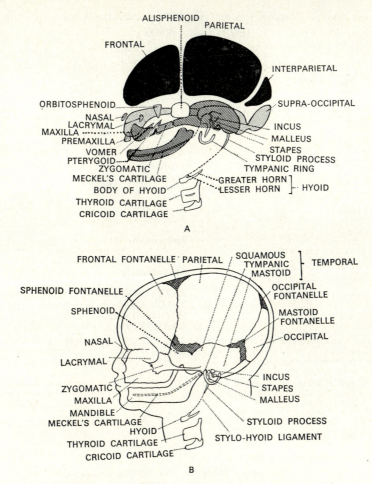

Fig. 15–14. Bones of the human skull (adapted from several sources):
  A. Lateral (left side) view of a scheme of the elements of the cranium: cartilagenous neurocranium, stippled; cartilagenous viscerocranium, blank; membranous neurocranium, solid black; membranous viscerocranium, cross-hatched.
  B. Diagram of the foetal skull to show the locations of the major fontanelles (cross-hatched).

brane and spread centrifugally. Soon the osteal mesenchyme becomes split into two limiting membranes, each consisting of an outer fibrous layer and an inner osteogenic layer (the periosteum). From the latter, trabeculae of spongy bone are formed in the manner previously described (p. 175). This spongy bone constitutes the diploe and the upper and lower bony plates become the outer and inner tables of the cranium.

The upper and lower osteogenic layers are continuous around and between the advancing edges of adjoining membrane bones and meet at sutures. A suture is a type of joint which has a "bone-fibrous tissue-bone" complex which allows active growth of membrane bones to continue during foetal life and childhood. When depositional activities of the osteoblasts of the two osteogenic layers (which are separated at the sutures by fibrous tissue) cease, the sutures ossify and further growth (spread) of the bones is terminated (see syndesmoses below). It is worth noting that the "bone-fibrous tissue-bone" complex found at the sutures corresponds to the "bone-hyaline cartilage-bone" complex (the epiphyseal plate) prevailing at the end of growing

TABLE 15–1. COMPONENTS OF THE SKULL AND THE ORIGIN OF THE
INDIVIDUAL BONES

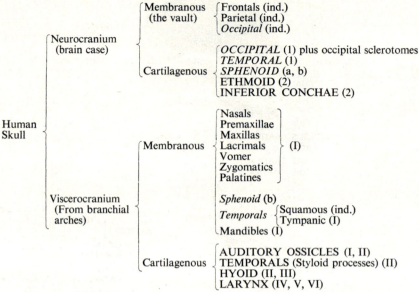

Origin of each bone is indicated in parenthesis: ind. = independent; I to VI, from branchial arches I–VI respectively; 1 from parachordal cartilage; 2, from trabeculae cranii cartilage; b, from alisphenoid (greater wing); a, from orbitosphenoid (lesser wing) (Fig. 15–12A).

The names of cartilage bones are printed in Capitals, those of membrane bones are in lower case letters. Mixed bones (partly cartilagenous and partly membranous) are printed in italics.

long bones (p. 178). In the latter, the elimination (by complete regression following atrophy) of the hyaline cartilage likewise brings an end to growth in length of the bones involved.

Bony derivatives of the branchial arches

Five pairs of branchial arches are formed in the human. They develop a cartilagenous skeletal element during the latter part of the 2nd month of development, without however attaining any considerable size. Most of the bones finally derived from them are of the cartilagenous type, although the jaw bones (the maxilla and mandible) derived from the first arch are primarily membrane bones developed from local branchial mesenchyme without the prior formation of cartilage (Fig. 15–15). Table 15–2 summarizes these derivatives (Fig. 15–15).

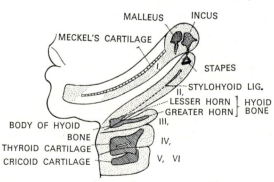

FIG. 15–15. Diagram showing the structures formed by the cartilagenous components of branchial arches 1 to 6.

TABLE 15–2. DERIVATIVES OF THE BRANCHIAL ARCHES

Arch	Portion	Derivatives
I	{ Maxillary process { Mandibular process	small quadrate cartilage →Incus* Meckel's cartilage ———→Malleus* (mostly degenerates)
II	{ Proximal end { Remainder	Styloid process————→Stapes* Styloid ligament
III		{ Lesser horn and body of hyoid bone { Greater horn of the hyoid bone
IV and V		Thyroid cartilages, arytenoid and other cartilages of the larynx

* Bones of the middle ear.

Bone articulations

Joints develop from the mesenchyme between adjacent developing bones, and are of two types, movable and non-movable.

1. Synarthrosis. This type of joint permits little or no movement. The intervening mesenchyme, the interzone, differentiates into a uniting layer of rigid connective tissue which may differ according to the type of joint, as shown in the list below.

Type of joint	Kind of connective tissue differentiated at interzone	Examples
Syndesmosis	Dense connective tissue	cranial sutures
Synchondrosis	fibro-cartilage	pubic symphysis
Synostosis	bone	epiphyseal line

2. Diathrosis. This type permits free movement of the joint, and is made possible by cavitation of the mesenchymal interzone (Fig. 15–16A). A diarthrosis is characterized by the presence of a prominent joint cavity filled with a fluid (developed in the 3rd month) between the movable skeletal parts, and a fibrous capsule at the periphery formed by the surrounding periosteum. The joint cavity is lined internally with a layer of vascularized mesenchyme, the synovial membrane. This membrane does not cover the free articular surfaces of the bones, which are formed by the articular cartilage (with a cap of persisting hyaline cartilage) of the two bones involved. Ligaments, developed in the capsule as local thickenings, hold the articular bones in proper relationship to each other and to some extent ensure their security (Fig. 15–16B).

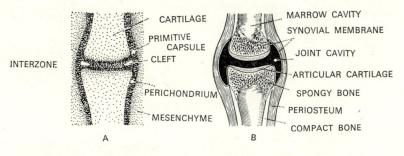

FIG. 15–16. Stages in the development of a diarthrodial joint (adapted from several sources):
A. Stage of early organization;
B. Completely formed joint.

Anomalies of the axial skeleton and associated bony structures

Many things can go wrong during the complicated process of the development of the axial skeleton, firstly during the formation of the individual vertebrae which involves union of bilateral halves, and subsequently in the fusion of successive vertebrae into a perfectly fitting vertebral column. Thus there are cases of asymmetrical fusion of successive vertebrae, absence of a half vertebra, an increase or decrease in the total number of vertebrae, and other imperfections.

One abnormality is called spina bifida (cleft vertebra); it results from failure of the neural arches to unite with each other (see Fig. 20–7). The defect is usually serious because it is almost always associated with herniation of the spinal cord through the cleft (see Chapter 20).

Abnormal ribs are usually secondarily associated with defects of the vertebral column; a missing vertebra (either whole or in part), for example, may lead to the absence of a corresponding rib, etc. When the ribs on the concave side of the chest are irregularly united or branched, the condition is known as scoliosis (crooked spine). It is congenital. When abnormalities occur in the skull, they are usually serious as they invariably involve the brain in one way or another, and often the combined defects (of bone and brain) are not compatible with life. Most of these cases will be treated in connection with the nervous system (Chapter 20). To give just one example here, microcephalus or acrocephalus will result if the sutures between the flat bones of the vault should close prematurely (Fig. 20–19).

CHAPTER 16

THE MUSCULAR SYSTEM

Classification and general considerations:

Type of muscle				Morpholagy			Mode of function
Visceral	.	.	.	non-striated (smooth)	.	.	involuntary
Cardiac	.	.	.	semi-striated	.	.	involuntary
Skeletal	.	.	.	striated	.	.	voluntary

The cardiac muscle is functionally more like the visceral muscles (both being regulated by the autonomic nervous system), but structurally more like skeletal muscle (both develop striations). Regardless of type, however, the unique feature of all muscular tissues is the development of "fibrils" or fibrillae, in the cytoplasm of the myoblasts. In all muscles, myofibrils are the ultimate units of contraction and their degree of differentiation determines the nature of the tissue.

A. SMOOTH MUSCLE

All smooth muscles are of mesodermal origin with the exception of the muscle of the iris which is ectodermal, the contractile cells of sweat glands, which are also ectodermal and the sphincter muscle of the perineum which is probably partly ectodermal and partly endodermal (pp. 193, 209, 246).

Smooth muscle develops from wandering mesenchymal cells of the splanchnic (hypomeric) mesoderm, which have migrated into developing viscera and the gastrointestinal and respiratory tracts. After arriving at their destination they begin to lengthen and orient themselves with reference to the direction along which future contraction will take place (Fig. 16–1A). During the 6th and 7th weeks of development, myofibrils are clearly recognizable in their cytoplasm

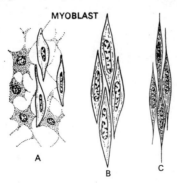

MYOBLAST

A

B

C

Fig. 16–1. Development of smooth muscle (adapted from several sources):
  A. at 13 mm. (45 days);
  B. at 27 mm. (60 days);
  C. Tunica muscularis of adult small intestine.

(Fig. 16–1B). Two weeks later, the young smooth muscle cells assume a characteristic spindle shape and their myofibrils have greatly increased in number. They do not develop any striations (Fig. 16–1C) and are, in fact, already functional and do not differentiate further.

B. CARDIAC MUSCLE

Muscles of the heart develop from the myocardium, the inner layer of the epimyocardium (p. 149); the surface layer, or epicardium, gives rise to the mesothelial covering of the heart.

Potential cardiac muscle cells are closely packed, forming a loose irregular mass (Fig. 16–2A, B). Some myofibrils appear in them, first at the periphery, gradually extending to the centre of the cell. A little later, cross-striations begin to appear, though to a lesser extent than those developed in skeletal muscles. The myofibrils increase in number through longitudinal splitting. In time, a characteristic structure, the intercalated disc, develops at the cellular junctions. The intercalated discs appear as short lines (0·5 to 1·0 micron thick) oriented at right angles to the long axis of the fibres, bounded on both sides by the Z lines. Sometimes the intercalated disc does not extend all the way across the fibre at one level, but stops suddenly only to continue one or more segments higher up. The repetition of these irregular shifts accounts for the assumption by these discs of the step-like appearance (Fig. 16–2C). Experimental evidence from tissue culture and electron microscopy supports the view that the intercalated discs represent specialized junctions between the cellular units of the myocardium, or simply the membranes of adjacent cells. It is suggested by some, however, that the intercalated discs may be sites of origin of new sarcomeres.

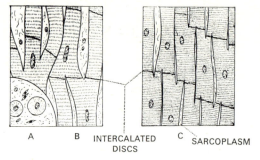

A   B   INTERCALATED   C   SARCOPLASM
                  DISCS

FIG. 16–2. Development of cardiac muscle:
    A. and B. Transverse section (A) and longitudunal section (B) showing the arrangement and
       characteristics of cardiac muscle;
    C. Adult cardiac muscle.

C. SKELETAL MUSCLE

Myogenesis of skeletal muscles

Regardless of their origin, whether from primary myotomes or from mesenchyme, all striated muscle fibres undergo the same process of histogenesis and exhibit the same definitive structural details at the end of differentiation. The embryonic myoblasts exhibit a fine granular cytoplasm as the cells increasingly elongate. At this early stage, the future muscle fibre has but a single nucleus, which is usually centrally located. Soon, however, the fibre becomes multinucleated probably by fusion of further myoblasts with the developing fibres; at the same time there is further elongation of the cell (Fig. 16–3A) and the alignment of the centrally situated nuclei. Young muscle fibres now become recognizable by virtue of both the increase in the number of fibrils and the beginning of regional differentiation (Fig. 16–3B). In the final phase of histogenesis, the myofibrils, now greatly multiplied in number, acquire the alternating band structure, which gives the fibre a cross-banded appearance. This is due largely to repeated concentrations of an anisotropic substance (Fig. 16–3c). The definitive myofibrils differentiate first close to the periphery of the fibre, a process which gradually continues towards its centre with the movement of the nuclei to their definitive positions beneath the sarcolemma. The muscles of the foetus at term, by and large, have already developed the histological characteristics of adult skeletal muscles.

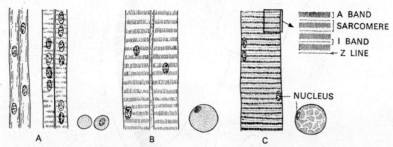

FIG. 16–3. Development of skeletal muscle (adapted from several sources):
  A. Longitudinal section (left) and transverse section (right) of 200 mm. embryos;
  B. From a human foetus at term;
  C. Adult. (A = Anisotropic, I = Isotrotic.)

The origin of skeletal muscles and their derivatives are tabulated below for reference.

1. Muscles derived from head mesenchyme (pre-mandibular). This is equivalent to the three pairs of cephalic myotomes present in the lower vertebrates. (The evidence for this statement is based partly on the innervation pattern of the extrinsic muscles of the eye). The head mesenchyme gives rise to the six muscles which move the eyeball (Fig. 16–5A), innervated by cranial nerves III, IV and VI as follows.

Extrinsic muscle of the eye	Cranial nerve innervation
Superior rectus	
Inferior rectus	
Medial rectus	III
Inferior oblique	
Superior oblique	IV
Lateral rectus	VI

2. Muscles derived from mesenchyme of the branchial (pharyngeal) arches. Muscles of this origin are called branchiomeric muscles; their derivation (Fig. 16–5A) and innervation (Fig. 16–5B) are listed below.

Arch No.	Branchiomeric muscles	Cranial nerve innervation
1	Muscles of mastication i.e. temporalis, mylohyoid, masseter, anterior belly of the digastric, pterygoids, tensor palati, tensor tympani	V
2	Muscles of facial expression; auricular muscle, occipito-frontalis, posterior belly of the diagastric, stylohyoid, stapedius, platysma	VII
3	Stylo-pharyngeus (upper pharyngeal muscle); Lower pharyngeal muscles;	IX
4, 5, (6)	Muscles of the soft palate; crico-thyroid and other intrinsic muscles of the larynx trapezius, sternocleidomastoid	X, (XII)

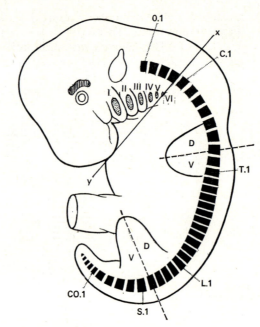

Fig. 16–4. Schematic representation of muscle masses in a 5-mm. human embryo (modified from Hamilton, Boyd and Mossman); The first occipital (O1), cervical (C1), thoracic (T1), lumbar (L1), sacral (S1) and coccygeal (CO1) somites are labelled. The somites giving rise to the muscles of dorsal (D) and ventral (V) halves of the fore and hind limbs are indicated. The derivatives of the cephalic somites (stippled), branchial arches and occipital somites (solid black) to the left of the line XY are shown in Figure 16–5A.

3. Muscles derived primarily from the myotomes. A total of 39 pairs of somites (4 occipital; 8 cervical; 12 thoracic; 5 lumbar; 5 sacral; 5 coccygeal) are developed in the embryo; they give rise to the following muscles. Contributions from the somatic mesoderm of the lateral plate (hypomeres) to the muscles of the appendages are also noted.

(a) The occipital myotomes. Intrinsic muscles of the tongue (mesenchyme in the floor of the mouth possibly also contributes to their formation); innervated by the XIIth cranial nerve.

(b) The cervical myotomes

Pairs 1–3. Infrahyoid muscles.

Pairs 3–5. Muscles of the diaphragm in part (later the diaphragm receives contributions from the thoracic body wall which are added to its periphery during its caudal migration).

Pairs 5–7. Muscles of pre-axial (dorsal) half of the upper extremities (with possible contribution from dermatomes of corresponding segments).

Pairs 7–8 and 1st thoracic. Muscles of the post-axial (ventral) half of the upper extremities (with similar contributions from dermatomes).

(c) Thoracic, lumbar and the first two sacral myotomes. These give rise to typical segmental musculature intimately associated with the vertebral column and the axial skeleton.

1. Intercostal and abdominal musculature, essentially the flexors of the vertebral column.

2. Musculature of the ventral body wall with contributions from unsegmented somatic mesoderm of the hypomeres.

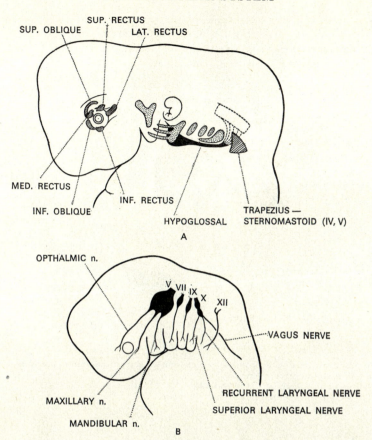

FIG. 16–5. A. Schematic representation of the developing musculature from the equivalents of cephalic somites (shaded), the branchial arches (stippled) and the occipital somites (solid black) in a 10-mm. human embryo (after Hamilton, Boyd and Mossman); B. The innervation of the branchial arches by cranial nerves (after Davies).

3. The first 5 pairs in the lumbar region form muscles of the pre-axial half of the lower extremities.

4. The 5th lumbar pair, and the 1st and 2nd sacral pairs together form the muscles of the post-axial half of the lower extremities.

The muscles of the lower extremities are complicated by the rotation of the extensors and flexors as an adaptation to weight bearing.

(d) The 3rd–5th sacral pairs form the pelvic diaphragm, the levator ani and the coccygeus muscles.

Major derivatives of the myotomes

During the 5th week of development, the somatic myotomes on each side split into dorsal epaxial and ventral hypaxial columns or muscle masses. The two groups are innervated, respectively, by the dorsal and ventral rami of the segmental spinal nerves.

The epaxial column subdivides further, giving rise to the muscles of the back, neck and trunk which form the extensors of the vertebral column. (The intervertebral muscles, representing a deeper portion, retain the primitive segmental arrangement.) The hypaxial masses migrate ventrally and laterally, and give rise to the prevertebral muscles which are primarily the flexors

G

of the vertebral column (Fig. 16–6A); some of the hypaxial masses also become the layered muscles of the chest and abdomen (Fig. 16–6B). The extensors and flexors, derived from the epaxial and hypaxial myotomes respectively, are well advanced in their specialization and differentiation by the seventh week of development.

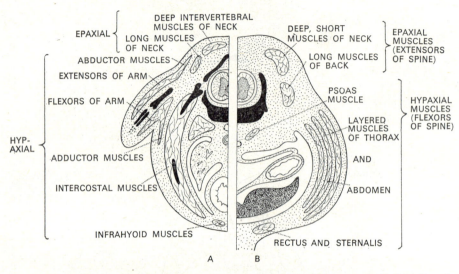

FIG. 16–6. The arrangement of primitive muscle masses shown diagrammatically in a 7-week human embryo (modified from Arey):
A. Half-section through neck and shoulders;
B. Half-section through the thorax and abdomen.

Muscles of the limbs

The innervation pattern of the appendages suggests that at the levels of the limb buds, the myotomes give rise to outgrowths, which extend into the growing appendage along with aggregations of mesenchyme migrating out from the hypomeric somatic mesoderm. These two masses of mesenchyme are grouped, respectively, as the dorsal (pre-axial) and ventral (post-axial) muscle masses with respect to the developing skeletal structures of the limb (Fig. 16–4). The muscles developed from the former are the extensors and those from the latter become flexors of the arms and legs. Primordia furnished by outgrowths from the dorsal mesenchymal mass give rise to abductor muscles; those from the ventral mass form adductor muscles (Fig. 16–6A).

Developmental mechanisms involved in the differentiation of muscles

These may be summarized under the following headings.
1. Rotation, involving changes from original cranio-caudal direction of muscle fibre orientation. Examples are the oblique muscles of the abdominal wall.
2. Splitting, which may be either:
    (a) Longitudinal splitting into two or more portions, as in the trapezius and sternocleidomastoid muscles.

    or

    (b) A tangential splitting of the original myotomal masses into two or more layers. Examples are the two oblique and transverse layers of the abdominal wall, and the intercostal muscles.

3. Fusion, where portions of successive myotomes fuse to form a single muscle. An example is the rectus abdominis, formed by fusion of the ventral portion of the last 6–7 thoracic myotomes.

4. Migration is the term used when muscle primordia, wholly or in part, migrate to segmental levels different from those of their origin. Examples are the latissimus dorsi, which moves from cervical to lower thoracic and lumbar levels, and the muscles of the face and musculature of the diaphragm.

5. Degeneration. In this instance a whole muscle or a portion of it may degenerate, resulting in the formation of fascia, ligaments and aponeuroses. Examples are the fascia iliaca and the dorso-lumbar fascia.

CHAPTER 17

THE ENDOCRINE SYSTEM

Introduction

The endocrine tissues and organs constitute a functionally independant system which has two important characteristics in common, firstly that the cells are capable of elaborating potent specific chemical substances, the hormones, which act selectively on certain " target organs " to bring about significant morphological and functional changes, and secondly that their secretion leaves the gland not by ducts, but via the vascular circulation. The integration and coordination of the body parts requires both quick action of the nervous system and effective sustained action of the various hormones. Some of these hormones are definitely indispensable to life while others are necessary for realizing the roles of genes (e.g., sex differentiation — see Chapter 13).

All three germ layers are potentially capable of giving rise to endocrine cells. In general, the hormones produced by endocrine tissues of mesodermal origin are steroids or steroid-like chemicals, whilst the hormones produced by glands of ectodermal and endodermal tissues are globulins or proteins. From an evolutionary point of view, endocrine tissues can be arranged in a series of increasing complexity with respect to their developmental mechanisms, as follows.

(*a*) Aggregates of cells located within an organ, which is not primarily endocrine in function.
(*b*) Endocrine glands derived from one germ layer.
(*c*) Endocrine glands having two distinct components, both developed from one germ layer.
(*d*) Endocrine glands involving two separate primordia contributed by two different germ layers.

These developmental relationships are presented in Table 17–1.

Pharyngeal pouches and endocrine glands

During the fourth week a series of folds or invaginations appears in the pharyngeal wall of both sides. At the same time the cranial end of the endodermal tube forming the fore-gut produces a corresponding series of protrusions (evaginations), each of which meets, face to face, with an ectodermal depression. This is the manner in which the " pharyngeal complex " is formed. Three components of this complex are readily recognizable (*a*) the ectodermal pharyngeal clefts (*b*) the endodermal pharyngeal pouches and, between these (*c*) solid pharyngeal or branchial arches, which are the mesenchymal cores formed inbetween the apposition of the respective clefts and pouches (see Fig. 9–3). (In the lower vertebrates, the apposed epithelial plates or closing membranes of the corresponding ectodermal clefts and endodermal pouches perforate to become the gill slits which alternate with the cartilagenous gill (branchial) arches. This does not happen in the Amniotes.) The main derivatives of the pharyngeal clefts and arches have already been discussed, but important endocrine glands originate from some of the endodermal pouches, the development of which will be briefly recapitulated.

At first, the pharyngeal pouches retain a spacious connection with the pharyngeal cavity, but soon this connection narrows down considerably, especially in pouches 2, 3 and 4. It is also significant that each of these pouches develops a dorsal and a ventral recess or wing. (A ventral recess of the first pouch never develops because of the hinderance given by the developing tongue.)

TABLE 17–1.   CLASSIFICATION OF ENDOCRINE TISSUES

Type		Examples	Germ layer Origin
Tissues within an otherwise exocrine gland or simply part of another organ		1. Certain epithelial cells of stomach and duodenum† . . . . . . 2. Interstitial cells of testes . . . . 3. Internal theca cells of ovary . . . 4. Islets of Langerhans* in pancreas . . 5. Trophoblast of chorionic villi . . .	Endodermal Mesodermal Mesodermal Endodermal Ectodermal (extra-embryonic)
Derived from one germ layer		Thyroid Parathyroid* Thymus (?)	All Endodermal
Initially having two separate primordia	from one germ layer	Hypophysis { Ant. lobe { Pars distalis / Pars tuberalis } Post. lobe { Pars intermedia / Pars nervosa .	Buccal ectoderm Neuro-ectoderm
	from two germ layers	Adrenal gland { Medulla—Chromaffin tissue of neural crest . Cortex*—Splanchnic mesoderm . .	Ectodermal Mesodermal

* Indispensable to life.
   † Producing the hormone, enterokinase, for stimulating secretion of the pancreatic enzyme, trypsinogen.

The ventral recess of pouch 4 is a diverticulum, the ultimobranchial body which, due to its continuous caudal movement, becomes the vestigial 5th pouch.

The dorsal recesses of the first and second pouches expand and merge into a common tubo-tympanic recess which remains connected to the pharynx by a narrow passage and meets with the first pharyngeal cleft; the combined recess has ectodermal and endodermal end plates which form the tympanic membrane (see Chapter 21). The adjoined and widened cavity next to the tympanic membrane becomes the middle ear cavity, connected directly to the pharyngo-tympanic tube (first pharyngeal pouch). The ventral recess of pouch 2, on both sides, forms the fossa and some of the tissue of the palatine tonsil. The right and left ventral recesses of the third pouch give rise to two masses of endodermal proliferations (shaped like the omental apron), which grow medially and meet with each other, thereby forming the bi-lobed primordium of the thymus gland. The dorsal recess of the same pouch, a solid endodermal mass, gives rise to one of the parathyroid (in fact, the definitive inferior) glands, and migrates caudally (beyond the origin of the fourth pouch) with the thymus (Fig. 17–1A) when the connection of the third pouch with the pharynx becomes lost. The dorsal recess of pouch 4 differentiates into the superior parathyroid, which, however, eventually becomes absorbed into the developing thyroid gland (Fig. 17–1B). Similarly, the ventral recess of the fourth pouch, which starts out as thymus tissue, is absorbed into the thyroid gland. Thus, out of the " caudal pharyngeal complex " (pouches 4 and 5), the whole of the fourth pouch and the ultimobranchial body (pouch 5) lose their identity after a brief association with the developing thyroid (Fig. 17–1B).

The thyroid

The thyroid gland makes its first appearance in the fourth week of development (Fig. 17–2A) as a median bi-lobed diverticulum, embedded in mesenchyme, from the pharyngeal floor at a

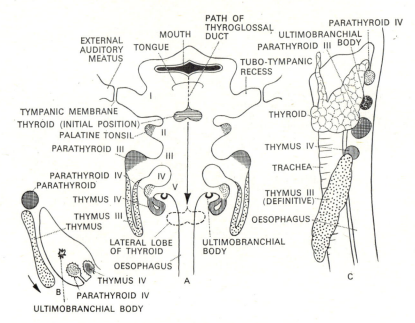

FIG. 17–1. Diagrammatic representation to show the derivatives of the endodermal branchial arches. (Note: the thyroid arises from the mid-pharyngeal floor, but it is conveniently considered here, together with the derivatives of the pharyngeal pouches) (adapted from several sources):
A. Ventral view of a 4-mm. human embryo;
B. Migration of thymus and parathyroid and their association with the thyroid;
C. Later disposition of the pouch derivatives, ventro-lateral view from the left side.

level between the first and second pharyngeal pouches. It soon loses connection with the pharyngeal floor, leaving its point of origin marked by the foramen caecum, and begins to migrate caudally ventral to the pharynx. By the end of the seventh week (Fig. 17–2B) it has come to lie at the level of the laryngeal primordium and its epithelium has become converted into solid epithelial cords and the intermingling mesenchyme has been vascularized (Fig. 17–2c). Follicles appear about the eleventh week (65 mm.) and colloid formation begins in them almost immediately (Fig. 17–2D). The thyroid secretion, thyroxine, (iodothyroglobulin) is an iodine-rich amino acid which has the following functions.

1. It regulates the basic metabolic rate.
2. It controls growth and differentiation in general, affecting:
    (a) the capacity of the nervous system, with especial reference to mental development
    (b) the development of the cardio-vascular system
    (c) the development of the skeletal and cardiac muscles and the haemopoietic organs.
3. It inhibits the growth hormone (somatotrophin, STH) of the anterior pituitary.

The parathyroids

Two pairs of primordia, parathyroid 3 and parathyroid 4, are formed respectively from the dorsal recesses of the third and fourth pharyngeal pouches (Fig. 17–1A). During the seventh week of development, the primordium of the thymus and that of parathyroid 3, (which arise together and remain closely associated) both become freed from the pharynx and begin to move caudad together. The rudiment of parathyroid 3 remains encased in the cephalic tip of the thymus for a while.

With further caudal migration of the thymus, parathyroid 3 becomes embedded in the adjacent capsular tissue of the thyroid, and comes to lie caudal to the rudiment of parathyroid 4 (thus reversing their original relative positions). The latter may assume some close relationship with the ultimobranchial bodies, but finally become adherent to the thyroid capsule and may even be embedded in the substance of the thyroid (Fig. 17–1B, C).

The parathyroids start out as solid cell masses, but soon break up into cords with large irregular capillary spaces (sinusoids) between them. (This is a typical pattern of endocrine gland development.) Young differentiating secretory cells, the principal cells, show a pale clear cytoplasm and are often vacuolated (Fig. 17–3). The final functional oxyphil cells are, however, not differentiated until the individual reaches 10 years of age; in an adult gland these cells contain numerous fine secretory granules (Fig. 17–3). The parathyroid hormone controls bone growth and is also essential for muscular contraction through regulation of serum calcium. The gland is indispensable for life.

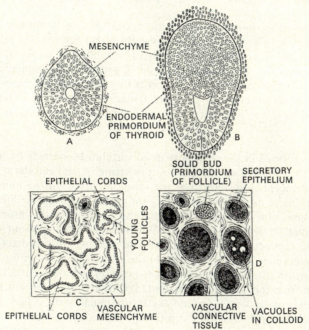

FIG. 17–2. Histogenesis of the human thyroid gland (projection drawings): A. 4-weeks; B. 6-weeks; C. 8-weeks; D. 19-weeks.

The thymus

The prospective definitive thymus arises in the 6th week of development as a ventral outgrowth from pharyngeal pouch 3. Because of its close association with the epithelial end plate of the third pharyngeal cleft it is possible that both ectodermal and endodermal cells participate in its formation. Soon the thymic rudiment loses its lumen and grows rapidly, approaching its counterpart from the opposite side and by the middle of the 8th week, the tips of both thymus primordia make contact as they slide down under the sternum into the mediastinum, along with other pharyngeal derivatives (Fig. 17–1C). There is superficial fusion between the left and right primordia but the definitive organ however, never entirely loses its paired character. In man a vestigial thymus rudiment from the fourth pouch migrates with the thyroid and becomes ultimately embedded in it, thereby losing its importance.

OXYPHIL CELLS

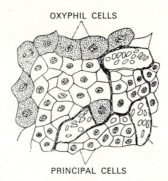

PRINCIPAL CELLS

FIG. 17–3. Section through human parathyroid gland showing the small principal cells and the large oxyphil cells containing secretory granules.

By the third month, the thymus assumes the appearance of lymphatic tissue with reticular cells and lymphocytes. It reaches a maximum weight about the time of puberty, after which it undergoes regression and is eventually involuted. The endocrine nature of this gland has never been conclusively demonstrated; histologically, it is primarily a lymphatic organ. The latest experimental evidence with regard to its function is that it acts as an organ of immunity during childhood by virtue of its developing lymphoid tissue. Possibly, the latter provides immuno-logically competent cells to the lymphatic system of the body for as long as the gland functions.

The hypophysis

The hypophysis is formed in the same way in all vertebrates, namely by fusion of two distinct primordia, which are (a) Rathke's pouch, an outpocketing of oral ectoderm, and (b) an evagina-tion of the floor of diencephalon, known as the infundibulum. In the human, Rathke's pouch begins to grow towards the infundibulum during the third week; by the 8th week (25 mm.), the pouch has lost all connection with the oral cavity, and approaches the infundibulum as a vesicle which retains a residual lumen (Fig. 17–4A). When the embryo is about 65 mm. C.R. length (11th week) intimate contact is established between the two primordia (Fig. 17–4B). These primordia soon differentiates into three parts (1) the pars distalis, the most rapidly proliferating ventral (anterior) portion (2) the pars intermedia, (which faces the neural lobe or pars nervosa, the only contribution from the infundibulum) and (3) the pars tuberalis, which is a small extension of pars distalis; it eventually wraps around the infundibular stalk. The pars distalis and pars tuberalis make up the anterior lobe of the pituitary (adenohypophysis); the pars nervosa and pars intermedia comprise the posterior lobe. When the gland is completely developed it becomes securely encased in the sphenoid bone (Figs. 17–4C; 7–5). The pars distalis is by far the most important component, so much so that it is called the " master gland ". This is not just because it elaborates more hormones than any other endocrine gland, but rather because its hormones control and regulate the functions of so many other endocrine glands. The following is a summary of its hormones.

1. Growth hormone (STH, somatotropic hormone), sometimes also known as the chondro-genic hormones. It regulates growth of long bones.
2. Lactogenic hormone (prolactin) — see p. 75.
3. Trophic hormones:
   (a) Thyrotrophin (TSH, thyroid – stimulating hormone).
   (b) Adrenocorticotropic hormone (ACTH).
   (c) The gonadotrophins (FSH, LH, and LTH) — see Table 7–2.

In the human, little is known of the functions of the pars tuberalis and the pars intermedia. The pars nervosa of the posterior lobe secretes two hormones (1) oxytocin, which acts on the

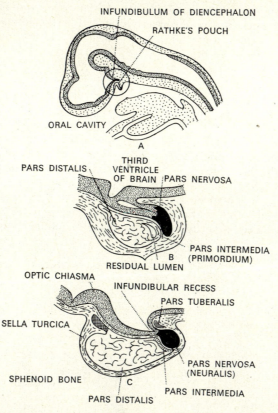

INFUNDIBULUM OF DIENCEPHALON

RATHKE'S POUCH

ORAL CAVITY

A

PARS DISTALIS

THIRD VENTRICLE OF BRAIN

PARS NERVOSA

PARS INTERMEDIA (PRIMORDIUM)

RESIDUAL LUMEN

B

OPTIC CHIASMA

INFUNDIBULAR RECESS

PARS TUBERALIS

SELLA TURCICA

PARS NERVOSA (NEURALIS)

SPHENOID BONE

C

PARS INTERMEDIA

PARS DISTALIS

FIG. 17–4. Development of the hypophysis cerebri (pituitary gland) (adapted from several sources):
A. Sagittal section of the cephalic part of a 6-week embryo showing the position of the two components (circled) of the gland: Rathke's pouch (blank); infundibulum (black);
B. 55-mm. embryo (about 80 days);
C. Newborn.

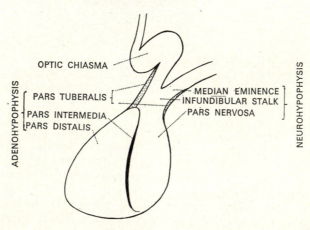

OPTIC CHIASMA

ADENOHYPOPHYSIS

PARS TUBERALIS

PARS INTERMEDIA

PARS DISTALIS

MEDIAN EMINENCE

INFUNDIBULAR STALK

PARS NERVOSA

NEUROHYPOPHYSIS

FIG. 17–5. Diagram of a sagittal section through the adult human pituitary.

smooth muscle of the uterus and facilitates child birth. This effect on the myometrial muscles is only observed after the latter have been properly prepared by the action of placental oestrogen (Table 7–2). (2) Pitressin (a vasopressor) has its effect on smooth muscles of arterioles and also has an anti-diuretic effect (see below).

Neuro-secretion

There is increasing evidence that the hormones, pitressin and oxytocin, which are supposedly secreted by the cells of the pars nervosa, are in fact produced by the hypothalamic nuclei. Such a claim is well grounded on an anatomical basis, namely the existence of a direct close physical connection between the posterior lobe and the hypothalamus (Fig. 17–6). Three such nuclei are shown in the diagram, the supra-optic, paraventricular and tuberal nuclei, the first of which is the most important of the three. Each of these nuclei has nerve tracts passing down into the pars nervosa. Theoretically, these tracts could be the pathway from the hormone-secreting neurons of the hypothalamus to the posterior lobe, and from there to the circulation. It has, indeed, been shown experimentally that cutting the supra-optic-hypophyseal tract produces diabetes insipidus; this is interpreted to be due to the stoppage or reduced output of the vasopressor hormone, pitressin.

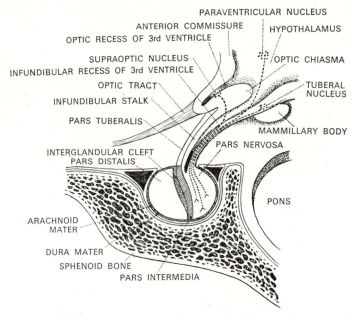

FIG. 17–6. Diagram to show the anatomical basis for neurosecretion; a sagittal section through the pituitary gland demonstrating the hypothalamo-hypophysial tracts.

The adrenal (suprarenal) gland

The adrenal gland, which is also formed by coalescence of two distinct primordia, consists of a central medulla and a peripheral cortex, much as in a developing ovary (p. 133).

Certain cells of the neural crest migrate, together with those destined to be the chain ganglia of the sympathetic system, and form a somewhat loose system known as the paraganglionic chromaffin bodies (so-called because they are stained brown with chromic salts). The largest of these, located just cephalic to the developing metanephric kidney, gives rise to the medulla of the adrenal gland (Fig. 17–7). The cortex is formed by cells of splanchnic mesoderm at the base of the dorsal mesentery near the cephalic pole of the mesonephros. By the end of the 8th week of development, a primary cortex is well established. It is of interest that the cells of the provisional cortex of this gland are assembled at the site first; the chromaffin cells then come along and penetrate the former to become the medulla, an " invasion " which occurs during the 7th week of development.

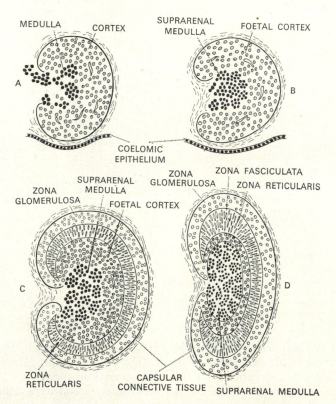

FIG. 17–7. Diagrams to show four successive stages in the differentiation of the suprarenal (adrenal) gland:
A. and B. 17 mm.; C. 35 mm.; D. 6 month.

In the third month the cells of this provisional cortex develop epithelial cords with vacuoles in them, suggesting that they may be already active in secretion (see below). Later, a permanent cortex is differentiated outside the primary cortex as the latter becomes involuted (Fig. 17–8A).

The primary cortex, however, shows very little further differentiation until toward the end of the foetal period when a process of replacement is evident. By the end of the first month of postnatal life, the degeneration of the primary cortex has far advanced. Its complete involution comes at about the end of the first postnatal year. The permanent or definitive cortex has, in the meantime, differentiated into three characteristic zones known as zona reticularis, zona fasciculata and zona glomerulosa (Fig. 17–8B). Of these, the reticularis (next to the medulla) is represented by degenerating cells; the middle layer, the zona fasciculata, is the functioning zone, whilst the outmost layer or zona glomerulosa, represents the regenerating zone. The latter shows active mitoses. On the other hand, the zona reticularis is the remnant of the provisional cortex, and as such, its cells appear to be secreting a substance. One theory is that this substance is a male sex hormone, the implication being that it is a mechanism whereby the large quantities of female sex hormone produced by the syncytiotrophoblast of the placenta may be counterbalanced. This theory receives some support from the observation that hyperplasia of the zona reticularis, such as is caused by a tumour, frequently leads to masculinization (cf. p. 142).

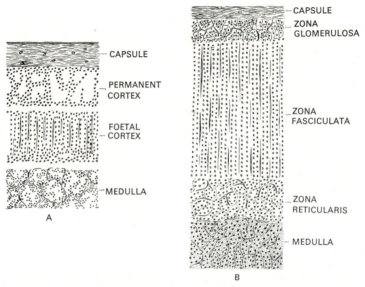

FIG. 17–8. A. Drawing of the developing adrenal gland of a 9-week (35 mm.) human embryo (from a photomicrograph);
B. Drawing of a section of the adult human adrenal gland; (cells of the zona reticularis are shown dark; cells of the medulla are light).

The adrenal is a very important endocrine gland, the hormones elaborated by its cortex being of such vital importance to life that an individual will not live without it. The cortical hormones produced by it are steroids and perform the following general functions.

1. Desoxycorticosterone regulates electrolysis between extra and intra-cellular fluids, acting especially on sodium and potassium ions.
2. Corticosterones stimulate glyconeogenesis with diabetogenic effect and increase the efficiency of muscles.
3. Cortisone (stimulated by ACTH) affects the connective tissue activity and regulates kidney functions.
4. A male-hormone-like hormone, may be produced under certain conditions and function as an androgenic hormone.

The adrenal medulla produces the hormone, epinephrine or adrenalin, which is a sympatho-mimetic agent whose actions resemble those obtained by stimulation of the sympathetic nerves. This is not surprising since the chromaffin tissue of the medulla and the sympathetic components of the autonomic nervous system are of the same derivation, namely from the neural crest.

CHAPTER 18

THE INTEGUMENTARY SYSTEM

The integumentary system may be represented as follows.

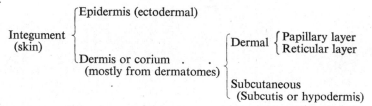

The papillary layer of the dermal portion of the dermis has two kinds of papillae. Some of them are vascularized and contain Meissner's corpuscles (Fig. 21–1); others are not supplied with blood vessels and nerve endings.

The reticular layer of the dermal portion of dermis contains both collagenous and elastic fibres. The subcutaneous portion of the dermis is highly adiposal, i.e., rich in fat (Fig. 18–1).

The development of the epidermis (Fig. 18–2) is summarized in the table below.

up to 4th week	5th week	3–4 months	Definitive (from 6th month onwards)
	Periderm*	(Periderm)	Stratum corneum (outermost layer)
a single layer of cuboidal cells	two cellular layers	stratum intermedium stratum granulosum	stratum lucidum stratum granulosum (spinosum) stratum germinativum (innermost or Malpighian layer)

Note: In the definitive epidermis, except for the soles and palms, the stratum lucidum and the stratum granulosum are either not easily distinguishable, or are not represented.

* a thin layer of flattened cells soon to be cast off.

The corium is derived from mesenchyme of two sources; these are (*a*) dermatomes from lateral wall of the somites and (*b*) somatic mesoderm of the lateral plate (Table 11–1).

Derivatives of the integument

1. Nails. The nail of primates is homologous with the claws and hoof of lower mammals. Its primordium in man arises during the third month of development as a thickened area at the end of the digit, the primary nail field. It is bounded by shallow lateral nail folds and a much deeper proximal nail fold (Fig. 18–3). Limited local cornification of the primary nail field gives rise to a false nail (of no significance); the true nail, however, is derived from the underlying epidermal layers of the proximal nail field. Active proliferations of the basal stratum germinativum cells in the nail matrix soon initiate keratinization in the cells of the stratum lucidum to form a nail plate. This process proceeds as far distally as the edge of the lunula, beyond which the nail plate migrates progressively over the nail bed until the tip of the finger is reached

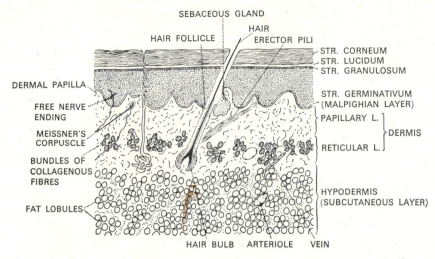

FIG. 18–1. Semi-diagrammatic drawing of a vertical section of human skin, showing its component layers and their derivatives.

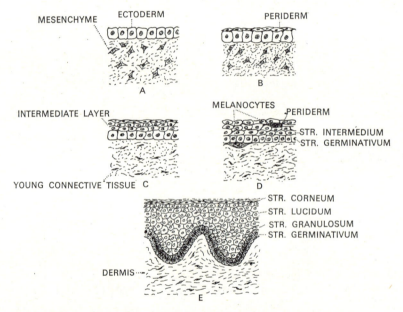

FIG. 18–2. Development of the human skin:
A. 4 mm.; B. 12 mm.; C. c. 30 mm.; D. c. 55 mm.; E. 145 mm.

some weeks before birth. At first, the corneum of the epidermis covers the free nail as the eponychium. The latter is lost during later foetal months except for a horny portion that persists and adheres to the nail plate only along the lateral borders. The epidermal cells underneath the free end of the nail differentiate into a horny substance, the hyponichium; this is not important in man, but the same substance forms the " sole " in hoofed mammals.

2. Hair. Hair first appears during the third month on the eye brows, upper lip and chin; it develops over the general body surface one month later. The fine hairs covering the entire

foetus constitute the lanugo; the latter, plus secretion from the sebaceous glands and desquamated epithelial cells, forms a peculiar mixture known as the vernix caseosa, which protects the delicate skin.

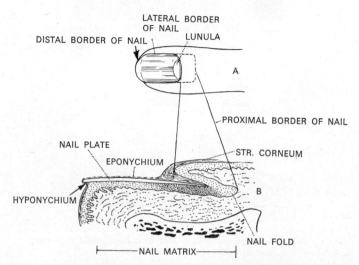

FIG. 18–3. Development of the human nail (adapted from several sources):
A. Diagram of the end of a finger and fingernail (dorsal aspect);
B. The developmental stage of the nail at birth, longitudinal section.

Development of hair

A hair starts as a solid ingrowth of stratum germinativum cells with a club-shaped bottom (Fig. 18–4A, B), which soon becomes indented to receive a mesodermal component, the dermal papilla (Fig. 18–4C). For the first generation, the entire hair shaft is composed of epidermal cells. Beginning from the second generation of hair growth, however, each new hair is differentiated from cells of the bulb and is arranged in layers around a central mesodermal core, the medulla. These epidermal layers may be listed from within as the cortex, hair cuticle, inner sheath cuticle, Huxley's layer, Henle's layer and external root sheath. Always associated with a hair are a sebaceous gland and an arrector pili muscle, both being attached to the follicular wall, the former slightly above the latter (Fig. 18–4C). The sebaceous gland represents a localized proliferation of epidermal cells, which secrete an oily substance (composed mostly of dead cells) into the follicular cavity (Fig. 18–4D). The arrector pili muscle is a strand of involuntary (smooth) muscle developed from the surrounding mesenchymal (dermatome) cells. The hair papilla, besides supporting blood vessels and nerves, also acts as an inductor for hair development. As in feathers, the dermal papilla is indispensable for regeneration of hairs that are shed or lost accidentally. Baldness is due to death of hair papillae.

3. Oral (salivary) glands. Three pairs of salivary glands develop between the third and sixth months, the earliest to appear being the parotid; the submandibular gland develops next and finally the sublingual (Fig. 18–5A). They are generally regarded as ectodermal, although the parotid glands could be both ectodermal and endodermal. Each of them starts as a primordium consisting of an epithelial bud (Fig. 18–5B) which grows by repeated branching into a bush-like system of solid ducts, the end twigs of which finally round out into berry-like secretory acini. The ducts are then canalized and the cells are differentiated for the secretion of saliva (Fig. 18–5B, C). A dense mass of mesenchyme finally furnishes an enveloping capsule, and the gland is subdivided into lobes. The same mesenchyme also supplies a stroma to support blood vessels

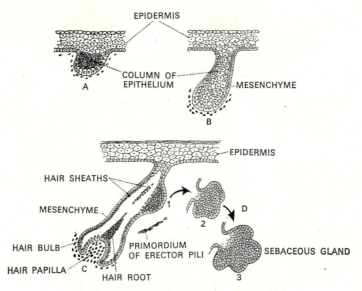

FIG. 18–4. Development of hair and sebaceous gland in human:
A. 3–4 month; B. 5-month; C. 6-month.

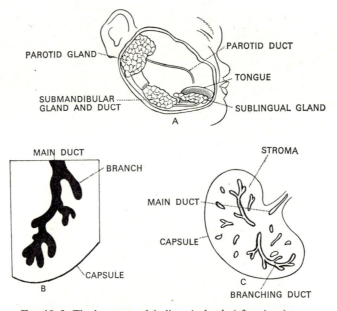

FIG. 18–5. The human oral (salivary) glands (after Arey):
A. Location of the major salivary glands in the newborn;
B. The submandibular gland at 2-months;
C. Diagram of the submandibular gland at 10-weeks.

and nerves. In addition to these main salivary glands, the oro-pharyngeal region (except for the hard palate) gives rise to numerous minor oral glands which are much smaller in size.

4. Sudoriferous (sweat) glands. These glands appear during the fourth month of development, first at the finger tips, palm and soles. Their mode of development is similar to that of

hair except that they are more compact and do not have a dermal papilla. During the sixth and seventh month the deeper portion of the ingrowth coils and acquires a lumen (Fig. 18–6A). In their final stage of development an inner layer of cells takes on the function of secreting, whereupon the peripheral cells differentiate into myo-epithelial cells which serve as the contractile elements (Fig. 18–6B) for the regulation of the amount of excretion.

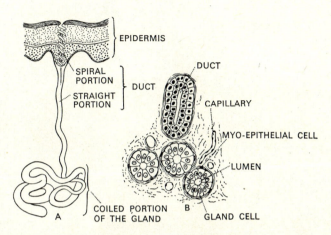

FIG. 18–6. Human sweat gland (adapted from several sources):
    A. Diagram to show the extent of an entire sweat gland;
    B. Drawing of a section through the lower portion of a sweat gland, including both the duct and glandular components.

5. Mammary glands. These are modified and greatly specialized sudoriferous glands. Their first appearance takes the form of a pair of longitudinal ridges (the milk lines) between the anterior and posterior limb buds (about 5–6 weeks); although continuous at first, most of this line later disappears (Fig. 18–7A). Of the two glands that ultimately develop in the human, each differentiates an areola (Fig. 18–8), a region devoid of hair and which surrounds the nipple. The glands are equally developed in the two sexes at birth (Fig. 18–7B, C, D), their subsequent development depending on the action of sex hormones (Chapters 7 and 17). At puberty, female sex hormone (ovarian oestrogen) excites the gland, with a consequent great enlargement due to an increase in the amount of supporting tissue and extension of the duct system (Fig. 18–8). During pregnancy progesterone and oestrogens (or the latter alone) cause further branching of the ducts and budding of the secretory end pieces (Fig. 7–7C). Such a gland is capable of secretion, but actual secretion of milk is withheld by the presence in the blood of placental oestrogen, oestriol, which inhibits the pituitary lactogenic hormone, prolactin, so preventing milk secretion. The latter hormone finally triggers milk secretion the moment the oestriol concentration falls, consequent upon the removal of the placenta at parturition.

Skin anomalies

    (1) albinism (complete absence of pigmentation) (2) melanism (over-abundance of pigments) (3) ichthyosis (rough, scaly skin) (4) " alligator " skin (an extreme case of (3)) (5) hypertrichosis (excessive hairyness) (6) amastia (absence of mammary gland (usually one missing) (7) macromastia (abnormally large mammary gland) (8) gynecomastia (development of female type of mammary gland in the male as the result of hormone disorder or inbalance) (9) hypermastia (supernumerary mammary glands — rare) (10) hyperthelia (accessory nipples).

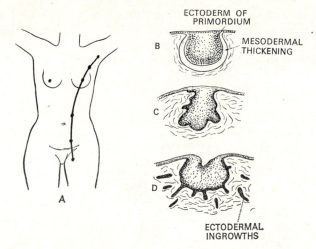

FIG. 18–7. Development of the human mammary gland (after Hamilton, Boyd and Mossman):
    A. Drawing to show the position of the mammary ridge (solid line, shown on left side only). Supernumerary mammary glands occur along this line;
    B–D. Drawings of photomicrographs of sections of developing mammary glands in human embryos;
    B. 24-mm.; C. 120-mm. female; D. 80-mm. male.

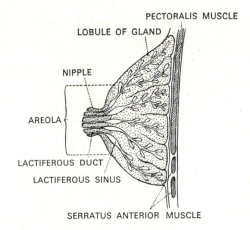

FIG. 18–8. Longitudinal section of the breast showing the virgin mammary gland.

Development of teeth

Teeth are highly specialized structures. They begin as areas of thickened oral epithelium, the dental ledges or lamina, in each jaw. As the ledge sinks deeper into the underlying mesenchyme, its basal end comes into intimate association with a dental papilla (cf. hair). As a result, the dental lamina is converted into a double-layered inverted " cup " known as the enamel organ, with its inner enamel layer directly apposed to the mesenchymal core of the indented dental papilla. The cells of the inner enamel layer in contact with the dental papilla differentiate into ameloblasts, which are specialized to produce the enamel of teeth (the hardest substance in the body). Meantime, the cells of the dental papilla lying immediately next to the ameloblasts give rise to odontoblasts, which produce the dentine (Fig. 18–9). The enamel (outer) and dentine (inner) so produced by the cells from two germ layers furnish a hard covering for the tooth (Fig. 18–10).   A total of 20 such tooth primordia are established by the end of the sixth week of development.

The space between the inner and outer enamel layers of the enamel organ is filled with a loose ectodermal mesenchyme, known as the enamel pulp.   At the base of each developing tooth, a third component surrounds the enamel organ and dental organ.   This is the dental sac, which is contributed by dermal mesenchymal cells (Fig. 18–9c).   Certain of these cells differentiate into cementoblasts (very similar to osteoblasts) and begin to produce a cement which covers the root of the developing tooth.   The remainder of the dental sac forms a peridental membrane. The function of this membrane is to produce characteristic ligamental fibres for the purpose of anchoring the root of the tooth to the cement on one side, and to the periosteum of the jaw bone on the other (Fig. 18–11).   Finally, as the tooth erupts, the central papilla lengthens to become the pulp of the tooth, sustaining blood vessels and nerves in it.

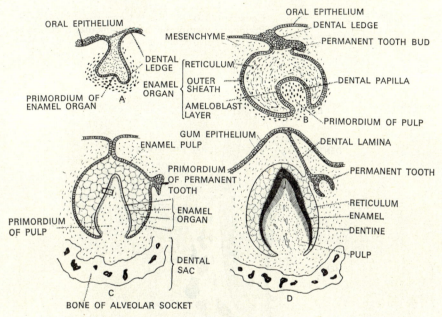

FIG. 18–9. Development of a tooth (adapted from several sources):
A. 9-week; B. 11-week; C. 14-week; D. 7-month.

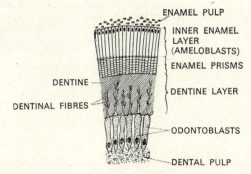

F G. 18–10. Diagrammatic drawing of histological details of the tooth-forming area indicated by a rectangle in Fig. 18–9c.

The primordia of permanent teeth are laid down beside the decidual (milk) teeth (Fig. 18–9c, D). Formation of dentine and enamel in the decidual teeth begins in the fifth month of development; this is followed by the first permanent molars during the sixth month, and after birth by the other permanent teeth. The three definitive components of a tooth and their respective derivatives are summarized below:

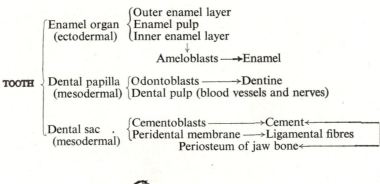

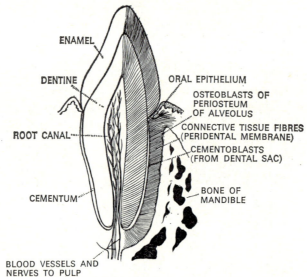

FIG. 18–11. Schematic diagram to show the topographical relations of a definitive tooth and its jaw bone as a result of the activity of the dental sac.

CHAPTER 19

THE NEURAL TUBE AND CREST

Introduction

The nervous system, plus the skin and its derivatives are derived mostly from ectoderm. Together, the two bring about coordination and integration of the different parts of the body, communicate with the environment, and achieve the level of mental development characteristic of *Homo sapiens*. In order to realize these functions the neurons have reached an exceedingly high level of morphological specialization, and the various components are closely knit into a working system. The nervous system consists of (1) the neural tube, which is subdivided into the spinal cord and has at its specialized anterior end, the brain, (2) the neural crest, a separate entity of nervous ectoderm, (3) the peripheral nervous system composed of ganglia and nerves of various origins, and (4) the sense organs, or receptors.

The establishment of the necessary connections between the central and peripheral stations and between the various receptors and effectors takes time. That is why, even though the nervous system starts to develop very early, it is the last system to be completed, especially when we take into account the cortical development of the cerebrum and cerebellum. The baby is born with its nervous system developed only to the degree which enables him to cope with situations necessary for life. Some coordination, however, exists long before birth as evidenced by such movements of the foetus as kicking, hiccoughing, and thumb-sucking. But, perfection in muscular control and the development of intellectual power only comes during postnatal years.

As previously stated (p. 83) the formation of the nervous tissue is a case of induction of the first order. The inductors involved are primarily the chordamesoderm, which directs the formation and morphogenesis of the brain and spinal cord, and the bilaterally arranged paraxial mesoderm, which induces the formation of the neural crest. In the former process, it is now evident that an actual transfer of a substance from the inductor to the cells of the medullary plate takes place (p. 85). This transfer is probably assisted by a close juxtaposition of the two tissues during the process of induction.

The neural tube

The neural tube first appears as a thickened band of ectoderm, the neural or medullary plate, which is formed along the mid-dorsal line of the embryo at the beginning of the third week of development and extends cranially from the primitive node. Two days later, the central line of this plate becomes depressed into a neural groove, whilst the two edges of the plate elevate to form the neural ridges or folds. These changes are well shown in Spee's embryo illustrated in Fig. 4–9. Next, the neural groove deepens and the neural ridges arch upwards, approaching each other until they fuse to form a tube, the neural tube (Fig. 19–1).

The fusion of the neural ridges begins at the level of the fourth somite, proceeding from there both in a cephalic and caudal direction until the closure of the tube is completed; this occurs first at the anterior end (about the 23rd day) and then at the posterior end (25th day). After the closure of the anterior and posterior neuropores the neural tube becomes the primordium of the central nervous system, with its anterior rounded end destined to form the brain and its posterior cylindrical portion to become the spinal cord. A cavity, the neural canal, runs throughout its length.

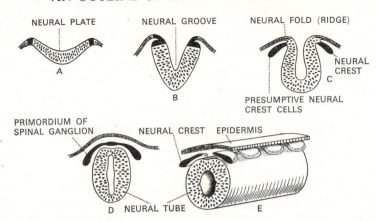

Fig. 19–1. Formation of the neural tube:
   A–D. Transverse sections from early human embryos to show the origin of the neural tube
        and neural crest;
   E. Drawing of a model of the early spinal cord and the segmented neural crest.

The primary vesicles of the brain

The prosencephalon, mesencephalon and rhombencephalon are three swellings at the anterior end of the neural tube which are known as the primary brain vesicles; they are established at about the 20-somite stage (Fig. 19–2A).

About two weeks later, further division of the prosencephalon and rhombencephalon takes place, the former giving rise to the diencephalon and the lateral telencephalon (or future cerebral hemisphere) on each side. The rhombencephalon subdivides into the metencephalon which is adjacent to the mid-brain and the myelencephalon which is continuous with the remainder of the neural tube (Fig. 19–2B), with the mesencephalon, however, remaining undivided. A small isthmus region marks the boundary between the mid-brain (the undivided mesencephalon) and the hind-brain, whilst a small diverticulum, the lamina terminalis, marks the most anterior point of the brain.

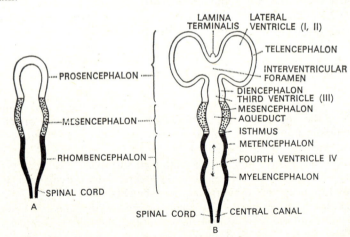

Fig. 19–2. Schematic drawings to show two stages in the development and regional differentiation of the brain (frontal section):
   A. 3-vesicle stage (about 25 days);
   B. 5-vesicle stage (about 40 days).

The cavities (ventricles) of the brain

The original neural canal is greatly expanded to form the ventricles of the brain; details about them will be given later in connection with the differentiation of each definitive division of the brain. The summary below provides the basic information on the locations and names of these ventricles and the infoldings of ependymal tissue or choroid plexuses which are contained in them.

Brain vesicle	Ventricle	Choroid plexus
Telencephalon (future cerebral hemisphere)	Lateral Ventricle (I, II)	anterior choroid plexus
Diencephalon	Ventricle III	
Mesencephalon	the aqueduct (of Sylvius)	
Metencephalon and myelencephalon	Ventricle IV	posterior choroid plexus

The lateral ventricles and the IIIrd ventricle communicate with each other via the interventricular foramen (the foramen of Monro).

Histogenesis of the neural tube

The epithelium of the neural tube is at first pseudostratified, but it soon gives rise to three recognizable zones, the ependymal layer, which is separated from the central canal by an internal limiting membrane, a middle mantle layer and a marginal layer which is bounded by an external limiting membrane (Fig. 19–3A, B, C). These layers remain distinct in the spinal cord, but in the brain their relative extent and positions are subsequently somewhat modified, especially in the fore- and hind-brain. This is primarily due to the fact that in these regions a secondary invasion of the marginal zone by the cells of the mantle will occur (see p. 225).

The ependymal layer, in its definitive condition, contains a single layer of ciliated cells which have no nervous function. Nevertheless, it starts out as the germinal layer and as such, mitotic figures are seen frequently in it during early development. This means that all definitive cells of the mantle layer (destined to be the future grey matter of the spinal cord and the brain) are the products of proliferation of this germinal layer. The axons of the neurons in the mantle layer run largely in the marginal layer and make up the white matter of the definitive spinal cord and brain.

When a cell of the germinal layer divides, the two daughter cells may both temporarily leave the internal limiting membrane, extending their processes into the mantle layer. Eventually, one of them remains in the germinal layer, ready to divide again, whilst the other becomes a permanent resident of the mantle layer from which neuroblasts and spongioblasts (precursors of the neuroglial elements) differentiate. The significant fact is that these cells do not divide further, but differentiate into the neurons and glial cells directly (Fig. 19–3D). It is also significant that the glial cells of the following types, protoplasmic astrocytes, fibrous astrocytes and oligodendroglial cells are of ectodermal origin.

The prospective neurons first appear as rounded neuroblasts, which become successively unipolar and multipolar as they differentiate into commissural neurons, motor neurons of the ventral horn, or motor neurons of the brain, e.g., the pyramidal cell of the cerebral cortex (Fig. 19–3D). Along with increase in the cell processes (dendrites and axons) distinct organelles (Nissl's substance, Golgi apparatus, neurofibrils* and an endoplasmic reticulum) begin to appear in the cytoplasm of the neurons. Losses of these highly specialized neurons of the central nervous system (whether on account of injury, degeneration or for any other cause) cannot be replaced.

The central nervous system has another type of glial tissue, known as microglia. These are small sustentacular cells always associated with blood vessels. The origin of these cells has not

---

* Recent research has shown that in the chick this is the first and earliest discernible organelle in differentiating neuroblasts of the tube.

been unequivocally established, but some workers believe they belong to the vascular adventitia (and are therefore a kind of pericyte) while others think that they may be derived from the neural crest.

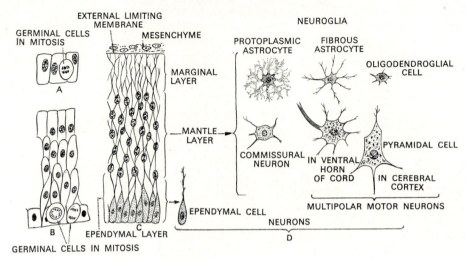

FIG. 19–3. Generalized stages in the histogenesis of the spinal cord; the diagram also shows the types of nerve cells and neuroglial cells derived from the mantle and ependymal layers of the wall of the neural tube:
A. Epithelium of medullary plate;
B. Wall of recently closed neural tube (5 mm.);
C. Transverse section of the spinal cord of a 6-week human embryo (10 mm.);
D. Neurons and neuroglial cells.

THE NEURAL CREST

Origin of neural crest

Before closure of the neural tube a longitudinal band of cells alongside each neural ridge is set aside from the prospective neural tube (Fig. 19–1B). During the closure of the neural tube these cells are left out, and form the discrete neural crest material which lies in the angle between the closed neural tube and the paraxial mesoderm (Fig. 19–1C, D, E). For this reason, the paraxial mesoderm is believed to have induced the formation of the neural crest. Immediately following its separation, the neural crest forms a cellular band extending the full length of the spinal cord and some distance cephalically on both sides of the brain. New crest tissue is then added progressively in a caudal direction along with the growth of the neural tube. Subsequently, however, a process of periodic attenuation sets in to cut the continuous band transversely into separate pairs of bead-like enlargements, one pair to each segment, corresponding closely to the somites. These discrete units of the initial crest material are the primordia of spinal ganglia. In the region of the hind-brain the neural crest gives rise to the ganglia of the cranial nerves, V to X, which supply the branchial arches (see Figs. 20–22 and 24).

Differentiation of the neural crest

The neural crest cells of the spinal ganglia primordia remain in their initial sites and differentiate into the somatic and visceral sensory neurons. These neurons are typical T-shaped unipolar cells (Fig. 19–5B, C), the axon of which migrates towards the spinal cord, stopping at the dorsal horn of the grey matter; the dendrite grows towards the periphery to become related to developing epaxial and hypaxial myoblasts (which will form the muscle masses of the shoulder, limbs and body wall) along the course of the dorsal root and main stem of the spinal nerves. Other cells of the crest move ventro-medially (Fig. 19–4). Along this path, they form the neurons of the sympathetic ganglia, cells of the preotic ganglia and organ plexuses and the cells of the medulla of the adrenal gland (Fig. 19–4). The latter cells are the most prominent members of a somewhat diffuse system of chromaffin tissue (so-called because they have a marked affinity for chrome salts); this tissue is capable of elaborating the hormone, epinephrine. Other chromaffin cells are scattered around the autonomic ganglia and plexuses as paraganglia which occur along the course of the aorta and possibly at other sites. Most of these paraganglia atrophy soon after puberty.

In addition, the neural crest also gives rise to the satellite cells, which form a capsule for the neurons of the spinal ganglia, and the neurolemma cells or cells of Schwann, which ensheath the axonal processes of these cells. Also, the melanoblasts are derived exclusively from the neural crest (Fig. 19–6). Meningeal cells of the pia-arachnoid are perhaps partly of neural crest origin (p. 220). A summary of the derivatives of the neural crest is given in Table 19–1.

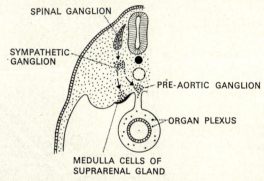

FIG. 19–4. Derivatives of the neural crest, schematic transverse section of a human embryo (approx. 6 weeks) to show ventro-medial migration of cells of the neural crest. This results in the formation of a sympathetic ganglion, a prevertebral ganglion, the medulla of the suprarenal gland and organ plexuses.

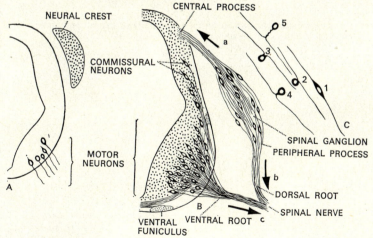

FIG. 19–5. A and B. Growth and differentiation of human neuroblasts in the spinal cord, seen in transverse section; A, at 4 mm.; B, at 5 mm.;
C. Stages in the transformation of bipolar (1) into definitive pseudo unipolar (5) neurons with intervening stages (2, 3, 4), which take place inside the differentiating dorsal ganglion root.

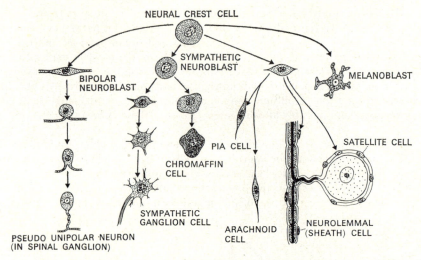

Fig. 19–6. Schematic representation of the possible developmental fates of neural crest cells.

TABLE 19–1.   DERIVATIVES OF THE NEURAL CREST

A. From the neuroblasts
    1. neurons of spinal ganglia
    2. neurons of cranial ganglia (possibly with contributions from placodes dorsal to the branchial grooves)
    3. neurons of ganglia of the autonomic nervous system with possible contributions from cells migrating out from the ventral plate of the spinal cord

B. From the spongioblasts
    1. Satellite (capsule) cells
    2. Cells of Schwann (sheath cells) of neurolemma, responsible for the formation of myelin in collaboration with the axon (another subsidiary source is cells from the mantle layer, passing out along the ventral root)
    3. The meninges (in part)

C. Other derivatives
    1. The chromaffin tissue including that which forms the medulla of the adrenal gland
    2. Pigment cells (chromatophores or melanocytes)

CHAPTER 20

CENTRAL AND PERIPHERAL NERVOUS SYSTEM

The origin and histogenesis of the neural tube, and the neural crest and its derivatives have already been considered. In this chapter we will trace the course of development by which the processes of the neuroblasts of neural crest origin become so linked with the brain and spinal cord as to be integrated into a closely knit system. This system comprises three components (1) the central nervous system, consisting of the brain and the spinal cord (2) the peripheral nervous system, consisting of the cranial and spinal nerves and the autonomic nervous system, and (3) the receptors (all types) which connect the nervous system with the external and internal environments. Parts of (2) and (3) plus the effectors (muscles, blood vessels, glands, etc.) comprise what is known as the action system.

I. THE SPINAL CORD

Cavity of the neural tube

An uninterrupted cavity runs the entire length of the neural tube. This cavity is filled with a plasma-like fluid, the cerebro-spinal fluid, the formation of which is credited to the secretory activity of the choroid plexuses. This fluid not only keeps circulating, but maintains a constant pressure. It flows from the ventricles of the brain to the subarachnoid spaces through special exits, the median aperture (foramen of Magendie) and the lateral apertures (the foramina of Luschka) in the roof of the fourth ventricle (Fig. 20–13).

The cavity of the spinal cord, which is quite spacious at an early stage of development, undergoes a substantial reduction, largely as a result of the development of the grey matter and finally reaches the size of the definitive central canal (Fig. 20–1). In the brain, however, considerable modification of this cavity takes place, the most significant feature about this modification being the formation of special vascularized structures, the choroid plexuses (p. 225).

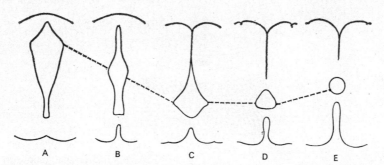

Fig. 20–1. A partial transverse section of human spinal cord showing the changes in the size and shape of the central canal (the dotted lines trace the approximate level of the sulcus limitans as a result of the changes): A. at 6 weeks; B. at 8 weeks; C. at 9 weeks; D. at 3 months; E. adult (adapted from several sources).

The meninges

Both the brain and the spinal cord are covered with connective tissue membranes, known as the meninges, which occupy a position between the nervous tissues and their bony enclosure. For this reason it is understandable that they have a composite origin, i.e., partly ectodermal and partly mesodermal. In the head their principal source is the head mesenchyme although possibly the neural crest in this region may contribute to it (Table 19–1). The meninges of the spinal cord are derived from the paraxial mesoderm, again with a possible contribution from the neural crest. Regardless of origin, all meningeal membranes have the same basic structure and develop in the same way. At first, the neural tube is surrounded by a highly angioblastic layer, the primi-

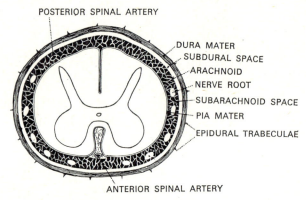

FIG. 20–2. Diagram of the spinal cord and meninges, seen in transverse section.

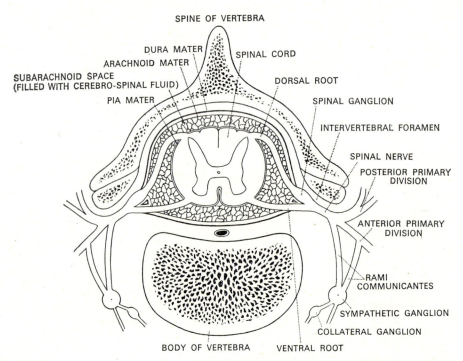

FIG. 20–3. Transverse section of the spinal cord, meninges, a vertebra and related structures.

tive meningeal layer. This layer gives rise to the capillary plexuses of the mantle layer of the neural tube and provides the vascular component (tela choroidea) of the choroid plexuses of the brain ventricles. The remaining cells of the primitive meningeal layer become the precursors of the definitive meninges. These consist of an inner thin endomenix (the pia mater, which is in contact with the marginal layer of the neural tube, separated by a space from the arachnoid mater) and an outer ectomenix, which is the much thicker dura mater with dural sinuses (Figs. 20–2; 20–3). The two inner layers are often referred to as the pia-arachnoid.

Regional differentiation of the spinal cord

The spinal cord is roughly uniform in diameter throughout its length except for two swellings, the cervical enlargement opposite the brachial plexus and the lumbo-sacral enlargement opposite the lumbo-sacral plexus (Fig. 20–22). The general shape of the cord and the size and shape of the neural canal undergo a series of changes until they reach the definitive condition in which the central cavity is reduced to a slit (Fig. 20–1). A dorsal median septum and a ventral median fissure are formed (Fig. 20–4). (The upper part of the slit-like canal is obliterated as a result of increases in the number of fibres of the posterior (dorsal) white column.) These changes may be attributed largely to an ever-increasing lateral expansion of the walls, particularly the mantle layer. During the process, a pair of lateral angles form a groove or sulcus limitans in the inner margin of the wall; this marks the division between the dorsal alar lamina and a ventral basal lamina of the neural tube (Fig. 20–4A, B). Both these plates contain all three layers of the wall; the various nuclei or cell columns develop in the mantle layer. The roof plate (above the alar lamina) and the floor plate (below the basal lamina), on the other hand, are devoid of a mantle layer and are therefore much thinner.

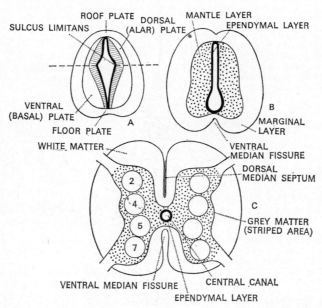

FIG. 20–4. Transverse sections through the spinal cord at three stages of development and differentiation of its gray matter. A. approx. 10 mm.; B. 25 mm.; C. at term, showing four columns of neuroblasts (nuclei) differentiating in the gray matter as follows;
     No. 2 — General somatic afferent (G. S. A.);
     No. 4 — General visceral afferent (G. V. A.);
     No. 5 — General visceral efferent (G. V. E.);
     No. 7 — General somatic efferent (G. S. E.).

Regression of the spinal cord

At about the third month (in 30 mm. embryos) the spinal cord extends throughout the entire length of the embryo. Subsequently, however, because of a differential growth rate of the vertebral column and the neural tube (the former extending far more rapidly than the latter), there occurs a progressive upward shift of the point of termination of the cord. At 6 months gestation the cord extends to the first sacral vertebra; at birth it is the third lumbar, and it terminates between the first and second lumbar vertebrae in the adult. During these positional shifts of the cord, the dura mater remains i.e., it extends throughout the whole length of the vertebral column throughout life whilst the inner meninges remain intimately related to the retreating cord. As a consequence, below the third lumbar vertebra the pia mater is reduced to a thread, the filum terminale; perhaps even more significant from a clinical point of view, a spacious sub-arachnoid space is left between segments L1 and L3. This space makes lumbar puncture for the withdrawal of cerebral-spinal fluid a safe procedure. Another consequence of this differential growth is that the spinal nerves become continually more slanted and extended farther from their segments of origin (Fig. 20–5).

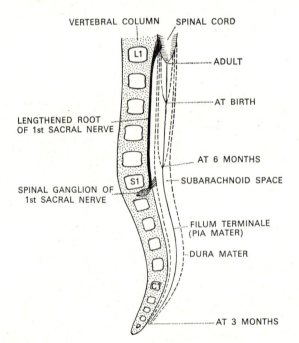

Fig. 20–5. Diagram to show the position of the caudal end of the neural tube in relation to the vertebral column at various stages of development. The vertebral canal is presented in the sagittal plane viewed from the left side.

Differentiation of nuclei in the grey matter

The mantle layer gives rise directly to the grey matter of the cord. Soon three thickened regions appear in it as centres of active proliferation and differentiation of neuroblasts into definitive neurons. These regions constitute the ventral (anterior) horn, the intermedio-lateral horn and dorsal (posterior) horn. The following four nuclei develop (Figs. 20–4c; 20–21). From the alar lamina

G.S.A. (general somatic afferent) receiving fibres from the exteroceptors in the skin and from proprioceptors (in tendons and joints) — No. 2, Figs. 20–4c, 20–6

G.V.A. (general visceral afferent) from taste buds and carotid sinuses — No. 4, Figs. 20–4c, 20–6

From the basal lamina

G.V.E. (general visceral efferent) to smooth muscle of blood vessels and viscera, and to glandular tissue, e.g., liver and salivary glands — No. 5, Figs. 20–4c, 20–6

G.S.E. (general somatic efferent) to skeletal muscles of trunk and extremities — No. 7, Figs. 20–4c, 20–6

The above four arcs are connected with commissural (association) neurons in the grey matter (Fig. 20–21). The four nuclei comprise the four components of spinal nerves. In the cranial region, however, additional nuclei develop e.g., a total of seven nuclei are present in the grey matter of the myelencephalon (Fig. 20–6). These additional nuclei (Nos. 1, 3 and 6 in Fig. 20–6) are to serve functions arising from special sense organs and from derivatives of the branchial arches. They include a special somatic afferent group from nose, eye and ear, which is situated just above the general somatic afferent nucleus; a somatic visceral afferent group just below the general somatic afferent nucleus, and a somatic visceral efferent group just above the general somatic efferent nucleus in the basal plate.

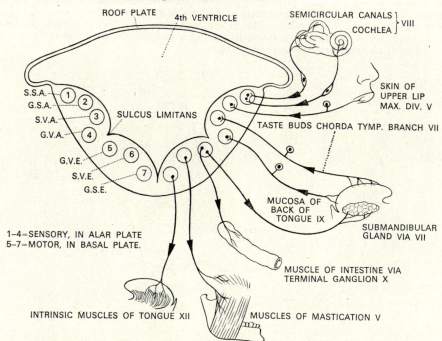

FIG. 20–6. A schematic composite diagram of a transverse section through the hindbrain after formation of the pontine flexure, showing the alar and basal laminae with their columns of neuroblasts. Examples of the various types of components found in cranial nerves are shown.

Development of the white matter

The marginal layer contains only the processes (fibres) of the neurons and constitutes the white matter of the spinal cord. At first, it is composed mainly of a network of processes from the neuroglial cells and ependymal cells, but later it receives axons of the neurons developing in the grey matter (the commissural fibres) and also axons from the neurons of the spinal ganglia.

Finally it is further thickened by additional fibres to and from the brain (the crossed ascending tracts and the descending corticospinal tracts arising in the cerebral cortex respectively). The white appearance of these fibres is due to their myelination which takes place in the fourth month of development. The fibres from these various sources become organized into bundles according to their place of origin.

Malformations of the spinal cord

A. Complete or partial rachischisis. By end of the fourth week the central nervous system is completely enclosed by bony structures (Fig. 20–3), and is thus detached from the overlying ectoderm. Occasionally, however, part of the neural tube (varying in extent) becomes exposed as a result of faulty closure of the neural groove traceable to either failure of the induction mechanism by the mesoderm or to intrinsic factors of the nervous system itself (Fig. 20–7D).

B. Spina bifida. Similar defects, if localized in the region of the spinal cord, are known as spina bifida, or cleft vertebra. The casual factor involved here is of a more specific nature, namely the failure of the neural arches of adjacent vertebrae to unite and fuse properly (cases of missing half-vertebrae or whole vertebrae are common). There are a number of categories differing only in the extent of the defect, the more severe cases involving hernia of the spinal cord. Some of these categories are listed below.

Spina bifida occulta (Fig. 20–7A). This is a case of failure of the dorsal portions of the vertebrae to fuse with one another, and usually is confined to the sacro-lumbar region. The defect is not externally noticeable except for a tuft of hair sometimes present over the surface of the bifid spine.

Meningocoele (Fig. 20–7B). When more than two defective vertebrae are involved, the meninges of the spinal cord bulge through the opening in the form of a sac covered with skin (cf. Fig. 20–20A).

Meningomyelocoele (Fig. 20–7C). This is a more severe case than meningocoele because the sac is so large that it contains, in addition to the meninges, also the cord and spinal nerves. The herniated parts are, however, still covered by skin.

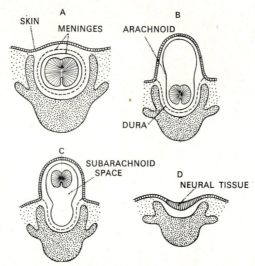

FIG. 20–7. Malformations of the spinal cord; various types of spina bifida: A. Bifida occulta; B. Meningocoele; C. Meningomyelocoele; D. Rachischisis.

II. THE BRAIN

The structural pattern of the spinal cord described above is modified in two basic ways in the brain. The first of these is by the formation of the choroid plexuses (Fig. 20–8). The roof plate which is devoid of mantle layer in the cerebral hemispheres (originally the telencephalon), diencephalon and rhombencephalon, becomes so thin that it consists of ependymal cells only.

The roof plate is in contact with blood vessels formed from the primitive meningeal layer described above; the two, being thus in close contact and growing at a rapid rate, fold repeatedly. This results in numerous invaginations, consisting of the ependymal cells on the outside and vascular capillaries on the inside being formed. These double-layered invaginations then project into the ventricle of the brain. (The formation of such composite structures may be compared to that of the renal corpuscle, which consists of Bowman's capsule and the glomerular capillaries, see p. 123). The term, tela choroidea, refers to the vascular roof of the brain ventricles in general. The other basic modification of the pattern of the spinal cord is the formation of the pallium in the cerebrum and cerebellum (Fig. 20–9). The great thickness of the cortex in both these divisions of the brain is the result of peripheral migration of neuroblasts of the mantle layer which produces the conspicuous thickened superficial layer known as the pallium. This enormous cortical expansion in three directions — anteriorly, laterally and caudally — may account, at least in part, for the

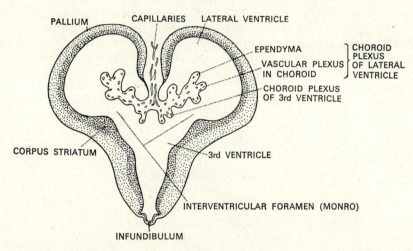

FIG. 20–8. Transverse section of the developing telencephalic vesicles (cerebral hemispheres) to show the invagination of the choroid plexuses into the lateral and third ventricles in a foetal brain (3-month).

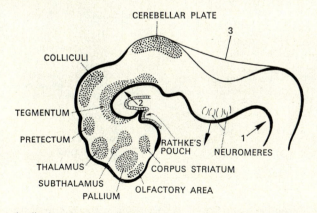

FIG. 20–9. Longitudinal section of the brain of a 7–9 mm. embryo showing the flexures indicated by arrows (1, cervical flexure; 2, mesencephalic flexure; 3, pontine flexure), and the principal areas and nuclear masses differentiating in the mantle layer of the lateral wall. The pallium is the future site of evagination of the cerebral hemispheres.

H

fact that in these regions there is an apparent reversal of the positions of the grey and white matters. The reversal is, however, not a real one but merely represents the outcome of a secondary translocation of the zones of the nuclei and fibre tracts, which are brought about largely by mechanical factors. Along with the pallium, other loci of nuclei differentiation are also shown in Fig. 20–9.

Brain flexures (Figs. 20–9; 20–10)

The primary brain vesicles (prosencephalon, mesencephalon and rhombencephalon) are established in 20-somite embryos. Soon after that the brain undergoes a series of flexures, which bend the initially straight brain into a number of intermediate positions leading to its definitive configuration. These flexures may be explained from a mechanistic point of view by assuming that they are designed to allow tremendous growth of the brain to occur within the limited space provided within the vault. The first flexure to appear is the cervical flexure, which sharply turns the brain ventrally at the junction of the hind-brain and spinal cord. The second flexure, also ventral but in the region of the mid-brain (mesencephalon), bends the future telencephalon downwards. In order to counteract the effect of these two flexures two flexures subsequently occur which bend the brain in the opposite direction; these are firstly the pontine flexure, followed very shortly by the telencephalic flexure. These two dorsal flexures have a telescoping effect on the developing brain, creating thereby a maximum possible room for its expansion.

The development of the human brain starts very early and the organ grows very rapidly

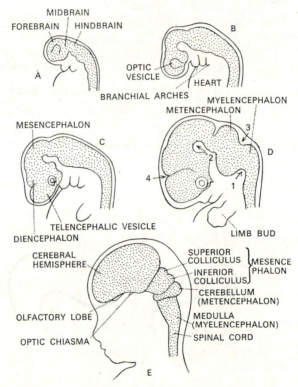

FIG. 20–10. Schematic representation of the changes in size and form of the embryonic and foetal brain (the area of the brain is dotted):
A, 20 somites; B, 4 mm.; C, 8 mm.; D, 17 mm.; E, 50–60 mm.
The arrows in D indicate the direction of bending of the four brain flexures (1, cervical flexure; 2, mesencephalic flexure; pontine flexure; 4, telencephalic flexure; see text).

By end of the 11th week of gestation (50–60 mm.) it has acquired the form of the adult brain and cerebral development is well advanced. Five stages in brain development (from $3\frac{1}{2}$ to 11 weeks) are presented in Fig. 20–10 to show the successive changes in shape, size and general contour of the human brain and its flexures.

Myelencephalon

The hind-brain, a derivative of the rhombencephalon, assumes a characteristic V shape, with its apex representing the pontine flexure. The definitive metencephalon and myelencephalon develop, respectively, from its cranial and caudal limbs, enclosing within them the thin-roofed fourth ventricle of the brain.

The myelencephalon extends from the first spinal nerve to the pontine flexure and becomes the medulla oblongata of the adult brain. Its roof is stretched thin and flattened out in the manner of a book being opened. The roof plate becomes thinned as the pontine flexure develops and is lined with a single layer of ependymal cells which are covered by the vascular pia mater (p. 225), the two making up the choroid plexuses of the diamond-shaped fourth ventricle (Fig. 20–14). The caudal and cranial angles of the fourth ventricle continue into the central canal of the spinal cord and the aqueduct of the mid-brain (Fig. 20–18). During the fourth month, three small apertures, two lateral foramina (foramina of Luschka) and a median foramen (the foramen of Magendie) are produced as a result of localized extreme thinning of the roof of the rhomben-cephalon (Fig. 20–13). These apertures make a free passage of the cerebrospinal fluid between the ventricles and the surrounding subarachnoid space possible.

The alar lamina gives rise, in part, to continuous columns of grey matter as in the spinal cord, and forms the following sensory nuclei (Fig. 20–6).

Type of nucleus	*Fibre source*
General somatic afferent	{from ear via stato-acoustic (VIII); from surface of head via bulbospinal (V).
Special visceral afferent	from taste buds (IX)
General visceral afferent	from intestinal tract (X).

In addition the alar lamina contains cells which migrate downward into the basal lamina as the bulbopontine extension to become the " olivary nuclei complex ".

The following motor nuclei arise in the mantle layer of the basal lamina (Fig. 20–6).

General somatic efferent (XII) — supplying muscles of the tongue derived from the occipital myotomes.

Special visceral efferent (nucleus ambiguus, IX) — supplying musculature derived from branchial arches 4, 5 and 6.

General visceral efferent (dorsal motor nucleus X) — supplying heart, lung and intestine bulbar portion of salivary nucleus (IX) — supplying glandular tissue.

The marginal layer of the myelencephalon receives longitudinally disposed myelinated fibres which form the conduction pathways between the spinal cord and the mid- and fore-brain.

Metencephalon (Cerebellum of the adult brain)

The metencephalon is located between the pontine flexure and rhombencephalic isthmus. If the roof plate is removed, the floor of the fourth ventricle will be exposed as the rhomboidal fossa. The cranial margin or rhombic lips of the latter, embracing the fourth ventricle, become thickened to form the primordium of the cerebellum. Cranial nerve V leaves its side.

The roof plate forms the roof of the anterior part of the fourth ventricle in which the choroid plexus develops in the manner described above. The alar lamina has the mantle layer of its dorso-lateral walls thrown into a series of folds, so forming the cerebellum (Fig. 20–11). The latter when completely developed, consists of three main lobes, a median vermis and two lateral hemispheres (Fig. 20–13). During its development, cells of the grey matter migrate peripherally to form the superficial cerebellar cortex. While other cells differentiate into definitive nuclei, the most important of which is the dentate nucleus, a second wave of migration takes place (Fig. 20–12). Cells derived from the latter, e.g., Purkinje cells, plus those developed from the first migratory wave, e.g., Golgi and granular cells, together form the substance of the definitive cerebellar cortex. Migration thus causes the greater part of the original roof of the metencephalon to become incorporated into the cerebellum, leaving only relatively small areas which remain thin as the velum (Fig. 20–12). The cerebellum contains synaptic centres involved in coordination of complex muscular movements.

Two groups of sensory nuclei develop in the grey matter of the metencephalon; these are general somatic afferent (contributions to the vestibular and cochlear nuclei of VIII and the pontine sensory nucleus of V) and a special visceral afferent component of VII.

The basal plate develops two groups of motor nuclei in its grey matter; a somatic visceral efferent nucleus for nerves V and VII — supplying muscles derived from branchial arches 1 and 2, and the secreto-motor salivary fibres of the VIIth cranial nerve, whilst the general somatic efferent nucleus of VI supplies the external rectus muscle of the eye.

The marginal layer of the basal plate expands into a ventral prominence, the pons (Fig. 20–11), which contains the pontine nuclei; these have migrated from the alar lamina of both the metencephalon and myelencephalon. The axons of the cells in these nuclei grow toward the cerebellum and give rise to the middle cerebellar peduncles. The pons and the cerebellar peduncles serve as a bridge connecting the cerebral and the cerebellar cortices with the spinal cord.

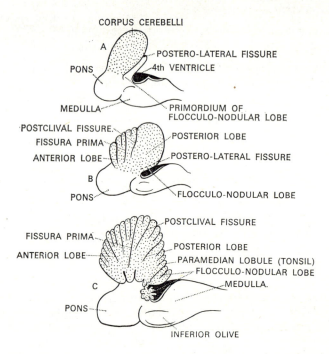

FIG. 20–11. Three stages in the development of the cerebellum (lateral view of left side): A, 95 mm.; B, 100 mm.; C, 150 mm.

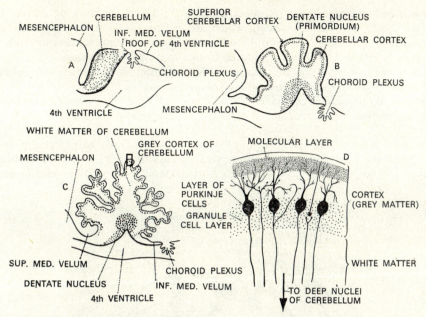

FIG. 20–12. Three stages (A, B, C) in the development of the cerebellum, seen in sagittal sections, which correspond, respectively, to those shown in Fig. 20–11. D. An area of the cerebellar cortex indicated by the rectangle in C is shown further enlarged.

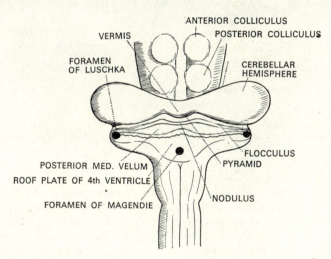

FIG. 20–13. Dorsal view of the mesencephalon and rhombencephalon in a 4-month human embryo (after Langman).

Mesencephalon

This is the least modified of the primary brain vesicles. It has thickened walls and contains a narrow lumen, the aqueduct of Sylvius, linking the third and fourth ventricles of the brain (Fig. 20–14).

The roof plate is represented only by a mid-line depression. Two pairs of rounded elevations develop from the mantle layer of the alar lamina or tectum, as it is called. They are the corpora

H2

quadrigemina, consisting of a pair of superior colliculi, which are synaptic centres for visual impulses, and a pair of inferior colliculi, which are centres for auditory reflexes (Fig. 20–13). Two other nuclei, the nucleus ruber and the substantia nigra occur in the mesencephalon. These nuclei either originate *in situ* or have migrated from a more dorsal position.

Two motor nuclei arise in the grey matter of the basal lamina or tegmentum. These are the Edinger-Westphal nucleus (general visceral efferent), supplying the sphincter pupillae muscle of the iris, and the general somatic efferent nuclei of cranial nerves III and IV — supplying, respectively, the internal rectus, lateral rectus, medial rectus, inferior oblique and the superior oblique muscles of the eye.

The marginal layer of the tegmentum gives rise ventro-laterally to prominent fibre tracts, the crus cerebri (basis pedunculi), which constitute pathways between the cerebral cortices and the lower centres of the pons and cord (e.g., the corticospinal, corticobulbar and corticopontine tracts).

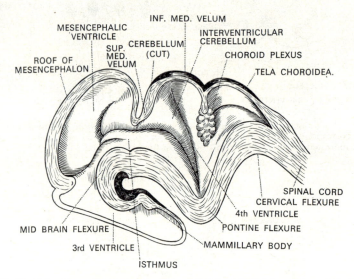

FIG. 20–14. Medial surface of a reconstruction of the right half (viewed from left side) of the mesencephalon and rhombencephalon of a 23 mm. human embryo (after Hamilton, Boyd and Mossman).

Diencephalon

This is the unpaired median portion of the original prosencephalon, in other words that part of the prosencephalon which does not participate in the formation of the cerebral hemispheres. It is characterized by a thin roof-plate and paired greatly thickened alar laminae, but lacks both floor and basal plates. It is bounded posteriorly by a plane passing behind the pineal and mammillary bodies, anteriorly by a plane just rostral to the optic chiasma encircling the foramen of Monro (Figs. 20–8; 20–15; 20–18).

The roof-plate gives rise to the anterior choroid plexus (plexus of the third ventricle) and the pineal body (epiphysis), which represents a dorsal evagination of its most caudal part with an obliterated lumen.

The mantle layer of the alar lamina develops on each side of the epiphysis a group of nuclei constituting the epithalamus. (Note: there is a possibility that the epithalamus is derived from cells of the roof plate, but in order to be consistent with the concept that the roof-plate is completely devoid of a mantle layer (see p. 221), it is treated here as a derivative of the alar lamina.) The marginal layer of the epithalamus gives rise to the habenular nuclei, which form a link in the olfactory conduction pathways and are connected to each other across the mid-line by the habenular commissure, the latter fibres being situated just rostral to the pineal stalk. Another group of fibres, the posterior commissure, which connect the two nuclei in a criss-cross fashion, are located caudal to this stalk.

The remainder of the alar lamina forms the lateral wall and the floor of the diencephalon as the thalamus and hypothalamus, respectively. The former bulges into the third ventricle and consists of dorsal nuclei having visual and auditory functions and ventral nuclei serving for relay stations. The hypothalamus has a distinct nucleus, known as the mammillary body. This is a round protuberance, forming a ventral boundary on each side of the middle line, concerned with the sense of smell. Other nuclei of the hypothalamus function as regulatory centres for sleep, digestion, body temperature control, and emotion.

A downward extension of the floor of diencephalon is the infundibulum. The hypophysis (p. 200) is derived jointly from the fusion of this nervous component and Rathke's pouch (Fig. 17–4).

Very early in development the optic vesicle arises as a pair of outpocketings from the ventro-lateral walls of the prosencephalon at the region of the future diencephalon.

The marginal layer also gives rise to prominent fibre tracts, the optic stalk tracts, and the optic chiasma which are closely associated with vision.

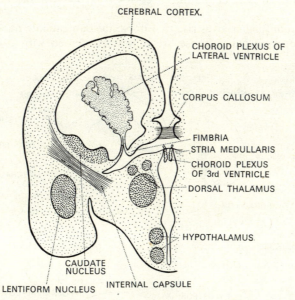

FIG. 20–15. Development of the cerebral hemispheres and their commissures. The hemisphere is drawn in transverse section, showing the corpus callosum and secondary fusion of telencephalon and diencephalon.

Telencephalon (Cerebral hemispheres of the adult brain)

The telencephalon begins to differentiate in 8 mm. embryos (about 5th week). The cerebrum comprises, in addition to the cerebral hemispheres, parts of the diencephalon and mesencephalon. The cerebral hemispheres develop as bilateral evaginations of the lateral wall of the prosencephalon as derivatives of the alar laminae. Beginning from the second month, they grow cranially, dorsally and caudally so extensively that eventually they overlap the diencephalon and mesencephalon. The formation of the frontal, temporal and occipital lobes results from this continuous expansion and growth of the cerebral hemispheres (Figs. 20–15; 20–16).

At the region where the pallium is attached to the roof of diencephalon, the choroid plexuses are formed in the usual manner (Figs. 20–7; 20–17). Sizeable tela choroidea project into the cavities of the telencephalon to form the choroid plexus of the first and second ventricles of the brain, more commonly known as the lateral ventricles, which communicate with each other and the third ventricle via the interventricular foramen (the foramen of Monro) (Fig. 20–8). Each lateral ventricle, assuming the shape of a reversed C, has an interior horn projecting into the frontal lobe, and a posterior horn projecting into the occipital lobe, and an inferior horn projecting into the temporal lobe (Fig. 20–18).

The cells of the mantle layer are differentiated into two portions, one of which migrates into superficial positions whilst the other remains deeply seated. The former, known as the pallium, (Figs. 20–8 and 9) is destined to give rise to the cerebral cortex, whilst the deeply situated cells of the latter give rise to the corpus striatum and other components of the basal ganglia (Fig. 20–8). The corpus striatum is recognizable by the middle of the second month of development as the mantle layer in the basal part of the hemispheres proliferates and bulges into the lumen of the lateral ventricle and floor of the foramen of Monro.

The pallium in turn, differentiates into two parts termed the palaeopallium, immediately lateral to the corpus striatum (7th week) and the neo-pallium. This latter is phylogenetically the most recent structure and constitutes that part of the cortex which contains such highly specialized neurons as the pyramidal cells of the motor cortex (Fig. 19–3D), and the granular cells of the sensory areas.

The corpus striatum further gives rise to a dorso-median caudate nucleus (Fig. 20–15) and a ventro-lateral lentiform nucleus. These are centres concerned with coordination of complex

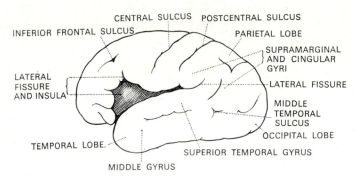

FIG. 20–16. Right cerebral hemisphere of a 7-month foetus, lateral view.

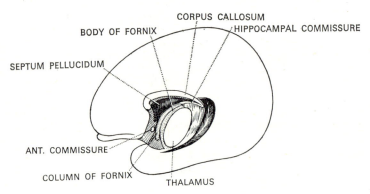

FIG. 20–17. A hemisected human brain at 4 months showing development of the commissures.

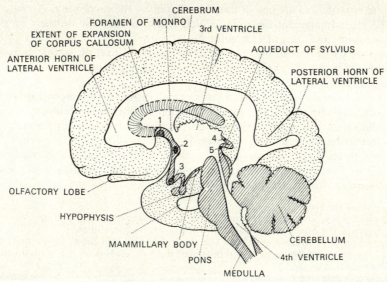

FIG. 20–18. Diagram of a hemi-section of human brain (over 4 months) showing the development and extent of cerebral ventricles and the sites of the various commissures: 1, corpus callosum; 2, rostral commissure; 3, optic chiasma; 4, habenular commissure; 5, posterior commissure.

muscular movements and their fibres, arranged in bundles, constitute the internal capsule which lies between the two nuclei (Fig. 20–15). In 10 mm. embryos some structures of the cerebral hemispheres and diencephalon come into very close association, e.g., the medial surface of the hemispheres meet and fuse with the lateral surface of the diencephalon, so causing the caudate nucleus and the thalamus to come into direct contact with each other.

The Commissures (Figs. 20–17 and 18)

These may be listed as follows.

1. Anterior commissures (part of paleopallium). They are visible in the lower part of the lamina terminalis by the 3rd month of development. (The lamina terminalis forms the anterior wall of the 3rd ventricle and represents the most anterior end of the neural tube; it is a natural bridge or commissural bed for fibre passage between the two cerebral hemispheres.) These commissures comprise fibres connecting the olfactory lobe and related brain areas of one hemisphere to the other.

2. The fornix (the part of paleopallium with olfactory functions). These are the dorsal or hippocampal commissures which arise in the hippocampus, pass anteriorly and converge on the lamina terminalis, thereby connecting the hippocampal areas to the mammillary body and hypothalamus, cross-connecting the two sides.

3. The corpus callosum (non-olfactory neo-pallial commissures). This starts to develop in the 4th month (later than the fornix); its fibres converge from all points onto the lamina terminalis, where they decussate dorsal to the hippocampal commissures, and then grow caudally and to the medial wall of the hemispheres. (The corpus callosum and the fornix system finally come to lie in the floor of the fissure between the cerebral hemispheres; between them lies a choroid fissure, which embodies the precursor of the anterior choroid plexus.)

4. The posterior or habenular commissures. These have already been described in connection with the diencephalon, see p. 231.

5. The optic chiasma. This lies in the rostral wall of the diencephalon and contains fibres from the medial halves of the retina which cross the mid-line on their way to the lateral geniculate body and the anterior colliculus.

The conduction paths interconnecting the cord and brain may be tabulated as follows.

(a) The dorsal funiculi of the cord, carrying impulses concerned with proprioceptive and tactile sensibility.

(b) Paths in the lateral funiculi, carrying sensations of pain and temperature to the brain and proprioceptive impulses from muscles, tendons, joints to be relayed to the cerebellum. These fibre tracts lie in the peripheral part of the white matter of the cord.

(c) Paths in the ventral funiculi, also carrying impulses of touch to the brain.

(d) The fibre tracts in the deeper portions of the lateral funiculi and much of the ventral funiculi, are occupied by descending paths transmitting impulses from the various levels of the brain to the efferent neurons of the cord.

Malformations of the brain

1. Micrencephaly, usually associated with a microcephalic head (Fig. 20–19A), is marked undevelopment of the brain which leads to very low level of intelligence.

2. Hydrocephaly (or macrocephaly). The condition is usually due to obstruction in the aqueduct of Sylvius; the impaired drainage of cerebo-spinal fluid distends both the brain and the yet unfused cranium (Fig. 20–19B).

3. Encephalocoele (see Fig. 20–20A). This is a case of herniation of the meninges and a part of the brain through an opening (usually at the base of the skull), resulting from faulty axial skeleton. This is particularly common at the weak spot where the skull joins the vertebral column.

4. Acrania (roofless skull) or anencephaly. This is usually associated with severe arrest of brain development. The brain consists of a mass of degenerative tissue exposed to the surface. The patient exhibits no neck and bulging eyes: face and chest form an almost continuous plane (Fig. 20–19C).

5. Cranio-rachischisis. This is a severe defect which combines acrania (see above) with an opened segment of the vertebral column (Fig. 20–19D).

6. Meningocoele (Fig. 20–20B). This defect consists of local herniation of the meningeal membranes through a defective portion of the skull (cf. Fig. 20–7B).

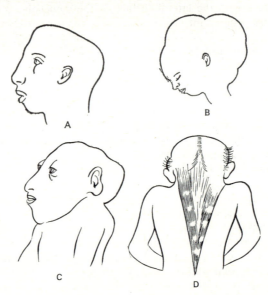

FIG. 20–19. Anomalies of the human brain (A, B, D modified from Arey; and C from Dodds):
    A. Micrencephaly (associated with a microcephalic head);
    B. Hydrocephaly, producing a macrocephalic head;
    C. Crainioschisis (acrania);
    D. Cranio-rachischisis (back view).

7. Meningo-encephalocoele (Fig. 20–20c) is a similar condition to encephalocoele, described above.

8. Meningohydro-encephalocoele (Fig. 20–20D), represents a modification of meningo-encephalocoele in that the protruded sac encloses not only part of the brain and its meningeal coverings, but also a part of the ventricle.

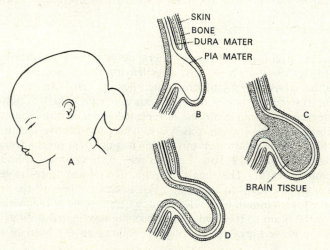

Fig. 20–20. Cranial bifida in various types of brain herniation due to faulty ossification of the skull (after Langman):
A. Profile of the head of infant bearing an encephalocoele;
B–D. Sections of such an encephalocoele to show the nature of the defect: B, meningocoele (cf. Fig. 20–7B); C, meningo-encephalocoele; D, meningohydro-encephalocoele.

III. THE PERIPHERAL NERVOUS SYSTEM

The action system

This is a useful term for introducing the peripheral nervous system. This system comprises all the necessary elements to complete an action circuit, the simplest of which may be represented by a simple reflex arc (Fig. 20–21), as follows:

A receptor
(carrying ascending impulse)
↓
afferent (sensory) neuron
↓
efferent (motor) neuron
↓
an effector
(receiving the descending impulse)

In more complex action circuits one or more internuncial or association neurons interposed between the afferent and efferent neurons may be involved, forming synapses at the junctions; these are the points at which nerve impulses pass from processes of one neuron to those of another.

The neurons

The neurons are the units of structure and function. Morphologically, each neuron has a cell body and cytoplasmic processes (Figs. 19–3D and 6). Of these processes the dendrites, usually terminating in an arborization within a receptor, convey impulses from the latter to the cell body of the neuron whereas the axon, which may possess collaterals (usually at right angles) transmits descending impulses away from the cell body to an effector. Thus, dendrites and axons of neurons are defined on a functional, rather than anatomical, basis. Besides the cell body and the processes, a neuron may or may not have a sheath that encloses its dendritic and axonal processes.

Myelin formation

As stated on p. 218, myelination of the peripheral nerve fibres is attributed to the sheath cells (cells of Schwann) (Fig. 19–6). These cells, after leaving the prospective spinal ganglia, wrap themselves around the axons, thereby becoming neurilemma cells. In this " strategic " position their cell membrane transforms into a fatty substance, myelin, which accumulates between the axon and the neurilemma by a unique process of repeated spiral coiling around the axon. This is not the case with fibres of the central nervous system where prospective sheath cells are not available. Instead, the fibres of the central nervous system acquire their myelin from a different source — the oligodendroglia cells (Fig. 19–3D). For this reason these fibres, although myelinated, do not have a neurilemma sheath. The time of myelination of any fibres is generally correlated with the time at which they begin to function. For instance, fibres of the spinal cord become myelinated during the fourth month of development, whereas some of the motor fibres descending from high centres of the brain to the cord do not become myelinated until as late as one or two years after birth. The nerve fibres are classified as follows on the basis of the nature of their sheath.

1. Medullated
   (a) With myelin, but no neurolemma (most fibres of central nervous system).
   (b) With both neurolemma and myelin (peripheral nerve fibres).
2. Non-medullated
   (a) With neurolemma, but no myelin (most unmyelinated fibres).
   (b) With neither neurolemma nor myelin (rare).

Receptors and effectors

These may be summarized briefly in the following manner.

Receptors	Effectors
1. Exteroceptive (pain, temperature, touch).	1. Those that terminate in skeletal muscles.
2. Proprioceptive (state of tension, of skeletal muscles and tendons; vibratory and deep sensibility).	2. Those that relay impulses to smooth muscle, blood vessels and glands by way of the autonomic system.
3. Interoceptive (impulses from internal organs).	

Functional classification of nerve fibres

The class of a nerve fibre may be described by three letters. Firstly, either G (general) or S (special); secondly, either S (somatic) or V (visceral), and thirdly, either A (afferent) or E (efferent). Only the first term requires further qualification. In case of afferent (sensory) somatic fibres, G stands for those originating in the integument whilst S is for those from special sense organs. In case of afferent visceral fibres, G stands for general viscera while S stands for special viscera innervated by mixed nerves (e.g., cranial nerve VII). In case of efferent visceral fibres, G stands for general viscera while S stands for smooth musculature derived from the branchial arches (i.e., branchiomeric). There is no S.S.E. nerve component because all somatic efferent fibres are of the general type (G.S.E.). For this reason we may designate them by S.E. (omitting the first letter, G).

Examples of nerve fibres according to this classification

Designation	No. of the nucleus used in Figs. 20–4, 6 and 21	Nerve fibres
from alar lamina { G.S.A.	No. 2 . . .	Fibres arising chiefly from the integument.
S.S.A	No. 1 . . .	Fibres arising from the sensory epithelia of eye and ear.
G.V.A.	No. 4 . . .	Sensory fibres from general viscera.
S.V.A.	No. 3 . . .	Sensory fibres from nose and tongue.
from basal lamina { (G.)S.E.	No. 7 . . .	Fibres terminating on skeletal muscles.
S.S.E. (non-existent)		
G.V.E.	No. 5 . . .	Fibres terminating about autonomic ganglionic cells, which, in turn, control smooth muscle, cardiac muscle and glandular tissues.
S.V.E.	No. 6 . . .	Fibres of cranial nerves terminating on striated musculature derived from the branchial arches.

THE SPINAL NERVES

Development

The spinal nerves are paired nerves arranged segmentally, and corresponding closely to the myotomes. They are characterized by a dorsal and a ventral root, the former bearing a con-

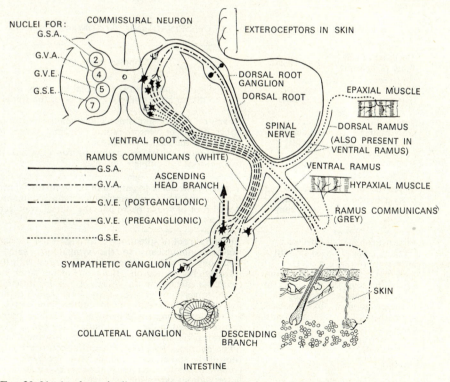

FIG. 20–21. A schematic diagram showing the development of the different functional groups of neurons and nerve fibres in the spinal nerves which are in close association with the sympathetic division of the autonomic nervous system.

spicuous ganglion (Figs. 20–3 and 21). During the fifth week of development the ventral roots grow out from the ventrolateral wall of the cord, at which time the prospective spinal ganglia are still in the form of repeated enlargements along the line of neural crest material (Fig. 19–5A). Later, cells of the primordial ganglia develop centrally-directed processes, which enter the marginal zone of the cord as dorsal root fibres whilst their peripheral processes extend in the opposite direction, and join the fibres of the ventral root (Fig. 19–5B). Beyond the point of union of the dorsal and ventral roots, the trunk of the spinal nerve gives off laterally its dorsal ramus and ventral ramus. The dorsal ramus contains somatic efferent and afferent fibres (Fig. 20–3); the former supply muscles, the latter end in the integument (Fig. 20–21). The ventral ramus, which is the stouter of the two rami, after receiving the gray ramus communicans (containing postganglionic sympathetic fibres) from an autonomic ganglion, divides into the lateral and ventral terminal divisions. (These branches of the ventral ramus are not shown in Fig. 20–21.) The efferent fibres of these two divisions supply muscles of the lateral and ventral body wall (also of the limbs) whilst their afferent fibres end in the integument of the same regions (Fig. 20–21). At the points where the ventral and lateral terminal divisions arise, fibres from adjacent nerves may form connections with them, thereby forming the distinct intermingling of fibres called nerve plexuses. These are especially pronounced at the levels of the limbs, forming the brachial and lumbo-sacral plexuses (Fig. 20–22).

Functional components

The motor (efferent) neurons (G.S.E.) differentiate in the ventral horn of the grey matter as typical bi-polar cells. Their axons form the ventral root of the spinal nerves (Figs. 19–5A; 19–5B,

TABLE 20–1. THE PERIPHERAL SYSTEM OF SPINAL AND AUTONOMIC NERVES

Component	Location of cell-body of neurons	End Organs	Impulse Pathways
Somatic sensory	Spinal (dorsal root) ganglion	Receptor, Integument	From skin via spinal nerve to spinal ganglion and its dorsal root to dorsal horn of the grey matter of the spinal cord
Somatic motor	Ventral horn of Grey matter	Effector, skeletal muscles	Via ventral root of spinal nerve to spinal nerve, from there to either dorsal or ventral ramus of spinal nerves to end in muscles of the back or front A communication or association neuron may link the above two neurons to complete the reflex arc
Visceral sensory	Spinal (dorsal root) ganglion	Receptor, Intestinal epithelium	Via autonomic nerve to ganglia of the sympathetic chain, from there via the white (preganglionic) ramus communicans and dorsal root of spinal nerve and the dorsal root ganglion to the dorsal horn of the cord's grey matter
Visceral motor (involving) two-chain innervation)	First neuron (Preganglionic, in lateral horn of grey matter) Second neuron (postganglionic, in the ganglion of sympathetic chain)	Effector to (a) smooth muscle, glands, blood vessels or (b) skin muscle, blood vessels, sweat glands	Via ventral root of spinal nerve, through white (preganglionic) ramus communicans to the sympathetic ganglia, there synapsing through a communication neuron with the second (postganglionic) neuron; the axons of the latter may either reach the effectors in the viscera (a) via the autonomic nerve or (b) traverse the grey (postganglionic) ramus communicans and the spinal nerve to effectors in the skin A third descending route involves yet another preganglionic neuron located in the ventral horn of the cord's grey matter, synapsing via an association neuron with the first preganglionic neuron. Its process (axon) also traverses the ventral root of the spinal nerve and the white (preganglionic) ramus communicans to enter the sympathetic ganglion, leaves the latter without synapsing, and passes to a collateral ganglion in which a second postganglionic neuron is located and whose axon ends on arterial walls

arrow c). The sensory (afferent) neurons, derived exclusively from the neural crest, are contained in the spinal ganglia (Fig. 19–5B, C). They are of two kinds, the somatic afferent (G.S.A.) and visceral afferent (G.V.A.) neurons (Nos. 2 and 4, respectively, in Fig. 20–21), but all of them undergo a process of morphological transformation from a typical bi-polar stage to the definitive T-shaped cells (1–5, Fig. 19–5C). These cells consequently have relatively short axons, which form the dorsal root of the spinal nerve and terminate at the dorsal horn of the grey matter (Fig. 19–5B, arrow a), and long dendrites (Fig. 19–5B, arrow b). These dendrites come from their respective receptors via the spinal nerve trunk from the integument. The remaining component to be discussed is a G.V.E. (No. 5, Fig. 20–21), the cell bodies of which are located in the lateral

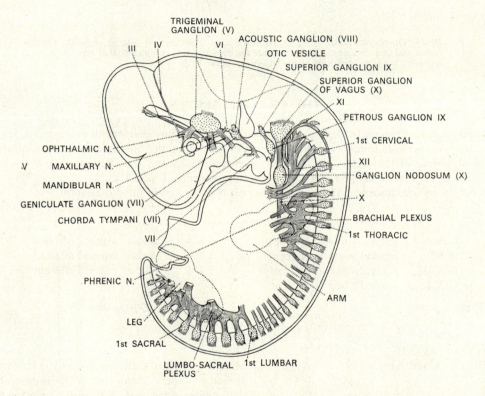

Fig. 20–22. Outline drawing of a 10 mm. human embryo (10 weeks) showing development of cranial nerves and associated ganglia (III to XII) and spinal nerves (c.n. I and II, not represented); all ganglia are shown in stipple.

horn of the grey matter. The efferent fibres (axons) traverse the ventral root, and branch off from the spinal nerve as components of the white rami communicantes (carrying pre-ganglionic sympathetic fibres). The white rami communicantes contain mixed visceral afferent and visceral efferent fibres whereas the grey rami communicantes (post-ganglionic) contain only visceral efferent fibres (Fig. 20–21). After synapsing with neurons in the autonomic ganglia (paravertebral and collateral) the visceral efferent fibres of the autonomic system terminate in the various effectors in the viscera. A summary of these spinal and autonomic nerves is presented in Table 20–1.

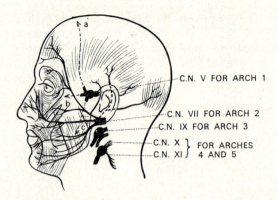

C.N. V FOR ARCH 1

C.N. VII FOR ARCH 2

C.N. IX FOR ARCH 3

C.N. X } FOR ARCHES
C.N. XI } 4 AND 5

FIG. 20–23. Diagrammatic drawing of the adult head from the left side to show the cranial nerves and their branches which innervate the derivatives of the branchial arches. a, b and c represent the three divisions of the trigeminal nerve (C.N. V).

THE CRANIAL NERVES

The cranial nerves have the following characteristics: (*a*) They have one or more, but never all, of the four components found in spinal nerves; (*b*) Their efferent fibres arise from neuroblasts in the basal lamina of the metencephalon and myelencephalon and (*c*) Their afferent fibres arise from cells in the cranial ganglia (with the exception of nerves I, and II).

A functional classification of the cranial nerves is presented in tabular fashion below.

Abbreviations

G.S.A. = general somatic afferent   S.S.A. = special somatic afferent
G.S.E. = general somatic efferent   S.V.A. = special visceral afferent
G.V.A. = general visceral afferent   S.V.E. = special visceral efferent
G.V.E. = general visceral efferent

Cranial nerves	*Designation*
I	S.V.A.
II and VIII	S.S.A.
III, IV, VI, XI, XII	G.S.E.
V, VII, IX, X and XI	Mixed, i.e., with both sensory and motor components. Note: cranial nerve XI is unique in that while it has a G.S.E. component, which supplies the shoulder muscles, its other components are of the special visceral kind supplying derivatives of branchial arches Nos. 4 and 5.

Group A. Nerves of the special sense organs

I. olfactory (S.V.A.)	Certain cells of the nasal epithelium lining the olfactory pit become sensory and grow into the olfactory bulb to establish contact with the sensory neurons of the olfactory tract.
II. optic (S.S.A.)	Both sensory cells and neurons develop from the retinal layer of the optic cup (originally a part of the brain wall). The axons of these neurons form the optic tract.

VIII. auditory (S.S.A.)	Typical bi-polar neurons develop in the acoustic ganglion, sending their axons into the myelencephalon, whilst their dendrites establish relationships with the epithelium of the otocyst. The nerve has two branches. (a) Cochlear — from the middle ear for hearing; (b) Vestibular — from the inner ear for maintenance of equilibrium.

Group B.   Somatic motor nerves (S.E.)

These develop from the basal lamina of the brain, and correspond to the somatic efferent components of spinal nerves.

III. oculomotor	This nerve supplies the internal rectus, lateral rectus, medial rectus and inferior oblique muscles of the eye-ball.
IV. Trochlear	Supplies the superior oblique muscle.
VI. abducens	Supplies the external rectus muscle.
XI. spinal accessory	This nerve has a G.S.E. component which innervates the muscles of the shoulder (see above).
XII. hypoglossal	This shows the least modification from a typical spinal nerve; its fibres supply the striated muscles of the tongue.

Group C.   Mixed sensory and motor nerves

Cranial nerves Nos. V, VII, IX, X, and XI have a developmental history in close relation to the branchial arches. Each of them may have one, two or three of the components of spinal nerves, but none of them contains a somatic motor (S.E.) component. This is because the striated muscles of the face and jaws are derived from the branchial arches (i.e., they are branchiomeric), not from myotomes. The visceral motor (V.E.) components of these nerves develop from neuroblasts in the lateral nuclei of the basal lamina of the metencephalon and myelencephalon whilst their sensory components arise from cells in their respective ganglia; most of these cells come from the neural crest, but it is probable that the ectodermal placodes in the cranial region also contribute.

V. Trigeminal	This is the nerve of the first branchial arch.
G.S.A. components:	the ophthalmic, maxillary and mandibular divisions contain fibres originating from cells in the trigeminal or semilunar ganglion (Figs. 20–22 and 24).
S.V.E. component:	the branch supplying the muscles of mastication.
S.V.A. component:	sensory fibres from the epithelium of palate and tongue.
VII. Facial	This is the nerve of the second branchial arch.
S.V.E. component:	supplies the muscles of facial expression.
G.V.E. component:	supplies secretomotor fibres to the submaxillary and sublingual salivary glands.
S.V.A. component:	These fibres grow out from cells in the geniculate ganglion and pass, via the chorda tympani nerve to the taste buds of the anterior $\frac{2}{3}$ of tongue.
XI. Glossopharyngeal	This is the nerve of the third branchial arch.
S.V.A. component:	fibres arising from the petrosal ganglion, supplying the middle ear, pharynx, and the posterior $\frac{1}{3}$ of the tongue.
G.S.A. component:	fibres from the external ear.

G.V.A. component:	fibres from general viscera, subserving visceral reflexes.
S.V.E. component:	this innervates the stylopharyngeus muscle of the pharynx.
G.V.E. component:	supplies secretomotor fibres to the parotid salivary gland.

X. Vagus . . . . . This is the nerve of the 4th and 5th branchial arches (in conjunction with XI)

S.V.E. component:	supplies voluntary muscles of the soft palate, pharynx and larynx.
G.V.E. component:	supplies smooth muscles, cardiac muscle and glandular tissue of the viscera via the ganglia of the parasympathetic autonomic system.
S.V.A. component:	this contains visceral sensory fibres from pharynx and larynx in conjunction with the parasympathetic autonomic system.
G.V.A. component:	This carries sensory fibres from the oesophagus.
G.S.A. component:	This contains somatic sensory fibres arising from the jugular and nodose ganglia to the skin of ear region.

XI. Spinal accessory

| S.V.E. component: | This supplies the muscles derived from the 4th and 5th branchial arches in general, i.e., muscles of the pharynx and larynx. |
| G.V.E. component: | This supplies the viscera of the thoracic and abdomen by way of the parasympathetic autonomic system (in conjunction with the vagus nerve). |

A summary of the components of the cranial nerves is presented in Table 20–3.

TABLE 20–3. THE COMPONENTS OF CRANIAL NERVES

Cranial nerves	Designation of components; Nos. based on Fig. 20–6	SOMATIC			VISCERAL			
		(1) S.S.A.	(7) (G.)S.E.	(2) G.S.A.	(6) S.V.E.	(5) G.V.E.	(3) S.V.A.	(4) G.V.A.
I. Olfactory							×	
II. Optic		×						
VIII. Auditory		×						
III. Oculomotor			×	×				
IV. Trochlear			×	×				
VI. Abducens			×	×				
XII. Hypoglossal			×					
V. Trigeminal				×	×		×	
VII. Facial					×	×	×	
IX. Glossopharyngeal				×	×	×	×	×
X. Vagus				×	×	×	×	×
XI. Spinal accessory					×	×		

CHAPTER 21

SENSE ORGANS

Evolution of receptors

Receptors are the first station in the chain of the " action system " referred to above. They have evolved from simple single sensory cells to highly complex organs of the special senses. Some of the sequences in this evolution process are summarized below.

1. The primitive condition. Certain superficial cells become sensory *in situ*, and send slender processes inwards. Typical examples are the sensory cells in *Hydra*.
2. Inward migration of primitive sensory cells. The primitive sensory cells segregate from the rest of the ectoderm and begin to migrate inwards, leaving their dendritic processes in contact with the epithelium. This condition is prevalent in the molluscs and arthropods.
3. Assumption of the typical vertebrate position of sensory neurons. The previous stage constitutes the forerunner of the situation in the vertebrates in which sensory neurons, derived from the neural crest, are aggregated in the spinal ganglia or cranial ganglia in close proximity to the neural tube. Their peripheral processes or dendrites assume new

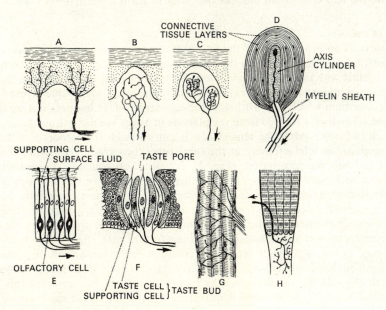

Fig. 21–1. Types of sensory nerve endings:
  A. Free nerve endings;
  B. and C. Two stages in the development of tactile corpuscles (B, nerve loops; C, definitive Meissner's corpuscle);
  D. Pacinian corpuscle;
  E. Olfactory sensory cells;
  F. Taste buds of the mammalian lingual epithelium;
  G. Neuromuscular spindle;
  H. Neurotendinous spindle (6 months).

relations by ending freely in the epithelium or connective tissue in manners typical of the sensory receptors.

4. Incorporation of specialized sensory cells into the afferent channel. In this last step certain epithelial cells become specialized into sensory (neuro-epithelial) cells, which receive the terminal arborization of the sensory neurons. Typical examples are the hair cells of the ampullae of semicircular canals and gustatory cells of the taste buds (Fig. 21–1).

Examples of various kinds of receptors developed in the human are illustrated in Fig. 21–1: they are A, free terminations of nerve endings (for pain, temperature, chemical senses); B, and C, tactile corpuscles of Meissner (for touch); D, lamellated (Pacinian) corpuscle (for pressure); E, bipolar olfactory cells; F, gustatory cells of taste buds; G, neuromuscular spindle (for muscle tension); and H, neurotendinous spindle (for relative position of body parts).

THE EYE

The development of the eye involves three processes of induction timed to occur precisely one after another in sequence. Firstly, the head mesenchyme that surrounds the wall of the prosencephalon at the level of the future diencephalon induces the formation of the optic vesicle. Secondly, before the latter invaginates to form the double-layered optic cup, and whilst its cells are in close contact with the head ectoderm, the cells of the optic cup induces the latter to form a lens vesicle. Finally, during the time when the prospective lens is closely adherent to the overlying ectoderm, the lens epithelium induces the latter to form a transparent cornea (Table 21–1).

Development of the eye

The eye starts as an evagination of the lateral wall of the future diencephalon region during the fourth week of development to form the optic vesicle (Fig. 21–2A). The head ectoderm, where it comes into contact with the optic vesicle thickens into a placode and soon both the optic vesicle and the lens placode invaginate together (Fig. 21–2B). The result is a double-layered cup, embracing the lens primordium which lies just below the ectoderm. This happens during the sixth week of development. The lens is formed from the placode in a very similar manner to the formation of Rathke's pouch (p.200). After the lens vesicle is cut off from the ectoderm, it loses its cavity and its cells specialize into lens fibres; at the same time, they gradually assume the shape of the definitive lens and become transparent (Fig. 21–2c; D). Subsequently, the ectoderm overlying the lens, together with head mesenchyme migrating in at the rim of the developing eye, also becomes transparent during the process of transformation into a cornea. Spaces in front of the lens (enclosed by the cornea) and behind it (enclosed by the optic cup) become, respectively, the anterior and posterior chambers of the eye. A semi-fluid substance produced by the mesenchymal cells fills each and is termed aqueous humour for the former case, the vitreous body in the latter.

The optic cup, as it doubles back into itself, creates a ventral trough in the future optic stalk. This trough is called the choroid fissure, and is, like the cup itself, also double-walled throughout its entire length (Fig. 21–3). Eventually, the trough closes off, but prior to this it serves as a pathway for head mesenchyme to migrate into the eyeball. This head mesenchyme gives rise to the hyaloid artery (Fig. 21–3B), the tunic surrounding the lens, and the vitreous body (Fig. 21–4). At the same time, the eyeball also becomes surrounded by head mesenchyme, from which is derived the connective tissue capsule of the eyeball. This capsule includes (a) the outer pigmented sclera, (b) the inner vascularized choroid immediately enclosing the eyeball. These tissues are homologous with, respectively, the dura mater and the pia-arachnoid coverings of the brain. The head mesenchyme also forms the mesodermal portion of the pars caeca, the blind or non-nervous portion of the optic cup which is in close relationship with the lens (Table 21–1). The

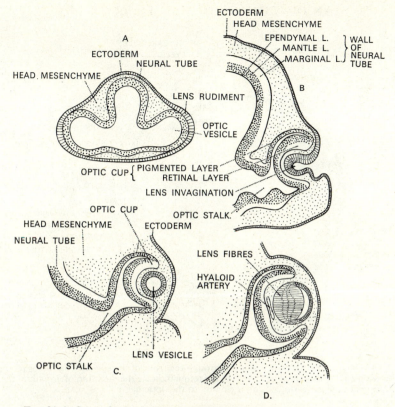

FIG. 21–2. Stages in the development of the vertebrate eye:
A. Transverse section through fore-brain of a 4-week human embryo;
B. to D. pig embryos (respectively, 6, 9, 12 mm.).

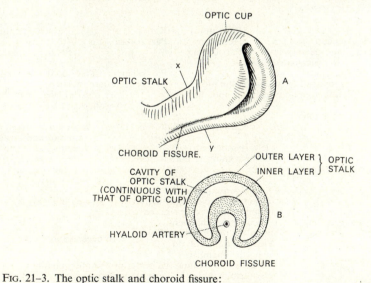

FIG. 21–3. The optic stalk and choroid fissure:
A. Ventro-lateral view of the optic cup and optic stalk of a 6-week human embryo;
B. Transverse section through the optic stalk at the level XY indicated in A, showing the position of the hyaloid artery in the chorioid fissure.

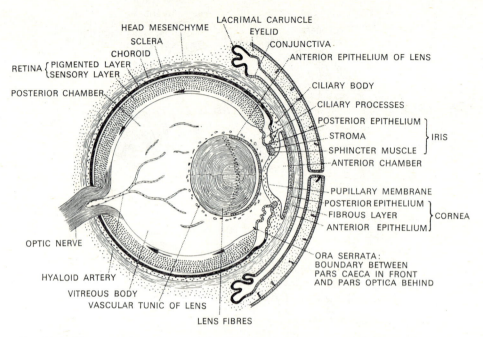

Fig. 21–4. Diagrammatic vertical section through the front of the eyeball in a foetus (composite between 16–19 weeks). The arrows in the retina indicate the direction of growth of the optic fibres from the ganglion cells on their way to the optic nerve.

TABLE 21–1. COMPONENTS OF THE EYE AND THEIR DERIVATIVES

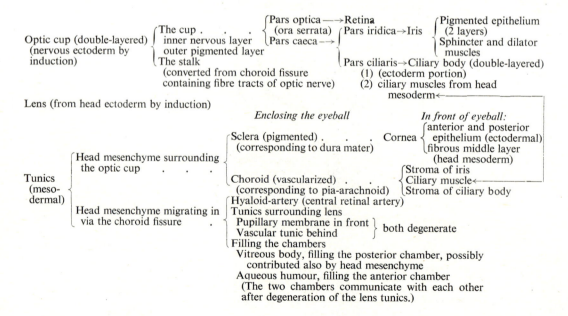

choroid fissure, when finally closed, becomes the optic stalk, which embodies the axons of the optic nerve (Fig. 21–4).

The optic cup, double-layered throughout, is divided by means of the ora serrata into two portions, the majority of which forms the pars optica, which roughly corresponds to the area posterior to the rim of the lens. Embracing the lens and partly covering it in front is the non-nervous pars caeca. The latter, jointly with the ectodermal elements, give rise to the iris and the ciliary body (Fig. 21–4). These are important structures because in them muscles will develop which will regulate the size of the pupil, and accommodate the lens.

Differentiation of the retina

The retina begins to differentiate from the centre to its periphery. In 12 mm. embryos it distinctly shows a nucleated layer next to the pigmented layer of the cup and is bounded by an external limiting membrane. The remainder of the retina facing the cavity of the cup is bounded by an internal limiting membrane (Fig. 21–5A). By the end of the second month of development three layers of the retina have been established (a) an inner neuroblastic layer, which roughly

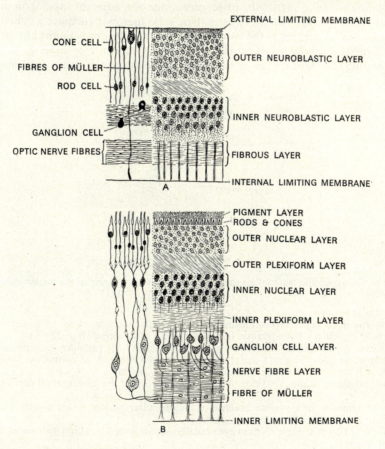

FIG. 21–5. Vertical sections of two stages in the differentiation of the human retina.
    A. At 3 months: on the left Cajal's analysis of the component elements using a silver impregnation technique is shown whilst the appearance with ordinary stains is seen at the right.
    B. At 7 months: on the left the chief neurons are shown by silver staining whilst the appearance with ordinary stains is seen on the right.

occupies the middle portion and is bounded by (*b*) an outer neuroblastic layer (next to the external limiting membrane) and (*c*) a marginal fibrous layer (Fig. 21–5A). By the sixth month the outer neuroblastic layer has given rise to the cone cells and rod cells, whilst the inner neuroblastic layer has developed into the ganglion cells. The marginal fibrous layer, by then, is loaded with the optic fibres, comprising the axons of all these neurons (Fig. 21–5B).

The unique feature about the retina is that its sensory cells (rods and cones) all develop from the mantle layer of the neural tube itself. This is because the eye, as a sense organ, is essentially a part of the brain wall which has been very early removed and set aside. The axons of the ganglion cells all converge towards the optic stalk and eventually those from the two sides unite at the optic chiasma, where some of the fibres decussate on their way to the brain.

Accessory structures of the eye

Eyelids. These are the folds of skin above and below the eye, which appear during the 7th week of development. Eye-lashes develop in them in the same way as any other hair (p. 209). The tarsal glands arise as ectodermal ingrowths at the edge of the eyelids.

The lacrimal glands are solid ingrowths of ectoderm into the adjacent mesoderm along the line where the upper lid and eyeball meet; later these solid ingrowths acquire a lumen (Fig. 21–6).

The naso-lacrimal duct originates as the naso-optical groove. Its epithelium sinks into the under-lying mesoderm as a solid cord of ectodermal cells. A lumen later develops in it to provide a duct connecting the inner corner of the eye with the inferior meatus of the nose.

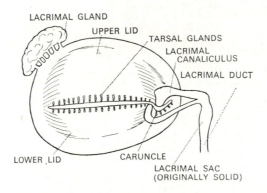

FIG. 21–6. The tarsal and lacrimal glands and the lacrimal duct system of the human eye.

Malformations of the eye

1. Coloboma iridis results from failure of the choroid fissure to close. The defect may extend from the iris to the ciliary body, retina, the choroid and optic nerve (Fig. 21–7C).

2. Persistent irido-pupillary membrane is due to failure of the pupillary membrane to disappear during intra-uterine life. The non-resorbed tissue forms a network of connective tissue in front of the pupil, which does not, however, disturb vision (Fig. 21–7B).

3. Microphthalmia is the condition where there is a small eye and eyeball (about ⅔ of normal size).

4. Anophthalmia is the complete absence of the eye, often accompanied by other serious cranio-cerebral abnormalities or defects.

5. Cyclopia. This is a single median eye (usually accompanied by abnormalities of craniocerebral origin) (Fig. 21–7A).

6. Cataract (opaque lens). This defect is known to be either genetically determined or caused by environmental factors, e.g., German measles contracted between the 4th–7th weeks of pregnancy. Babies born by mothers who contract the disease after the 7th week of pregnancy have normal eyes, thus strongly indicating that the sensitivity of the developing eye to cataract-causing agencies decreases sharply after this time.

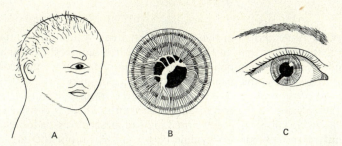

FIG. 21–7. Anomalies of the human eye (after Arey):
  A. Cyclopia of a newborn with a single eye ball but partial doubling of the lids, and a proboscis-like nose above it.
  B. Persistent pupillary membrane in an adult.
  C. Coloboma of the iris.

THE NOSE

In 4 mm. embryos a pair of ectodermal thickenings, the olfactory placodes, appear on the antero-ventral part of the head surface. Shortly afterwards, these placodes sink inwards to form the olfactory pits (Fig. 21–8A) which extend dorsally towards the telencephalon (Fig. 21–8B), thus progressively deepening the pit. The formation of the palate (p. 48) finally separates them from the mouth after which, the upper part of the nasal pit develops into the olfactory region of the definitive nose. The olfactory epithelium lining this region gives rise to two kinds of cells (a) olfactory cells and (b) supporting cells (Fig. 21–1E). The former send axons into the brain, establishing relation with the neurons of the olfactory tract. It is interesting to note that the olfactory cells, while behaving like nervous cells, are nevertheless derived from ectodermal epithelium instead of from the neural tube (cf. p. 244). In fact, the nose is the only sense organ in which the sensory cells are transformed into neuron-like cells. Consequently, the olfactory nerve (first cranial nerve) is the only cranial nerve whose fibres arise as outgrowths from sensory cells (instead of neurons). In most other cases (except the eye, see p. 247) the fibres of the sensory nerves grow from distant nervous cells into the sense organ where they come into relation with the sensory cells (e.g., organs of touch, taste, etc.).

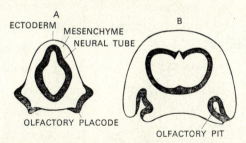

FIG. 21–8. Development of the olfactory organ (generalized):
  A. Section through head of a 6 mm. pig; note the olfactory placode.
  B. Section through head of a 9 mm. pig; the olfactory placode has now invaginated.

THE EAR

The ear begins as a thickened patch of head ectoderm, the otic placode, in the region of rhombencephalon in 9-somite embryos, prior to the closing of the neural tube (Fig. 21–9). The placode then invaginates and becomes pinched off as the otic vesicle, much as the lens placode is converted into a lens vesicle (Fig. 21–9; cf. Fig. 21–2B, C).

The inner ear

The entire inner ear is derived from the otic vesicle. Each vesicle differentiates into a dorsal component, which is the primordium of the utricle, the three semi-circular canals and the endo-lymphatic duct, and a ventral component, which constitutes the primordium of the saccule and the cochlear duct. The latter is the primordium of the organ of hearing, sometimes termed the organ of Corti. By the 9th week of development all these structural units are established (Fig. 21–10); together they constitute the membranous labyrinth (which is completely ectodermal in origin). At first, this entire labyrinth is embedded in head mesenchyme, a loose connective tissue, which is subsequently transformed into hyaline cartilage. At about the end of second month this cartilage becomes ossified to form the bony labyrinth, which is found in the petrous part of the temporal bone. During this process a ring of soft perilymph is left out to separate the inner membranous labyrinth from the outer bony one. The inner ear is of adult size at birth.

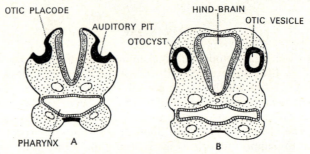

FIG. 21–9. Development of the human otocyst, transverse section (after Arey):
  A. at 16-somite stage (3 weeks);
  B. at 4 mm. (4 weeks).

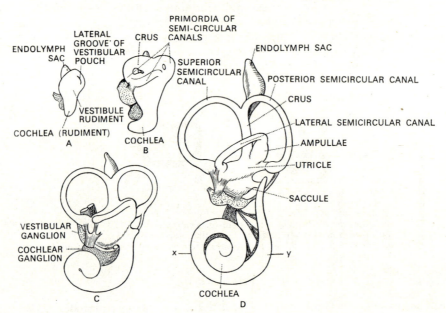

FIG. 21–10. Development of the left membranous labyrinth, left side view of a model (A, 6.6 mm.; B, 13 mm.; C, 20 mm.; D, 30 mm.). The stippled area indicates vestibular and cochlear division of the acoustic nerve (c.n. VIII) and its accompanying ganglia. The line XY in D indicates the plane of the section shown in Fig. 21–11.

Organ of hearing

In the meantime, a limited number of cells become segregated from the otic vesicle and give rise to the stato-acoustic ganglion. This ganglion further divides into a dorsal vestibular portion, which supplies the sensory cells of the saccule, utricle, and semi-circular canals, and a ventral cochlear portion, which supplies the organ of Corti. The proximal processes of the neurons join to form the stato-acoustic nerve as they grow toward the brain.

The saccular portion of the otic vesicle gives rise to the cochlea through a continuous process of spiral coiling (Fig. 21–10c, D). A schematic plan (sectional view) of the cochlea is shown in Fig. 21–11. Impulses arising from the neuro-epithelial cells (hair cells) and the tectorial membrane of the cochlear duct pass on to the auditory fibres of the VIIIth cranial nerve via the spiral ganglia. The mesenchyme into which the spiral cochlear duct penetrates differentiates into a thin fibrous basement membrane, which surrounds the ectodermal epithelium lining the cochlear duct, and a cartilagenous shell outside it. (Fig. 21–12A). During the tenth week of development, this cartilagenous shell dissolves to form two large perilymphatic spaces, the scala vestibuli and scala tympani (Fig. 21–12B), which are permeated, however, by a loose fibrous tissue. Ossification of the surrounding cartilage to form the petrous part of the temporal bone completes the development of the bony labyrinth (Fig. 21–13C).

Further differentiation of the epithelial cells lining the cochlear duct results in the formation of an inner and an outer ridge, followed by the appearance in each of specialized neuro-epithelial cells, the hair cells, and a tectorial membrane to connect the latter (Fig. 21–12C). The hair cells

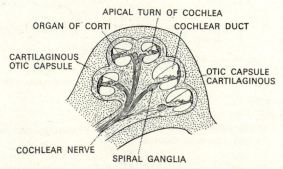

FIG. 21–11. A schematic plan of the cochlea is shown to indicate the relation of the supporting tissue and perilymphatic spaces to the development of the membranous labyrinth in a 4-month foetus.

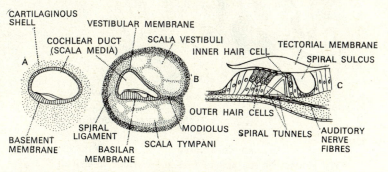

FIG. 21–12. Development of the scala timpani and scala vestibuli:
    A. Cochlear duct surrounded by a fibrous basement membrane and cartilagenous shell;
    B. Large perilymphatic spaces appearing in the cartilagenous shell (10-week);
    C. Development of the organ of Corti at full term.

and the tectorial membrane comprise the components of the organ of Corti. Impulses received by this organ ascend to the central nervous system by the auditory fibres of cranial nerve VIII.

The utricle and the semi-circular canals, which are also derived from the otic vesicle, constitute the organs for maintianing the proper position of the body. The neuro-epithelial cells lining their wall convey impulses of changes in position of the body to the brain via the vestibular branch of the auditory nerve (Fig. 21–10c, D).

The middle ear

The Eustachian or pharyngo-tympanic tube, the tympanic cavity and the auditory ossicles housed in the latter comprise the middle ear. Unlike the components of the inner ear, which are completely ectodermal, the middle ear is of branchial origin. The first pharyngeal pouch, lined with endoderm, appears in the third week of development and extends laterally to meet with the

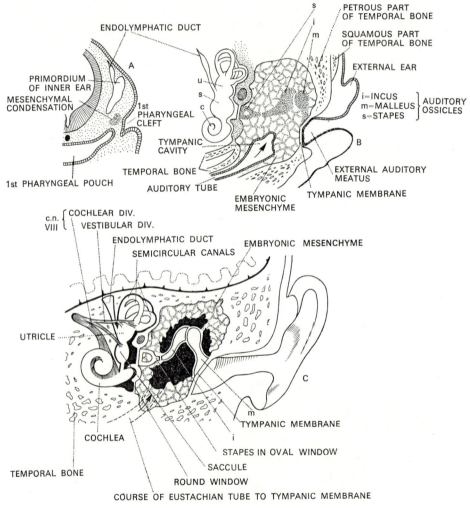

FIG. 21–13. Stages in the development of the middle ear chamber and the auditory (otic) ossicles: A and B early; C, Schematic representation to show the ear at term. The cochlea is turned medially in order to show its spiral course. m and i and s represent the malleus and the incus and stapes respectively.

first pharyngeal cleft (Fig. 21–13A). The distal end of the pouch expands to become the tympanic cavity (Fig. 21–13B) whilst its proximal end remains narrow, forming the Eustachian tube. The latter connects the future middle ear with the naso-pharynx.

Beginning from the 7th week, proliferations from branchial arches 1 and 2 result in the formation of a number of mesenchymal condensations. These condensations (Fig. 21–13A) are closely associated with the distal tips of the skeletal elements of the first and second pharyngeal arches; they are the precursors of the auditory ossicles, the malleus and incus (from arch 1) and the stapes (from arch 2) (Fig. 21–13B, C) (see also Fig. 15–15). They begin to ossify during the 5th month of development and have attained adult size at birth. The malleus is in contact with the tympanic membrane while the stapes rests directly on the fenestra vestibuli leading to the bony labyrinth of the inner ear, with the incus bridging the two. They constitute the medium for transmission of sound waves (Fig. 21–13B, C).

The auditory ossicles are at first embedded in head mesenchyme (Fig. 21–13B). The latter, however, soon degenerates and completely disappears from the scene. At the same time as these changes an expansion of the primitive tympanic cavity occurs (arrow, Fig. 21–13B). This expansion is accomplished by means of mesenchymal-like cells of endodermal origin (of pouch 1) becoming detached from the bulging pharyngeal pouch, pushing its limit upwards and laterally so that eventually the newly enlarged tympanic cavity becomes filled with this mesenchyme-like tissue. For a time, the auditory ossicles are also invested with this tissue. Eventually, however, they become free and their epithelium finally forms a mesentery-like (double-layered) membrane which connects the ossicles to the wall of the definitive tympanic cavity. The supporting ligaments of the ossicles develop later in these membranes as well as the tensor tympani muscle of the malleus (from arch 1) and the stapedius muscle of the stapes (from arch 2). These muscles are innervated, respectively, by the Vth and VIIth cranial nerves.

External ear

The external auditory meatus is derived from the first pharyngeal cleft. As this tube grows inward towards the endodermal lining of the tympanic cavity (first pharyngeal pouch) a thickened epithelial plate develops, which however shortly dissolves and is replaced by epithelial lining in the floor of the enlarged meatus. It is these cells that ultimately form the definitive eardrum, tympanic membrane.

The auricles (Fig. 21–14A) originate from a number of mesenchymal proliferations formed during the sixth week of development by the dorsal lips of the first and second pharyngeal arches, three on each side of the external meatus. A summary of the components of the ear and their derivatives is presented in Table 21–2.

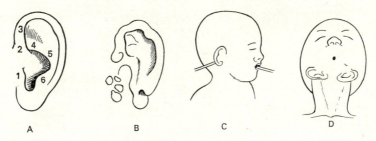

FIG. 21–14. Anomalies of the human ear (auricle) (after Arey):
    A. Normal auricle (adult);
    B. Malformed auricle;
    C. Fistula auris, probed to show its relations;
    D. Synotia, combined with microstomia and agnathia.

TABLE 21–2. COMPONENTS OF THE EAR AND THEIR DERIVATIVES

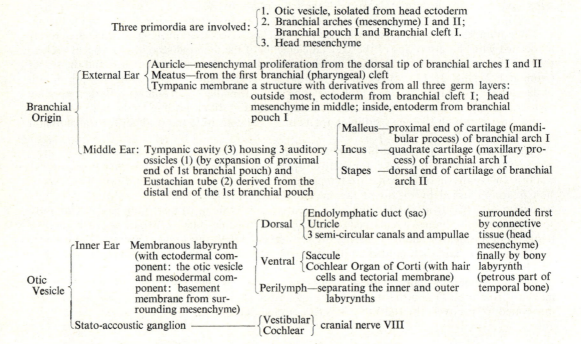

Three primordia are involved:
1. Otic vesicle, isolated from head ectoderm
2. Branchial arches (mesenchyme) I and II; Branchial pouch I and Branchial cleft I.
3. Head mesenchyme

Branchial Origin

External Ear
Auricle—mesenchymal proliferation from the dorsal tip of branchial arches I and II
Meatus—from the first branchial (pharyngeal) cleft
Tympanic membrane a structure with derivatives from all three germ layers: outside most, ectoderm from branchial cleft I; head mesenchyme in middle; inside, entoderm from branchial pouch I

Middle Ear: Tympanic cavity (3) housing 3 auditory ossicles (1) (by expansion of proximal end of 1st branchial pouch) and Eustachian tube (2) derived from the distal end of the 1st branchial pouch

Malleus—proximal end of cartilage (mandibular process) of branchial arch I
Incus —quadrate cartilage (maxillary process) of branchial arch I
Stapes —dorsal end of cartilage of branchial arch II

Otic Vesicle

Inner Ear   Membranous labyrynth (with ectodermal component: the otic vesicle and mesodermal component: basement membrane from surrounding mesenchyme)

Dorsal
Endolymphatic duct (sac)
Utricle
3 semi-circular canals and ampullae

Ventral
Saccule
Cochlear Organ of Corti (with hair cells and tectorial membrane)

Perilymph—separating the inner and outer labyrynths

surrounded first by connective tissue (head mesenchyme) finally by bony labyrynth (petrous part of temporal bone)

Stato-accoustic ganglion ——————
Vestibular
Cochlear } cranial nerve VIII

Malformations of the ear. The most severe cases involve the absence of a tympanic cavity and external auditory meatus. Certain defects of the ear are transmitted genetically while others have been recently linked to many teratogenic agents as possible causal factors. Among these are the *rubella* virus of German measles, poliomyelitis, erythroblastosis foetalis, diabetes, and toxoplasmosis (see Chapter 8).

Malformed auricle (Fig. 21–14B).

Fistula auris (rare) connected with mid-ear cavity (Fig. 21–14C).

Synotia (or fused ears) which occur near the mid-ventral line in the upper part of the neck (Fig. 21–14D).

INDEX